The New
NUTS
Among the
Berries

The New
NUTS
Among the
Berries

Ronald M. Deutsch

P.O. Box 208
Palo Alto, CA 94302

Design: Jill Casty

Copyright 1977 Bull Publishing Co.

ISBN 0-915950-08-1 (cloth)
      0-915950-09-X (paper)
Library of Congress Catalog No. 77-70401
Printed in the United States of America

This book is for
my son, Jeff
as he enters a world which,
though often flawed
by absurdity and deceit,
is nevertheless
always full of wonder.

Books by the Author

Nutrition
The New Nuts Among the Berries
Realities of Nutrition
Nutrition Labeling (with the National Nutrition Consortium)
The Family Guide to Better Food and Better Health
The Food Counter's Guide (in press)

Psychology and Physiology
Pairing (with G. Bach)
Key to Feminine Response in Marriage

Fiction and Humor
The Grass Lovers
Is Europe Necessary?

Contents

1

The Magical Feast

As usual, Daisie Adelle Davis Sieglinger was up by 4 A.M. Switching on some of her favorite early-morning music, Tschaikovsky's *1812 Overture,* to set a proper mood for the day, she sat down to breakfast.

Each food was chosen for what she believed were extraordinary properties. The fruit was "organic." The milk was raw and certified. The cereal was her own home-made design, with such ingredients as unrefined sesame and sunflower seeds, organic honey, and wheat germ.

Setting out a dish of yogurt (covered with undiluted frozen-orange juice concentrate) for her husband, Frank Sieglinger, Jr., she opened her unique plastic fishing-tackle box. In each compartment was a different high-potency pill or capsule. For example, among not less than a score of supplements there were single tablets containing three million *acidophilus bacteria,* others of compressed desiccated liver, and capsules containing the vitamin E of nine pounds of wheat germ. Quickly choosing and swallowing, Adelle felt herself ready to serve the millions who loved and trusted her.

With the *Overture's* cannon and bells still at full cry, she sat down at her accustomed workspace, her dining-room table, and began to deal with the hundreds of letters which, in hope and in desperation, asked her what to eat.

These appeals were not addressed to Daisie Sieglinger. For one thing, she was known as Daisie Adelle only to such intimates as her elder sister, who still kept the family farm (in Union Township, Indiana) where Daisie had been born in 1904. Early in life, that first name had been dropped. Daisie said there were too many cows and horses who shared it. Nor was she known much as Mrs. Sieglinger, for in this second marriage she kept her private and professional lives quite separate—except for working at home.

To the world, the lady at the dining table was simply Adelle Davis, the earthy food crusader whose opinions were as strong as her voice—a voice so firm and low that, in her Church of Religious Science choir, she sang not with the soprano or alto ladies, but with the tenors. People believed in that voice. They believed in its threats—of a national wave of "slow murders in the kitchen"—and in its promises—of a healthy longevity for all those who ate as Adelle taught. Indeed, in all of history, probably no other person has been so closely identified in the minds of so many with the gospel of food and health.

Adelle's reputation was built through multimedia promotion. In the introductions to her $2,000 lectures, in the billboard openings of television talk shows (from Dinah Shore to Merv Griffin and Johnny Carson), in newspaper and magazine articles and on the covers of the more than ten million books she sold, she was "the nation's most noted nutritionist," and "America's most celebrated nutritionist." In public opinion, Adelle Davis was at once the immaculate scientist—she did indeed hold the master's degree in her field—and the feisty, but caring, Earth Mother.

Small wonder that they wrote to her by the thousands. And true to her image, she answered every call for help—all except what she called "the dumb ones." For she truly cherished her public.

Yet Adelle had a practical side, too. For example, while she would rise before daylight to deal with the mail (and later in the day use two secretaries to help), generally, before giving any advice, she requested that a dietary-history sheet be filled out When the sheet came back, she promptly gave her opinion, provided that the sheet was accompanied by a check for $50.

Her complex personality was clearly stamped on the Palos Verdes Estates, California, home which she and Frank had designed themselves. For instance, where the normal front yard should have been, there stood instead a hodge-podge of organically-growing vegetables. The living quarters were almost always described as "homey" by visitors. But the doorknobs and chandeliers were sculpted in fantasy shapes by Adelle, from lumps of plastic. And the walls were hung with her own flamboyantly-painted canvases, inspired by LSD trips with such of her Hollywood friends as Aldous and Laura Huxley.

Not many of her nutrition faithful knew that she had written works which did not deal with eating. Under the pseudonym of Jane Dunlap, she authored *Exploring Inner Space.* It described her "miraculous" experiences while dropping acid, revelations which she said had inspired her religious life and shaped her philosophy.

Adelle did not work steadily through the day. She took a morning tennis break five days a week. And whenever she began to feel really frazzled, she would tighten the topknot wound from her waist-length hair, strip to the buff and head for her pool, which lay between the living room and the bedroom.

She always said that pool was her second best investment, next only to her three kinds of psychoanalysis, Freudian, Jungian and Reichian. This was saying quite a lot. For not only had the analyses freed her, but it was through their mutual psychiatrist that she had met Frank.

Adelle liked to invite visitors to swim with her, despite the house custom of dipping in the raw. And she liked to ask guests what they were reminded of by the pool's shape. It was in the form of a fat lozenge, leading to a narrow neck.

A reporter from *Cosmopolitan* magazine guessed—with reasonable logic, considering Adelle's main interests—that the pool represented a stomach. But she shook her head in disgust. "It's a *womb,*" she retorted, "all the way to the vagina."

She also pointed out that the water was kept quite warm, to provide a proper "uterine" sensation. Asked why she wanted this, Adelle explained that it was necessary to recreate the peaceful feeling of life before birth. It was this feeling which she sought to ease the stresses of life. As she summed up her quest: "When we reach the feeling of total acceptance, as we felt in the womb, we feel love, don't we?"

Such were the directness and simplicity of Adelle Davis' applications of science. She flatly believed that good food meant good health, and she tolerated few reservations or complications. For example, she affirmed repeatedly that if only one ate the right food, one could prevent or cure such ills as kidney disease, warts, eye troubles such as glaucoma, allergies, bad nerves, infections, menstrual cramps, multiple sclerosis, muscular dystrophy, hemorrhoids and literally hundreds of other ailments. But she did not stop there; she said that, "Alcoholism, crime, insanity, suicide, divorce, drug addiction and even impotency are often merely the results of bad eating."

The answers to all these problems, Adelle said, could be found in any kitchen or health-food store. They just needed a little putting together in one of the condensed-nutrition potions for which she was famous, such as *Tiger's Milk*. As one example, Adelle believed that most illness called for the regular drinking of her "Pep-up" concoction. This was made from egg yolks, oil, lecithin, calcium salts, magnesium oxide, yogurt, granular kelp, milk, yeast, wheat germ and soy flour. Blended without cooking, "Pep-up" was supposed to make almost anyone recover better and faster, provided he drank about two-thirds of a cup six times a day.

But many of Adelle's cures and preventives were even simpler. Consider menstrual cramps. She said that these resulted from the lack of calcium in the body. To stop them, one had only to drink an hourly glass of milk, bolstered with calcium powders, and to help things along, blend the shell of a boiled egg into the brew.

Even so baffling a medical puzzle as cancer was not beyond Adelle's nutritional ken. As she wrote in her book *Let's Get Well,* "I have yet to know of a single adult to develop cancer who has habitually drunk a quart of milk a day."

Such simple nutritional cures and preventives had been

Adelle's hallmarks since her training days of the early 1930's. Her student nickname was "Vitamin Davis."

But few of her faithful knew that most of the dietary nostrums of "America's most celebrated nutritionist" were flatly rejected by nutrition science. She was not invited to professional meetings, given membership in the key professional societies or published in the journals of science. At the 1969 White House Conference on Food, Nutrition and Health, the panel on deception and misinformation agreed that she was probably the most damaging single source of *false* nutrition information in the land.

Professors of nutrition and medicine are normally both conservative and genteel in their public statements. But in recent years, they characterized Adelle's work with such phrases as "hogwash" and "garbage" and "potentially dangerous." Typical of many such comments is that of Dr. Leo Lutwak, professor of medicine at UCLA and an internationally-known nutrition authority. "Her books," he said, "are phony, and her quotations are deliberate distortions of facts taken completely out of context."

But what is doubly ironic is that even those of Adelle's faithful who knew of these criticisms tended to dismiss them. Adelle had the answers they liked. They wanted to believe.

Such insistent belief in the magic of food is the theme of this book. And this belief is largely founded upon a single human truth. It is that when we are confronted with the fear of pain and death, even the wisest of us may suspend our judgment and common sense.

The first great American health fad began in 1796, when Dr. Elisha Perkins discovered the secret of perpetual good health. Surprisingly enough, it was quite simple. Dr. Perkins fabricated two metal rods, each three inches long and each of specially compounded materials. By placing the tractors—as they came to be known—over the area of the body that suffered from pain, heat, or disease of some kind, then drawing them out to one of the extremities, Dr. Perkins could remove the illness.

Eventually Dr. Perkins found that his own healing hands were not needed to guide the tractors. Anyone could do it. Quite understandably, Americans rushed to buy tractors from their benefactor. No price was too large for such a boon. It is recorded, though not well documented, that one Virginian, in selling his home, accepted tractors enough to total the entire value of his estate.

Elisha Perkins had become the first great American quack.

Of course, action was taken by the authorities at once. President George Washington immediately bought tractors for his entire family. And Supreme Court Chief Justice Oliver Ellsworth, after calm judicial reflection, took an even more foresighted course. Having purchased tractors from Perkins and tried them, he took care to introduce the good doctor, with the highest recommendations, to his successor, Chief Justice John Marshall.

Medical historians are convinced that Perkins was sincere. To this conclusion they adduce the evidence of the great yellow fever epidemic that struck New York City in 1799. Dr. Perkins rushed to the very heart of the plague and tended the stricken. But he soon realized that tractors alone were not enough. He decided that vinegar, quaffed in judicious combination with the magical tractors, was the answer. Confidently, fearlessly, he applied his cure. Three weeks later Dr. Elisha Perkins was dead of yellow fever.

In so dying, Perkins at once advanced and refuted the first important American food fallacy. He also left the heritage of the tractors to his son Benjamin, who cynically plied his tractor trade in both the new world and the old, was honored wherever he went, and in building a fortune never for a moment gave credence to his father's medical faith. It is a pattern we shall see again and again.

The story has a moral. Quaint? A wry vestige of a distant past? Not quite. For recall Dr. Perkins' finest hour, his ultimate discovery—vinegar to cure yellow fever. And then look at a more recent episode of healing.

In 1958, Dr. De Forest C. Jarvis burst upon the literary scene with a book called *Folk Medicine, A Vermont Doctor's Guide to Good Health*. The book said that Vermonters knew how to get relief from headache, arthritis, diabetes, vague physical weakness, a tired mind and other scourges. They simply knew how to use two ancient nostrums. One was honey. And the other—shades of Elisha Perkins—was vinegar. In a short time, 500,000 copies were swept from the shelves, and its precept still persists as one of the chief "natural" remedies for arthritis today. Both this book and a sequel, *Arthritis and Folk Medicine,* are still on the paperback racks.

Even more recently, vinegar has been part of one of the most popular theories of weight-reduction. *Family Circle* offered it to some eight million readers in an article called "My Amazing Cider Vinegar, Lecithin, Kelp, B-6 Diet." After all, the author pointed out, "oil and vinegar don't really mix. Maybe vinegar and my fat wouldn't either, and vinegar might just win out." Apparently, this logic, supported by the labeling of vinegar as "an old folk remedy," was convincing to *Family Circle* readers.

The public response to the concept was so impressive that the magazine hastened to advertise its effectiveness in an advertising trade journal called *Media Decisions.* The ad featured testimonials from the health-food world. As a vice president of General Nutrition Center's 250-store chain was quoted: ". . . the last two weeks have been hectic ones with all the calls we have been getting from our store managers for additional stock. . . ."

The ad closed with a straightforward sub-headline: *"Family Circle.* Who else is doing what we're doing?"

The lamentable answer to the question is, which magazine is not? With very few exceptions, the nation's media have responded to a sharp growth in nutrition interest with one volley after another of scientifically invalid ideas for weight control and better health through eating.

One cannot really measure the result very accurately, but clearly the overall impact is enormous. Recently, the U.S. Department of Health, Education and Welfare made a comprehensive attempt to assess nutrition in America, in its Ten-State Survey. The report concludes: "The results . . . indicated that a significant proportion of the population surveyed was malnourished or was at high risk of developing nutritional problems."

There were obvious vitamin and mineral shortages in the dietaries studied, and these were generally confirmed by the HANES (Health and Nutrition Examination Survey) study which was subsequently conducted. Iron deficiency was indicated for more than 90 percent of American women aged 18 to 44, as well as for most children under the age of six. Obesity is one of the major nutrition-related health problems. The Ten-State Survey found that over 20 percent of white males from 14 to 60 (with incomes greater than 150 percent of poverty maximums) were obese. Obesity among women in this same group ran as high as 41 percent.

Still more recently, in late 1974, the Federal Trade Commission, studying food advertising and looking for the causes of this malnutrition, found that: "A variety of data indicates that a significant portion of the malnutrition . . . arises from consumers' lack of awareness of the health significance of food choices . . . and lack of information."

Turning to the White House Conference on Food, Nutrition and Health, certainly the most comprehensive and large-scale analysis of nutrition problems in America, the FTC staffers found the same theme repeated by various study panels: "The White House Conference Report repeatedly attributes malnutrition not to an overall shortage of available nutrients, but rather to, among other reasons, a lack of nutrition knowledge on the part of consumers and *actual misinformation disseminated in advertising and other communications media.*" (Emphasis added.)

As the Conference's panel on deception and misinformation summarized: "No other area of the national health probably is as abused by deception and misinformation as nutrition. Many travesties cheat the public of enormous sums of money, and of good health as well . . . In many cases, the lie is a promise of extraordinary health value in some special food or system of eating . . . Those who cannot afford poor food choices are especially exploited. The poor, in particular the old, the ill and the least educated are cruelly victimized . . . [by] needless high-priced supplements and 'health' foods. Or they are lured by advertising that suggests falsely that certain cheap, widely-sold products, because they contain a few added vitamins or minerals, can replace usual foods or even whole meals."*

*To be candid, the author must admit that he wrote this report. But he expressed the opinions of his five authoritative colleagues on the panel, an expert legal consultant from FDA, and several hundred Conference participants who participated in various sessions of the panel. And this expression was tightly reviewed.

The economic implications of false nutrition teaching and marketing are very great. One has only to note the evidence presented at the 1974 U.S. Senate Nutrition Policy hearings to get some idea of the financial meaning of misguided food choices. Even the Department of Agriculture's data showed that food was taking more than a sixth of the typical American budget. And most of the discussants at these meetings were more persuaded by data that showed the number to be something more like 30 percent of the budget, rising as high as 60 percent for millions of the poor.

In this light, consider the Ten-State Survey conclusion that, "Consumers are paying substantially more than is necessary to obtain needed nutrients."

And this is scarcely a problem only for the poor. Speaking to the American Association for the Advancement of Science, the Commissioner of the Food and Drug Administration, Dr. Charles Edwards, said: "While the potential for fatal consequences may be remote in the United States, nevertheless the incidence of nutritional deficiencies . . . is provable and numbers in the millions. And these millions are not counted among the poor alone. It is a problem crossing all social and economic boundaries, *often because of our national penchant for fads.*" (Emphasis added.)

"Food," wrote the Federal Trade Commission staffers, "is of central importance to consumers' health and finances."

What do we know about the financial impact? Looking at just one corner of the problem, we find that one conservative study, by J. D. Power and Associates of Los Angeles, is reported to show a billion-dollar-a-year market in health-food stores alone. It also indicates that these stores have 13 million homemakers as customers. If this is an accurate estimate, some 40 million Americans are eating foods from these stores.*

People who use these stores tend to be militantly opposed to many ordinary food products. They tend to be firm believers in the needs for special foods to sustain health.

And health foods are far from cheap. Many studies have

*The author would question some of this data, for it would imply that the average expenditure per person in families which patronize these special stores is only $25 a year, or $2 a month. All indications are that the typical health-food buyer spends many times this amount.

shown that one cannot eat cheaply and eat "health" foods. They can cost from 30 percent to 500 percent more than ordinary foods. The averages are reflected in a recent study by the U.S. Department of Agriculture. It found that, in the Washington, D.C. area, a shopping list of 29 standard foods cost $11 in a supermarket. The same list, filled in a "low-profit" food store which was declared to be "natural" (along the lines of a number of food cooperatives) cost $17.80—some 70 percent more. In the "natural" and "organic" sections of a supermarket, the cost was $20.30—93 percent more. And when the same foods were bought in a health-food store, the tab was $21.90, just about double.

The annual billion-dollar-plus take of the health-food stores does not include the similar food items sold in other establishments, from supermarkets to gift shops that sell organic fudge, herb teas or "natural honey"—the latter presumably made by bees which are not artificial and which have dined on blossoms which are not synthetic. It is hard to estimate the dollar volume of all these products.

To these we must add conventional grocery products which are consumed on the basis of spurious health theories. A Department of HEW study indicated, for example, that some 35 million Americans took nutritional supplements—usually as vitamin-mineral preparations—without a doctor's advice. There is at least a $600 million annual bill for these, the very vast majority of which, according to all true authorities, are unnecessary.

For example, take the "natural" cereals put out by major companies. At last look, these had taken more than seven percent of the cereal market, some $100 million a year. Most cost at least 50 percent more than conventional cereals, and they have far less nutritive value, since their boast of "no additives" means that they lack the vitamins and minerals added to most conventional cereals.

We shall see that many such products are involved in our total bill for weight control—which is variously estimated, but surely runs into the billions. Most of the money spent here is for dollar-grabbing plans with little or no worth.

Add to this the questionable nutrition plans offered in the nation's many gyms and salons, together with the nutrition books and magazine articles, most of which are based on well-meaning fantasies or cold-blooded deceptions, and the bill continues to mount. And it is going up fast.

By 1971, *Time* magazine, in an article on *The Profitable Earth,* interviewed Marshall Ackerman, then executive vice president of Rodale Press, the source of such journals as *Prevention* and *Organic Gardening,* along with whole libraries of similar literature on "natural" eating: "I've been in this business for 16 years," said Ackerman, "and nothing happened for the first 13. Since then [1968], it's become phenomenal."

The total sales ticket is probably at least $5 billion annually (though *Newsweek* guessed the weight-control business to be $10 billion a year, all by itself). Moreover, Dr. George Briggs, of the University of California, told a congressional hearing that between $30 billion and $75 billion of America's total medical bill could be traced to poor nutrition, most of this caused by misinformation.

As a seemingly minor example, but one typically meaningful in everyday human terms, consider the mother who laboriously prepares her own baby foods with a blender, to retain such nutrients as vitamin C, only unwittingly to generate far more destructive heat and air-exposure in cooking and handling, and ends with a dish from which most of the vitamin C has been removed; consider also the mother who switches her child from ordinary breakfast cereal to a "granola" and unwittingly steals 24 percent of her child's iron supply for the day.

And we shall see also some bitter cases, like those cited by Dr. Hilde Bruch, professor of psychiatry at Baylor College of Medicine. She notes, for example, author John Gunther's tale of his 16-year-old son's fight against brain cancer. "This intelligent, sophisticated and well-informed family used the best neurologists and brain surgeons in a renowned medical center and, at the same time, turned to whatever hearsay remedy seemed available, including health foods, vegetable juices, freshly squeezed juice of calves liver, and so on."

Aside from such stories of useless, meaningless treatment, Dr. Bruch observes that, "Quackery and food fads become dangerous, unmitigated evils when their false promises keep people from seeking medical treatment that might have saved their lives, or spared them unnecessary pain and suffering."

We are all at least a little vulnerable to such foodism. As Dr. Bruch concludes, "Even in a society dominated by the scientific method, magic is not as far away as we would like to think. It is a background to which we are all heir and which we may be tempted to use in situations that are high in ambiguity and fraught with great threat."

How much are you protected by reason and education from this susceptibility? Virtually all of us—whether we are consciously aware or not, whether our ideas were planted in childhood or chosen in maturity—are affected by *foodism,* the attribution of illusionary good or bad qualities to foods and how we eat them. On the chance, however, that you might have been lucky, there is a simple test. You are entirely free of the influences of foodism, and its legacy of both foods and ideas, if you:

Do not think "organic" food is more healthful.
Have never eaten a Graham cracker.
Have never worried about the refining of flour or sugar.
Have never drunk bitters in a cocktail.
Have never believed that "natural" foods were better foods.
Have never taken gelatin to strengthen your fingernails.
Do not take vitamin C to cure a cold.
Do not believe that eating more protein makes more muscle.
Do not believe that hard work demands more protein.
Do not believe that chemical fertilizers deprive you of important vitamins and minerals in foods.
Have never eaten peanut butter or yogurt.
Have never exercised on a mechanical horse.
Do not believe that fatness is caused by eating carbohydrate.
Think that milk cannot cause cavities in teeth.
Have never drunk blackstrap molasses for health.
Are not afraid to eat any two foods or drink any two drinks together, or at almost the same time.
Have not taken laxatives to be "regular."
Have not tried vitamin E to improve your sexual potency or to prevent heart disease.
Have not eaten bran to "save your life."
Have not drunk hot water on arising.

Have not starved either a cold *or* a fever.

Have not chewed your food once for each tooth in your mouth.

Have not believed that oysters or any other food aroused sexual passions.

Have not thought that toast was less fattening than bread.

Have not thought that steak was better for weight control than was a potato.

Have not thought that margarine was less fattening than butter.

Have not worried about hypoglycemia (low blood sugar).

Have not worried that hormones in beef would cause cancer.

Have not believed that salt would make you fat, or that sweating would make you thinner.

Have not eaten raw foods as more healthful.

Have not eaten *granola* because it was more healthful than ordinary cereals.

Have never believed that pills could supply all your vitamin and mineral needs.

For all of these ideas are the result of mistaken reaches into food magic. And most of them have been conceived, at least in part, to drain dollars from our purses—often into the purses of the light-fingered and agile-minded.

Are we not protected from frauds of this kind, even if they are naive but well-intended? As the White House Conference found in one of its reports, "The American people falsely believe that they are well protected, both by Government and by the ethics of commerce."

Clearly, we shall see, the public is not protected. "They" *can* say that in print, even if it isn't true. And we shall see that the most reputable magazine and book publishers *will.* We shall see also that advertisers can still, at this writing, mislead and deceive with impunity, if only they know the law.

A generation ago, Frank Voorhees, Jr., then director of the Division of Food, U.S. Food and Drug Administration, wrote that: "Good, cheap wholesome food products, that are nothing more than that, are recurrently exploited as modern miracles . . . are peddled as boons to mankind; and worthless nostrums are extolled as lifesavers . . . Conscienceless fakers ply their trade in such as these with all the trappings of last century's 'medicine man.' Their pitch is obviously directed to the weak and the ill, those most to be harmed by their vicious deception."

How has protective law been handcuffed? What might it, wisely administered, do? Where did our melange of nutritional nonsense come from? We shall soon see.

No attempt is made here to catalog fully every quack, every faddist, every unusual thinker who has affected the American dietary. Rather, the author has attempted what he hopes will be informative glimpses into an overpopulated pageant. For while the supply of intriguing characters in that procession is virtually inexhaustible, the author, sadly, is not.

As a final word about a final irony, let us return for a moment to Adelle Davis. It is 1973, and as the autumn comes, the word is out. Adelle is not well. She has *multiple myeloma*—cancer. She has drunk the quart of milk a day, and it has done no good. The lectures had quietly been cancelled, ever since her surgery in June.

She is sure that she knows how the protection of her good nutrition was overcome. In 1972 her sponsors had decided to insure her, and there had been x-rays. She is sure that the x-rays caused her cancer. "I was just dumbfounded," she says. "I just couldn't believe it. Cancer is a disease I was sure I would never get."

At first, hearing the verdict, Adelle was "shocked . . . fearful . . . panicky . . . I couldn't even think straight." Then she began a new nutritional analysis of her problem, and came up with some new solutions. "I'll tell you this," she told one interviewer, "I am trying some pretty unconventional things. Frankly," she lifted the strong chin, "I'd be very surprised if I die of cancer. I'm eating better than ever."

Adelle had promised a longer life to those who ate as she divined that people should. She had dismissed the Bible's statement about man's proper lifespan being 70 years. But early in 1974, Adelle died, victim of the cancer she had always said she could prevent. She was exactly three score years and ten.

2

Of Cabbages
and Things

In the second century before Christ, Marcus Porcius Cato, better known as Cato the Elder, became enthralled by cabbages. The famed Roman censor and agriculturist (noted for his pastoral classic, *De Re Rustica)* wrote long treatises in which he concluded that man could indeed live by cabbages alone. He grew them in profusion on his farm just outside Rome, and offered them as curatives to any of his workers and neighbors who fell ill.

Often the cabbage diet seemed to work. Nutritionally, there is one reason why it might. For there seems to have been a fair amount of scurvy in Rome. Scurvy is the disease which results from a dietary shortage of vitamin C. Cabbages have a goodly content of vitamin C, and when scurvy is treated with vitamin C, the results are dramatic; the seemingly moribund are soon up and about.

Two kinds of diets predominated in Rome, one for the rich and one for the poor, and paradoxically, both disposed to scurvy. For the wealthy favored diets of meat and fish. The legendary Roman banquets consisted of such foods as the venison of Gaul and the cured meats of Andalusia, of eel, skate, lobster and octupus from the Mediterranean, of African ostrich and gazelle. Meats were even assigned to each banquet guest according to his particular zodiacal sign—for example, the belly of a virgin pig for a Virgo, and for the Gemini (who was seen to have need of twinned comestibles) such paired meats as kidneys and testicles.

For the poor Romans, bread and barley gruel were the staples. At one point, some 25 percent of the Romans were receiving the *tessera*, a kind of early food stamp, with which to buy bread.

Since neither meats nor grains have much, if any, vitamin C, the cabbages may have filled a real gap in nutrition. Hence they may have alleviated some symptoms.

Medically, there is another reason why Cato's cabbages might have seemed to heal the sick. And this factor is what makes many deceptions about food and health so convincing. For most physicians are agreed—as was evidenced in one survey by the AMA—that *left untreated, perhaps as many as 80 percent of human illnesses are healed by normal bodily defenses.* This impressive percentage has always been the mainstay of the quack, and supported the otherwise unsupportable theories of the faddist. For it means that no matter what you recommend for your patients—provided you are careful not to poison or cripple them—a majority will get well and confer upon you both money and gratitude.

Thus any food or nutrient, when prescribed for the ill, appears to be effective most of the time. For example, a common cold which gets no special attention is usually gone in from three to five days. If one follows Dr. Linus Pauling's advice to dose the cold with perhaps 1,000 milligrams of vitamin C every hour—thus in half a day consuming the amount of the vitamin recommended for the adult male for 267 days—the cold is usually gone in from three to five days.

But here and there the nutritional cure is put to a more severe test. In time, Cato's own wife and son fell ill with a mysterious fever, the nature of which cannot be guessed from the information we have. Cato fed them cabbage. Tragically, both died. Cato was deeply saddened. But, typical of the history of health-foodism, this misfortune did not change Cato's thinking about cabbages. It is an axiom of the health-food school, through history, that no dedicated health-foodist is disturbed by mere fact.

Such early medical beliefs about food permeate every known culture. They are so old that there is rarely history early enough to tell us how they began. And in every culture, along with the magical "good" foods, there are bad ones.

It is not hard to see how such beliefs must have begun. For early man had no supermarkets and no Food and Drug Administration. He had only his own experience and legend to guide his choices for dinner. To understand, we have only to picture ourselves foraging for something to eat in forests and meadows. Which plant is edible and which is the foxglove with its heart stimulant? Which mushroom do we dare try? Food myths guided these choices, and the primitive forager had no way to know when the warnings were inspired by incidents of sudden death and when by some unfounded taboo. The unfamiliar was always a threat.

We of the age of science are not so different. Americans wince at the idea of sitting down to a nice, juicy horse steak. Yet in France, horsemeat is widely sold as a delicacy, while the Indian is repelled by the meat of the cow.

We cannot understand tribes which find eggs and chicken disgusting food, but who love a good mouse or dog. To touch upon the ultimate in civilized repugnance, we are certainly loath to dine on one another. Yet before 1250 A.D., certain Tibetans ate the dead bodies of their parents. As William of Rubruck, who in the 13th century made a journey into the Orient, put it, the eating was done "out of piety, in order to give them no other sepulcher than their own bowels." Curiously, while most of us think of cannibalism as directed toward enemies, there are records of many cultures in which only the eating of loved ones was acceptable.

Spix and Martius, two early 19th century anthropologists, once asked a chief of the South American Miranhas why he practiced cannibalism, and got an answer with real insight into the phenomena of food prejudice: "You whites will not eat crocodiles or apes, although they taste well. If you did not have so many pigs and crabs, you would eat crocodiles and apes, for hunger hurts. It is all a matter of habit. When I have killed an enemy, it is better to eat him than to let him go to waste."

Much taboo about food is related to ancient beliefs that, since food gives man its nourishment, it also conveys other qualities. So we find that some Australian aborigines believe that to eat the flesh of the parrot or cockatoo is to risk developing, like the birds, a hollow in the top of one's head and a hole under one's chin. And because the fox is long-winded, some tribes feed fox lungs to those with asthma. Believing the liver to be the seat of mercy, others forcibly feed the organ to the sly or mean of their tribes. Some are afraid to eat deer or snake because to do so might make them timid or sneaky, and there are still Chinese who prescribe a dish of bats for the weak of eye and the hard of hearing.

To some primitives, the magic of food has been so powerful that it can actually be transmitted when someone else eats it. For example, the Blackfoot Indians sometimes ate rosebuds, but would not eat them when trapping an eagle. For some of the Indians had itched after eating rosebuds, so they feared that the eagle, being stalked by a rosebud eater, might also itch, and would merely sit and scratch himself instead of taking the bait.

Sir James Frazer cites a number of such beliefs in his 1921 book, *The Golden Bough*. At the time, soldiers of Madagascar were forbidden to eat hedgehog, "as it is feared that this animal, from its propensity of coiling up into a ball when alarmed, will impart a timid, shrinking disposition to those who partake of it." Frazer also mentions that the Malagasy soldier "must eschew kidneys, because in the Malagasy language the word for kidney is the same as that for 'shot'; so shot he would certainly be if he ate a kidney."

Some of these beliefs have been carried to appalling extremes. For example, in 1899, Spencer and Gillen, studying the Central Australian primitives, found that in the Luritcha tribe: "It is not an infrequent custom, when a child is in weak health, to kill a younger and healthy one, and then to feed the weakling on its flesh, the idea being that this will give to the weaker child the strength of the stronger one."

It is apparently from such beliefs that foods became medicines, good and bad, for the ancients. In fact, in virtually every developing civilization food *was* medicine—the cause and cure for most disease. For example, the great physician of the Greek Island of Cos, Hippocrates, whose oath is still taken by physicians and who is revered as the "father of medicine," based his whole scheme of treatment and prevention on what his patients ate. "Thy food shall be thy remedy," he maintained, and for some 2,000 years this advice was followed by Western civilization.

As Galen, reputed to be perhaps the next greatest of the Greek physicians, wrote more than half a millennium after Hippocrates: "Let those who refuse to admit the efficacy of food in making men better or more dissolute, more unrestrained or more reserved, bolder or more timid, more barbarous or more civilized, or more given to disputes and fighting, let them on thinking better of it inquire in order to learn from me what they should eat or drink."

And as late as 1747, the physician Gaubius was quoting these same words to advise his readers on health.

In China, another school of medicine arose, quite separate from the influence of the Greeks. Yet it, too, sought in food the answers to suffering. The Chinese attitude is exemplified by the ancient god Shen-Nung, portrayed in clothing of leaves. Interestingly, this deity had three related roles—as god of medicine, god of pharmacy and god of agriculture—symbolizing the concept that to be well one had to know what to eat.

What kinds of medication resulted from these beliefs? In the Orient, it was held that the drinking of red wines would make blood, as would the dark meat of the duck. Dark foods were highly recommended for women who were nursing boys. (And to this day, they are still.)

In Greece, Discorides (of the Hippocratic school) laid down principles of treatment which were respected for 1,500 years. These included such remedies as eating grasshoppers for bladder disorders, the liver of an ass for epilepsy and alleviating fevers by ingesting seven bugs in the skin of a bean.

Certainly Rome's medicine was derived from the Greek school of food-healing. Pliny reports that Nero ate leeks seven days each month to clear his voice. Lettuce was sure to cleanse the senses. And beans were eaten only with care and ceremony, since the Romans believed that the souls of the dead reposed in them. In Egypt, which shared some of the Roman and Grecian ideas, beans were entirely forbidden to the priests, along with garlic, leeks and onions, and any meat except goose and beef.

It is not surprising that the Romans came to think that eating garlic gave one physical strength. But it must have taken considerably more research to learn that truffles provided greater sexual potency. Pliny swore by them and ate them often. Considering the recreational interests of Rome in Pliny's time, it is logical that truffles commanded quite a price in the markets. And only recently the author was assured by a learned truffle grower in Perigueux that everyone who has good access to the truffle knows the truth of Pliny's contention.

Another important tradition of foodism also began in the ancient world: the idea that self-deprivation at the table was the key to health. Some Romans, despite wealth, tried to survive mainly on barley gruel and water. Fasting was a method of physical purification.

This rejection of food was also notable in the Chinese medical tradition, which reached the medical school at Salerno in the Middle Ages and there combined with Graeco-Roman-Egyptian thinking to form the nub of Western medicine for seven centuries. The Salerno physicians said, for example, that, "A large supper imposes the greatest punishment on the stomach." And they advised that "Cheese and bread are good food for those in good health—if a man is not healthy do not add the cheese to the bread."

The merging of east and west did not really change the nutritional approach to medicine very much from Hippocrates' day. Foods continued to be the basis of the pharmacopeia. But the cures began to be more exotic. Medieval physicians fed their patients dung in wine, worms for lung disease, deer fat for nerves and such curiosities as the moss growing on the skull of a hanged man for illness they could not diagnose.

Understanding of human physiology and the origins of disease were still very limited at the time, and continued so well into the 18th century. Aromas were commonly blamed for contagion, so that in time of plague the gentry carried perfumed handkerchiefs. Handkerchiefs tucked into the lacy sleeve or held artfully in the hand in the French courts of the Louis' were as much preventive medicine as they were foppery.

European physicians searched constantly for new foods from the further corners of the world, much as we watch for new antibiotics. Pregnant women adopted a Chinese custom of eating pigs' feet to guard against demons and ill humours. When it was learned that the Sultan of Turkey ate a special clay from the Island of Lemnos, the product became a health-food import on the European continent.

Each new food from explorations was regarded as a possible pharmaceutical or poison. When in 1632 a grocer displayed the first banana in London, the pharmacists objected, saying that it was a powerful drug which should be dispensed only by the trained druggist.

Even spices were given medical meanings. When coffee first came to Europe, its berries were ground and eaten with fat as a laxative. Later it was cooked with wine and used to treat fevers.

As the 1700's began, physicians turned even more to the writings of the ancients for health secrets. Aphrodisiacs were of the keenest interest. Pliny's advice about truffles was revived, as was a belief that sexual prowess derived from eating the foot and snout of the hippopotamus.

European doctors healed the pain of love with Horace's prescription of pigeons and turtledoves. They wooed the mood of love with pistachio nuts, radishes, celery, dates, mint, parsley, quinces and walnuts. We probably have some of these foods still because of their early cultivation as drugs.

When the tomato reached Europe, it was at first sold as a decorative plant and known as the *lycopersicon,* or wolf of the peach, and sometimes as the love apple. Then the Italians began to say that tomatoes had amorous effect, and the red Italian sauces became popular.

For a century, lettuce was thought to be a sexual stimulant. Then suddenly, it was looked upon as a repressor.

When the potato was brought from South America to Spain, peasants marveled at its lush growth but somehow came to think that it poisoned the soil, spread the plague and could cause diarrhea and leprosy. This poor reputation may have stemmed from the strict Spanish clergy, who decided that there was no authority in the Bible for the potato's existence.

Some governments intervened, seeing the potato as an answer to periodic famines But even though it was soon a staple in Ireland, the potato was thought by some to be immoral, since it was easy to grow and left the hands of farmers idle.

By the middle of the 18th century, the new rational science began to take hold. Everywhere in the West, researchers began to catalog and categorize natural phenomena, from plants to animals and diseases, in the first step toward true scientific method. Soon the circulation of the blood was revealed. Soon Lavoisier understood the principles that made nutrition science possible. Before he went to the guillotine he wrote what may be the first real line of biochemistry: "Life is a chemical function." Soon Descartes declared that medicine was the best hope for the perfection of man.

But in 1744, Dr. Leonard Lynch published a most respected treatise for the public, his *Guide to Health.* Spelling out what medicine then knew of nutrition, he wrote:

"Plumbs purge Choler, extinguish Heat, take away Thirst in Fevers; but they are bad for weak and cold Stomachs and for phlegmatic persons, and such as are subject to Colics . . . Currants are good in spitting of Blood, extremely cooling and somewhat astringent . . .

Oranges that are sweet are more replacing than the Seville Oranges; but these last are an excellent remedy for the hot Scurvy. The Sweet Oranges increase Choler . . . Grapes . . . help the Appetite and Digestion; but in great Quantities, they dissolve the Gall too much and produce fluxes . . ."

By the time of the American Revolution, the medical view of foods was much more rational. The potato was no longer suspect. It was seen as a "stomachic." For example, whenever his Colonists would act up, King George III, having flown into rage and frustration, followed by dyspepsia, would sit down to an unkingly dinner of a single boiled potato. And in the height of the great French Empire, Napoleon was also basing his diet on potatoes, prescribed not as a stomachic, but to deal with his embarrassing obesity.

By the 1830's modern medicine had truly begun to take shape. But foodism remained. When cholera broke out on the eastern seaboard of the U.S., several cities banned the sale of fruits, thinking they were the cause, along with salads and uncooked vegetables. In Washington, D.C., on August 16, 1832, the Board of Health issued this order:

"The Board of Health, after mature deliberation, has resolved . . . that the following articles are . . . highly prejudicial to health at the present season . . . They hereby decree that the sale of them . . . be prohibited . . . for the space of 90 days.

Cabbage, green corn, cucumbers, peas, beans, parsnips, carrots, egg plants, squashes, pumpkins, turnips, watermelons, canteloups, musk melons, apples, peas, peaches, plums, damsons, cherries, apricots, oranges, lemons, limes, cocoanuts, ice creams, fish, crabs, oysters, clams, lobsters or crawfish.

The following articles the Board have not considered it necessary to prohibit the sale of, but even these they would admonish the county to be moderate in using. Potatoes, beets, tomatoes and onions."

While the cholera epidemic continued, scarcely anyone seemed to object to this ruling. Indeed, a generation later, in 1849, the *Chicago Democrat* reported that two boys "partook freely" of oranges and coconuts and went to a circus. "In a short time," said the *Democrat,* "one was a corpse and the other reduced to the last stage of cholera."

In 1867, the *Chicago Tribune* told of a man who passed a stand of spoiled peaches and got an attack of "the gripes." Warned the *Tribune:* "If bare proximity to those peaches caused him so much pain, the eating of them would have been certain death."

These are not isolated incidents. They reflect the typical thinking of the time. As we can see, they stand in a long line of foodism which stretches back to primitive days. That line continues into the early part of our own century, when we find an advertisement which was regarded by most as perfectly sensible. It was placed by Charles W. Post, who had started a cereal company in Battle Creek, Michigan, using secrets which Mr. W.K.

Kellogg and his brother John Harvey felt Post had stolen from them.

The offer was in the mode which Mr. Post had used to establish his coffee substitute, *Postum*. He had flatly promised that *Postum* would "make red blood."

Post, who wrote the ad himself, had a medical reason why people should buy his new cereal: "There are no blotches on the face of Beauty when fed on Grape-Nuts."

In the short space of time since that ad first appeared, nutrition has become a true science. And while all is, of course, not known, a great deal is understood. Yet at this writing, the periodicals are still cluttered with such ads as: *"You can now command your body to Melt Away Fat."*

Were Cato the Elder to come suddenly to life again, he might well read this ad and hundreds of others, and with equal sense decide, "I still prefer cabbages."

3

Mr. Graham
Bakes a Cracker

From his birth in 1794, Sylvester Graham was a sickly youngster. It is uncertain from the records, but he was either the 12th, 14th or 17th child of aging parents. It is agreed, however, that his father was 70 at the time, and that from the age of two, Sylvester was an orphan and an object of charity.*

This third generation Connecticut Yankee child was to become what some histories still call the father of the public health movement in America. At the very least, Sylvester certainly can be dubbed the father of what we now call food consumerism, and something of his style is still seen among many of his modern counterparts.

*These circumstances may be worth noting, for an early loss of parents is part of the lives of many noted foodists, suggesting a psychological pattern. As an example, Adelle Davis' mother suffered a stroke within 10 days of Daisie Adelle's birth, and died before the baby was two.

The son and grandson of minsters of the Gospel, Sylvester had a strong religious bent, probably strengthened by the seeking of divine help during his childhood illnesses. In any case, he used religious authority all through his life to advance his health opinions. In fact, he said flatly that he bore the word of God to the nation. In his missionary efforts for health, he likened himself to the prophet Isaiah.

Little is known of Sylvester's life until the age of 29, when he entered Amherst College as an unusually old undergraduate. He was soon known for the fanaticism of his ideas. The frequency with which he made long, emotional speeches about these ideas soon earned him a campus nickname, "The Stage Actor." His classmates were so skeptical of his sincerity and so annoyed by him that they conspired to have him dismissed from Amherst, and eventually succeeded. Immediately, Sylvester had a nervous breakdown, of which he carried a memento for many years—his nurse, Miss Sarah Eads, whom he married after he regained his health.

Children soon appeared, and Sylvester, now 32, began to seek work. Since his only assets were his oratory and his theological upbringing, he turned to religion. Despite his lack of education, he persuaded the Presbyterian Church to ordain him a minister. And in 1826, the Church began to send him out as a substitute preacher and roving evangelist, based in Newark, New Jersey. Impressive in his evangelism, he soon was an agent for the Pennsylvania State Society for the Suppression of the Use of Ardent Spirits.

Sylvester was good at expounding on the mix of hellfire and ill health that menaced the tippler. But Sarah Graham sneered a bit, and not always privately. She liked to take a nip of gin herself now and then, refused to pledge abstinence and took few pains to conceal either fact.

Then on trips to Philadelphia, Sylvester came in contact with some brother evangelists whose style was so close to his own that, perhaps for the first time in his life, he made some real friends. These were elders and emissaries of the young Bible Christian Church.

The Church had been formed in the 1790's, in Manchester,

England, by a young Anglican curate named William Cowherd. The name was perhaps ironic, for Cowherd had begun his religious thinking with vegetarianism—troubled by lines in the Bible which seemed to forbid the killing and eating of animals.

Various religious injunctions to abstain from meat have been claimed since earliest Greek and Hindu times. But they are hard to substantiate from Judaeo-Christian scripture. For there are bald contradictions of the idea, as in the line from Deuteronomy: "These are the beasts ye shall eat; the ox, the sheep and the goat . . ."

But Cowherd was so convinced of the Christian necessity for vegetarianism that he felt he could not continue in a Church of England whose clergy relished a nice joint of beef or plate of chops. At first he thought that he might be able to manage as a Swedenborgian. But conscience troubled him here as well, and more and more he felt that theology should be based upon care of the body and man's proper mode of living, as revealed in Holy Writ. He gave up the Swedenborgian cloth and set out with a small group of followers, the Bible Christians, to build a new church.

The evangelical style of the Bible Christians was not, however, popular with their neighbors. The British at this time were relatively tolerant of others' religious feelings, far more so certainly than in the Puritan and Carolean days, when Church and State were closely joined and the Pilgrims were driven off to the Colonies. But to badger an Englishman to accept a choice between his immortal soul and his dinner was foolhardy. By 1809, the Bible Christians had engendered a violent hostility.

It was in this year that William Metcalfe joined the new church. His strength and persuasiveness soon made him a leader. When mounting intolerance made it clear to many Bible Christians that they could not flourish in Britain, Metcalfe was chosen to lead them in perhaps the last religious exodus from England to the New World.

The voyage took 11 weeks and had sad consequences. A pained and bewildered Metcalfe always blamed the sea air. But whatever the cause, before land was sighted again, half the Bible Christians had succumbed to meat.

The new church was founded in Philadelphia. But it was so small and so poor that there was no money to pay Pastor Metcalfe. So he taught school a bit, and then, putting to work his religiously-inspired views of health, began to treat the sick by homeopathy.

Because homeopathy is closely linked to the ideas of "natural" living and medicine which Sylvester Graham was to promulgate, and which were to have a powerful influence on current American ideas of health, a brief look at this concept may be useful. It began in the late 1700's, in the mind of a Philadelphian named Samuel Hahnemann.

Just before the nineteenth century Hahnemann, a physician, noticed that a drug he was using produced symptoms much like those of malaria. Leaping to a series of conclusions—quite permissible under the rules of *Naturphilosophie*, a rising German school of scientific thinking—Hahnemann produced his *Law of Similia*.

This law states generally that "like cures like." In other words, if you have malaria, you take the drug that produces symptoms like those of malaria. Presto! You are cured. Nature has provided a specific for every ailment. Diseases, said Hahnemann, are really just different kinds of *psora*, or itches.

In homeopathy it is the symptoms which count, not the disease. And you can't rush homeopathic medicine, Hahnemann said. Thirty to sixty days may pass before the results can be seen.

One extremely important concept had to be added, however. For example, consider the problem of food poisoning, with vomiting. The *Law of Similia* indicates that one should deal with vomiting by finding an herb in nature which *causes* vomiting. It is easy to see how this could cause trouble. But Hahnemann had a modification which prevented making bad situations worse.

As he explained in his basic work, *The Organon*, the real art of homeopathy was *dilution*. The reasoning goes like this: The more diluted the medication, the less the symptom worsens; therefore, the more we dilute medicine, the more curative, the more powerful it gets!

By this method, Hahnemann found that he could make medicines of incredible power, soon reaching dilutions to one *decillionth* of the original concentration—that is, diluting until the medicine was one part substance and 999,999 parts water, then taking this powerful potion and using one part of *it* to 999,999 parts water, then repeating this same process eight more times. If we follow Hahnemann's reasoning, we can see that the power of such dilution must surely be awesome.

Hahnemann found such new drugs as the tears of a young girl, the aromatic essence of skunk and powdered bedbugs. Costly homeopathic medicines were much used throughout the 19th century. In fact, by 1901 there were 21 schools of homeopathic medicine in America.

The idea survived, but it had begun to have much less acceptance among physicians after 1842, when Oliver Wendell Holmes had written "Homeopathy and Kindred Delusions." Some suggestion of the one-time influence of homeopathy may be seen in the statue to Samuel Hahnemann which stands at Scott Circle in Washington, D.C., and in the fact that one of the nation's eminent medical schools today (though its philosophy is changed) is Philadelphia's Hahnemann Medical College.

Thus we have some idea of the kind of teaching which Bible Christian Pastor Metcalfe conveyed to an eager Sylvester Graham. Homeopathy, however, was not what appealed to Sylvester. What he liked was the idea that there was a "natural" kind of living for mankind, and an "unnatural" kind, especially in terms of eating. Moreover, Graham was deeply affected by the idea that God had left clues about which was which. Where specific instructions were omitted from the Revealed Word, a righteous man's intuitions would point out the right path.*

Thus Sylvester began to think of himself as a prophet, revealing God's intentions in Nature. And he perceived the core of these intentions in food. After all, it was with vegetarianism that the Bible Christians had begun.

In Sylvester's mind, the right food would save not only man's life but also his soul. The idea struck fire in the popular mind, and soon Graham's lectures were packed, as he moved up and down the Atlantic seaboard.

*This thinking was bolstered by German scientists, who, frustrated in their attempts to penetrate the secrets of the physical world, had about 1910 formed the school called *Naturphilosophie,* which held that philosophy was the way to breakthroughs in medicine.

He lectured on cholera, on fresh air, on taking baths. He was one of the first to offer lectures containing blunt sexual advice to young men. Chastity was a subject on which he could thunder terrifyingly, and thunder he did, to an extent that may have had considerable effect on the birth rate. But his greatest success lay with lectures on food.

Where Graham's ideas about eating came from, other than those on vegetarianism, seems to be a matter of speculation. But he expressed them with such force and bluster that he became a popular lecturer. Before long he left the Pennsylvania Temperance Society to barnstorm, soon picking up fees of $300 per lecture.

In 1830, indigestion occupied a place of popularity in the American mind equalled today only by neurosis and allergy. The American diet was a pork fat, pie-rich fright, to be sure, out of which eventually grew a patent-medicine empire. Dyspepsia was the byword, and it was out of dyspeptic bondage that Sylvester promised to lead the faithful.

Dyspepsia, Graham said, was the product of too concentrated a diet. And the way to break up that diet was to put the bran back into wheat flour. Naturally, nothing was then known of the vitamin or mineral content of the bran. Graham's protest was against the loss of bulk.

But some years before, millers had begun to run flour through bolting cloth, to try and whiten it. "Put back the bran," thundered Graham. The plainer and more natural a man's food, he said, "the more perfectly the laws of his constitution are fulfilled . . . the more health will be in his body . . . the more perfect his senses . . . the more powerful his intellectual and moral faculties be rendered by suitable cultivation."

It all hung together. The right food could end by saving a man's soul. Graham trudged up and down the Atlantic Seaboard, growing rich and famous. Any man who expressed scientific interest in his food was called a Grahamite.

The lectures quickly became the focal point of a crusade. One of Graham's assistants said alcoholism killed 50,000 Americans yearly, "folly in dress" killed 80,000 and "down-right gluttony" killed 100,000. Considering the size of the American population of the time, these figures should have left the continent empty of all but Grahamites in a decade; so the reader is advised not to rely upon them.

Graham pushed on. Meat excited vile tempers and habits. It drove men to sexual excesses and it was sexual excess that was filling the insane asylums. People did not bathe enough. They needed external applications of cold water at least once a week. They needed to open their windows in the morning, exercise, and breathe the icy air.

From these few concepts alone, it may be seen that Graham's advice was not ignored, and perhaps there was even some good done thereby. Saturday night bathing habits are directly traced to Sylvester's lectures, as are hard beds and the setting-up exercises before open windows which are only just now going out of fashion. Even women, he said, needed exercise. And the Grahamites established Ladies' Physiological Reform Societies throughout New England, to work for emancipation from tight lacing.

The *Graham Journal of Health and Longevity* came into being, to say, among other things, that, "Every farmer knows that if his horse has straw cut with his grain, or hay in abundance, he does well enough. Just so it is with the human species. Man needs the bran in his bread." And the *Journal* joined Graham in saying bread should be baked in the home, if not for health reasons, then as an almost sacred rite.

Contrary to the belief of many modern foodists, white bread is not new. In ancient Rome, the most prized bread was made from *alica,* a processed product of *emmer* wheat. So important was its whiteness that a kind of white chalk called *creta* was blended with the wheat.

Graham was also the first of many to compare man physiologically to the orang-utan and to conclude that like the apes, his natural food was vegetable. He added that food should never be eaten hot, that it should be chewed slowly and energetically and that water should never be taken with meals. Tea, he said, could produce delirium tremens. Condiments, like sexual excess, caused insanity. Like most health prophets, his program grew with his enthusiasms, his enthusiasm grew with his audience, and his audience grew bigger as his statements grew wilder. It was a vicious circle.

Excessive lewdness and chicken pie were the causes of

cholera, he decided. And the more energy he devoted to the problem of lewdness, the larger crowds he drew to hear about unbolted Graham flour.

When he arrived in Boston in 1835 for a speaking engagement, the city was divided into two ardent camps. On one side were the rabid reformers of the day. On the other were such as the newspaperman who dubbed him the Peristaltic Persuader. The faithful lavished gifts upon him, and the commercial bakers lavished epithets. The Boston Physiologic Society had become a Graham meetinghouse.

When Graham prepared to speak in the main dining room of the Marlborough Hotel, having been barred from Amory Hall out of fears of violence, the bakers and butchers took arms. So violent and many were the threats that Boston's mayor apologetically warned that he did not believe that his police force could manage the situation.

At last the time for the lecture arrived. Inside Graham shouted to the faithful. Outside, a butcher-baker-incited mob muttered darkly. There were arguments, then threats. The mob moved forward. But on the roof of the Marlborough Hotel were ready guards. In wooden troughs they had great quantities of slaked lime. In their hands were shovels. When the threat seemed earnest, the guards began to hurl down clouds of lime. Sylvester Graham was saved.

Such incidents helped to spread the fame of Grahamism, and Sylvester was encouraged to make bolder and bolder claims—such as that tuberculosis was curable by vegetarianism, and that if a meat eater and a Grahamite were both "shot down and killed in warm weather," the vegetable-eater's body would last two or three times as long.

By 1837, one of Dartmouth's most noted professors, Dr. R. D. Mussey, was a Grahamite lecturer. The American Physiological Society was formed to publicize Graham ideas. And Graham teas were held for ladies, to allow discussion of intimate female problems over bran tea and Graham milk toast, perhaps the first U.S. sessions in consciousness raising.

Graham boardinghouses appeared in Boston and New York. Newspaper editor Horace Greeley, soon to be a candidate for

President, took his meals in a New York Graham hotel. Williams College instituted a Graham Club, and Wesleyan University offered its students Graham board, chiefly of rice, beans, pudding and harsh Graham bread. (The situation was not much different from that of the late 1960's and early 1970's, when a number of American schools, even Yale, began to offer "natural" and "organic" cafeteria lines as alternatives.)

In 1837, Graham's polemics appeared in two thick volumes as *Lectures in the Science of Human Life*. These became the prime health books of the day's progressives. Progressives and reformers of every kind flocked to the Graham movement. Some were wholly acceptable to him. The Abolitionists were an example. Others horrified him. Among these was an early feminist named Mary Gove, who ran a Massachusetts school which taught girls the benefits of Graham bread, loose corsets and, appallingly, free love.

Some of Graham's effect may be seen in the 1838 meeting of the American Health Convention. It resolved to advocate the teaching of anatomy and physiology in the schools. It also condemned the use of medicines, pledging itself to the support of "natural" hygiene. As a corollary, it resolved that the vegetarian diet was superior.*

Medicine was in its infancy. Pierre Louis, for example, was just beginning to apply statistical methods to treatments, counting how many patients who were treated by any particular therapy lived or died. His efforts actually outraged many physicians, who did not care to be evaluated.

In the early 1800's, the care of infants was still being left to the untrained. As a London physician of the time, Dr. Cadogan, wrote: "A general practice is, as soon as a child is born, to cram a dab of butter and sugar down its throat. . . a little oil . . . or some such unwholesome mess . . . It is a custom of some to give a little roast pig to an infant which, it seems, is to cure it of all its mother's longings."

---

*Scientifically, it is not. The vegetarian diet is workable, but nutritionally precarious—partly because proteins are of varying quality, and wheat is not a source of high-quality protein. No single plant is. So plant foods must be knowledgeably combined to keep vegetarians healthy. Graham's food plan would have made protein intake questionable.

The measuring of pulse and temperature did not begin until about 1835, when some French physicians started the practice. Oliver Wendell Holmes said that even by the Civil War, there were scarcely a dozen clinical thermometers in use. Until 1887, there was no device for measuring blood pressure, and none was widely used until our own century. As late as 1850, the signs of appendicitis were treated with morphine and purging, with consequent high risk of death. Not until 1848 had London's Henry Hancock, defying scoffers, performed the first surgical removal of an appendix.

As for nutrition, the word carbohydrate was not coined until 1844, when Schmidt first showed that certain natural products, on hydrolysis, yielded sugar. The concept of the vitamin was unknown until our own century. Where were the doctors? Scratching their heads, wondering, performing a little surgery when there was no other choice and without anesthetic, administering emetics, laxatives, and dangerous drugs, offering bloodletting for fevers, and casting a skeptical but curious and uncertain eye toward the Grahamite camp.

Their patients? Did not bran make as much sense on the surface of things as the leech? Was it not possible that three meats at a company dinner, finished off with three kinds of potatoes and three desserts really *was* a cause of dyspepsia? And if Graham was right about that, could he not also be right about bran, about lewdness causing cholera, about bathing, about meat leading to sin? Where, after all, was the criterion to divide sense from nonsense?

As he neared sixty, Sylvester Graham retired from the lecture platform to live in Northampton, Massachusetts, which was becoming a center for popular water cures. Harriet Beecher Stowe sought the help of the waters there, as did Jenny Lind. Almost everyone took to a little of Grahamism—with the possible exception of Mrs. Graham, who spread a groaning board, to Sylvester's everlasting shame.

Graham began to write poems and grow a little senile. He amplified his interest in Indian clubs and exercise. He took an ice bath every morning, ate old dark bread. And he suffered dismally as the press twitted him without mercy. In 1851 he was sick and tired. He tried a rice diet to alleviate his difficulties, but it failed him. He died in September of that year, after stimulants, a tepid bath, and a dose of Congress waters, at the age of fifty-seven.

We shall see Sylvester's ideas live on and on, into our own day. But to most Americans, the name of Sylvester Graham is virtually lost, except for one last ironic vestige, the Graham cracker.

4

Little Men, Little Women, Little Food

It is dawn on a frosty New England day. Young Louisa May Alcott—one day to be known as the authoress of *Little Women*—stands naked behind a curtain in her childhood home. With her are her three naked sisters, who will be immortalized in the book. Enter their kindly father, Amos Bronson Alcott, known to many as the Seer of New England, well-remembered both as a philosopher and a pioneer of progressive education. He has trudged through the snow to a nearby stream, broken the ice and drawn a bucket of numbingly cold water. With a cheery smile, he dumps the bucket behind the curtain. The girls shudder, and when they can speak again, thank him.

The time is about 1840, and the ceremony is a daily one. For Amos is a staunch Grahamite.

He had grown up a big, hard-working farm boy, but one who

did not care much for meat. Even in a day when there was no replacement, Amos would leave his salt pork on his plate. In midwinter, this difficult child would ask for vegetables. And neighbors spoke in low tones of the common knowledge that he wanted to try living on apples.

Amos had a cousin of about the same age, William, who shared his tastes. The boys grew up on neighboring farms, shared books and helped each other learn to write by conducting a very formal correspondence on boyish matters. Neither had any interest in taking over the family farms.

Amos and William reached early manhood in a day when a young man's fortune might be made by putting a pack of Connecticut-manufactured oddments on his back, putting a box on a coastal steamer and heading for the southern states to become that familiar folklore figure, the Yankee Pedlar. Amos made several such trips. He sold barely enough to pay for them, because he kept getting interested in conversations and forgetting his merchandise. At last Amos' pleasure in the trips tempted William to go along, but he hated it. Buying for less and selling for more offended his stern moral sense. The experiment ended when Amos Bronson came down with typhus in Norfolk, Virginia, and William had to nurse him for five weeks in an attic room.

Right after this trip, William went on to college in Boston. Amos stayed on the farm and taught school. But soon he began to move from town to town. For he had odd ideas. He would hold theological discussions with his little pupils and write down their ideas. He even published them, a cause of so much outrage that eventually he had to give up his career as a headmaster in Boston, barely managing to slip away from a mob that had come for his scalp.

Following this, Amos was unable to get another teaching job. Today his ideas of education are widely accepted. But then they were seen as outrageous. Wherever he went, his reputation as a crackpot went before him—getting children to discuss life's meaning and think about it was certainly a madman's scheme. Always jobless, moneyless, with strange ideas and stranger friends, Amos was destined to be an outsider. For him, respect was to come largely as a posthumous reward. It is hardly surprising that he felt at home with every outcast and reformer.

Cousin William had chosen a more acceptable field for reform. A vegetarian writer on health, in contact with the Bible Christians and William Metcalfe, who gave him encouragement and Biblical quotations to prove that meat was sinful, William was making a name. It was William who, partly through his *Vegetable Diet as Sanctioned by Medical Men and by Experience in All Ages,* convinced Dartmouth's Professor Mussey of the need for a vegetarian crusade. It was through William that some of the key doors in New England were opened to Sylvester Graham. For example, it was William who persuaded Mussey to invite Graham to Dartmouth, and also to Bowdoin College in Maine.

William demanded an even tougher bread than did Sylvester himself. For William's bread must be made without yeast even, chock full of bran and unleavened. As for baking soda and baking powder, William pronounced them deadly poisons. His was probably the first important American diatribe against "additives" of any kind.

Amos gave close attention to his learned cousin. He stopped eating meat in 1835, the year of the Boston Butchers' and Bakers' Riot. Not only had he never much cared for meat, but he had been reading the Greek, Pythagoras. And Pythagoras, in addition to propounding that theorem which bears his name—and solves the problems of the right triangle—also demanded that his followers have nothing but vegetables and conversation for dinner.

Soon Amos Bronson also gave up eggs, cheese and butter. But a kindly soul, he long forebore to ask his wife, Abigail, and Louisa May and her sisters to do the same. Even while William was founding the monthly magazine, *Moral Reformer,* and following this with publication of his *Library of Health,* writing that "Eating of the flesh of animals is a violation of the first dietetic law given to mankind by the Creator," Amos Bronson found himself out shopping for meat.

He did it for Abigail and the children, when there was money. But returning from one such harrowing expedition, he wrote: "What have I to do with butchers? Death yawns at me as I walk up and down this abode of skulls. Murder and blood are written on its stalls. Cruelty stares at me from the butcher's face. I tread amongst carcasses. I am in the presence of the slain. The death-set eyes of beasts peer at me and accuse me . . . Quartered, disemboweled creatures suspended on hooks plead with me . . . I am a replenisher of graveyards. I prowl, amidst other unclean spirits and voracious demons, for my prey."

Although Amos Bronson could not get a job, he had a strong following among New England's intellectuals. In fact, in one financial low, Amos and the family went to Concord to accept the help of their good, though meat-eating, friend, Ralph Waldo Emerson.

Emerson often got them through bad times with loans which became gifts. He helped them to settle in a house called "Dove Cottage," where Amos Bronson was determined that they should live an idealistic "Pythagorean life." Thus began Louisa May's icy baths, as prescribed by Sylvester Graham, and endorsed by Cousin William.

Graham had instructed that bread should be made in the home, and this Amos Bronson did himself, serving it now with nothing but water and apples. He was a little torn between indulging his family, and, as their spiritual leader, giving them the discipline which would save their bodies and souls. But in the end, he always favored the discipline; by 1843, the Alcotts were to keep a strict vegetarian home.

Life at Dove Cottage was not, however, joyless. There were plenty of guests. The much loved Emerson dropped in regularly. And Henry Thoreau would come down periodically from his hermitage at Walden Pond to break bread—no mean feat with these sturdy, unleavened loaves—with the Alcotts.

Meanwhile, Bronson—who more and more was becoming known without the *Amos,* and rather liked the new name better—continued to write about education. In both the U.S. and in Britain, his work was known and appreciated only by small in-groups of intellectuals. The Americans reacted mainly by buying his books and, like Emerson, trying to help him in his poverty. But his English admirers, Bronson was learning, were more moneyed.

They had even formed a pioneering school at an estate which they called Alcott House. Money was raised to send Bronson to see it.

Commending his "little women" to Emerson's kindness, Bronson prepared for the trip by baking himself a large store of coarse, unleavened cottage bread from Graham flour. Then, taking some of his Dove Cottage apples and even some Concord water, he set sail for England.

Bronson had a number of introductions, for part of his mission was cementing relations between intellectual kin on either side of the Atlantic. But his most prized note was from Emerson to the moody prince of Scotland's historians and philosophers, Thomas Carlyle.

Knowing of Alcott's vegetarianism, Carlyle had his wife, Jenny, prepare strawberries and potatoes for the visit. But Carlyle was appalled when Bronson, being served, pulled the two together on his plate so that, "The juices ran together and fraternized." Carlyle could not then eat a bite, but rose and, in disgust, "stormed up and down the room instead." There followed a testy exchange, and Bronson left the next day, despite an effort by both men to patch over the discord.

Bronson hurried to London, in the hope of finding people who, while less brilliant, could at least see no harm in combining strawberries and potatoes. On route, he toured London, seeking the pubs where Boswell and Dr. Johnson had discoursed. But finding such as *The Cock* and *The Cheshire Cheese* to be full of meat, he hurriedly withdrew.

Arriving at Alcott House, in London's near countryside, he was astonished by the wealth and beauty implied by the big halls and the sweeping views of the estate. And he was comforted to be again in the company of those who ate nothing but vegetables, a little fruit and Graham bread, and who shared his joy in the cold bath.

But soon Bronson felt something was wrong. In New England the cold bath did not seem to penetrate to the heart. Here it did. For while the American reformers were full of bright hopes, their English cousins instead tended to withdraw in cynicism, viewing society as depraved. One heard less of Christianity and

more of self-deprivation. Any physical contact between individuals was loathsome. Sex was seen as disgusting—even for the
purpose of guaranteeing a future membership.

Coldest and most dour was the leader of Alcott House,
Charles Lane. Bronson was soon anxious to leave. But he was so
concerned about seeming ungrateful that he resorted to urging
Alcott House's most extreme believers to return with him to Dove
Cottage. We have reason to believe that Alcott was dismayed
when Charles Lane not only accepted, but offered to lead a
delegation of four himself.

When the group arrived, something of gloom descended on
Dove Cottage. The cold morning bath was no longer just a
sloshing; beginning at 6 A.M. sharp, Lane led the ritual of a careful
icy *sponging,* following which all dried themselves by scrubbing
with special coarse towels.

Alcott himself continued to prepare breakfast. It was always
hard Graham bread, stored apples, cooked potatoes and ice water.
Dinner at noon was just the same. So was supper. There was,
howver, more conversation at dinner and supper, as had been
prescribed by Pythagoras.

Charles Lane wrote: "Thus have passed away many happy
days—happy to me, and I believe none of us would like to return to
a more complicated diet of molasses, milk, butter, etc., all of which
are given up. The discipline we are now under is that of abstinence
in tongue and hands. We are now learning to hold our peace and to
keep our hands from each other's bodies."

Lane's last statement was aimed directly at Abigail Alcott.
He did not care much for females. And he was appalled by any sign
of physical affection between her and Bronson. He tried his best to
crowd her out, and eventually he succeeded in getting Bronson to
sleep away from her.

Abigail did not take kindly to this. Her health had declined,
and she needed at least some consolation. She wrote: "My diet is
. . . obviously not diversified, having been almost exclusively
coarse bread and water—the apples we have not being mellow and
my teeth very bad."

Let us speculate about this statement. "Bad teeth" might have
to do with calcium loss, and there was precious little calcium in the

Dove diet. Note, for example, that milk was banned. Bread is a poor source of calcium. Of the 1,000 mg. daily which are now recommended, a slice of wheat bread furnishes only about a fiftieth.* Bran adds virtually no calcium. As for apples, a medium-sized one (about three to a pound) offers only a third the calcium in a slice of bread. So Abigail may well have been short of calcium after years of dietary shortage. Small wonder that her teeth were bad and that the Alcott girls were not in good health. Similar shortages would probably have occurred among other nutrients.

One cannot say how much damage was done to the public health by Grahamite ideas. But it may have been considerable. And more and more, the Graham diet became linked to a wave of many kinds of reform.

Both Bronson and William became ceaselessly involved in meetings advocating reform, in food, health, education, sex and religion. Each group, regardless of its primary objective, began to incorporate the reforms of the others.

For example, Bronson spent much time with Come-Outers and Millerites, religious reformers. Bronson Alcott was at the Groton Convention when William Miller predicted the advent of Christ in 1843. While the Alcotts did not accept this, many of their friends did. Thousands in the Northeast readied ascension robes, painted their carriages to ride to heaven and closed their houses neatly. When nothing happened, Miller recalculated the day, naming October 22, 1844. The fervor was great, and many moved to the hilltops. Some brought laundry baskets in which to be carried up and away. As night came, and with it disappointment and disillusion, Yankee restraints crumbled. There were angry fights and sexual orgies.

Among those who sought social change, there was not only open-mindedness but also a determination to live their ideas. So it was that Alcott and Lane planned Fruitlands, a communal family, and established it at Harvard, Massachusetts.

Ralph Waldo Emerson endorsed the plan, lending some money to help buy a house and eleven acres. He described it as:

*Throughout this book, "recommended amounts" refer to U.S. RDAs (U.S. Recommended Daily Allowances), the recommendations upon which food labelings are based, unless otherwise specified.

". . . a Concordium, or Primitive Home, which is about to be commenced by united minds who are desirous . . . with simplicity in diet, dress, lodging &c, to retain the means for the harmonic development of their physical, intellectual and moral natures. The institution is to be in the country, the inmates . . . of both sexes, they are to labor on the land, their drink is to be water, and their food chiefly uncooked by fire . . ."

The Fruitlands' Graham bread was to be supplemented by growing maize, rye, oats, barley, potatoes and beans. Cotton was forbidden for clothing; for the Abolitionists were friends of the Alcotts, and cotton was grown with slave labor. Wool was forbidden because its use exploited sheep. Linen was acceptable, and the ladies, in support of that first thrust for feminine freedom, would reject corsets and wear linen bloomers. Even if rabbits molested crops, they would not be killed, and honey could not be stolen from bees.

Fruitlands was fairly near two other communities which existed as living expressions of reform. One was a colony of Shakers, who also lived very plainly and left us symbols of their simplicity in the clean, clear lines of their classic furniture. They, too, were Grahamites in diet. Charles Lane admired them because they housed men and women separately, a system which was to some extent instituted at Fruitlands. The two communes were harmonious.

The Oneidans also kept the simple life and supported the reforms of the day. In the family concept of their commune, they were actually closer to Fruitlands than were the Shakers. But one reform of the Oneidans appalled the Fruitlanders. Oneidans took literally the commandment to love one another. *Coitus interruptus* prevented unplanned populating. The method was taught to young men at puberty, in practice sessions with older women. Mature men demonstrated the method to the adolescent girls. It was the one freedom Fruitlands could not tolerate.

Fruitlands failed within a year. It had laid down too many strictures on the already harsh business of farming. Returning to Concord, the Alcotts were now impoverished indeed. Bronson was depressed, but eventually began to go again to the endless meetings in Boston. He was the only after-dinner member of the

Saturday Club there. He came late, for the nuts and apples, which he declared "the best part."

The Alcott women began to loosen their diets again, but Bronson never relented. One evening, Emerson had them to dinner and served a roast, which he knew the ladies would share, and which he believed they needed. As Ralph Waldo carved, he told some horrifying stories about cannibals. "But Mr. Emerson," quipped Alcott, who always kept his humor, "if we are to eat meat at all, why should we not eat the best?"

When Fruitlands failed in 1844, Bronson was 45 and Louisa May 12. Slowly, during the next decade, Bronson came to be regarded as less of an educational radical. He found some work, but the family remained woefully poor until 1854, when Louisa May's first book, *Flower Fables,* began to bring in some money. She also helped by working as a servant.

While Bronson lived out the rest of his life apart from the mainstream of food crusading, Cousin William became a food-reform leader. With Bible Christian Pastor William Metcalfe, he formed the first American vegetarian society. "A vegetarian diet," he steadfastly held out, "is at the basis of all reform."

William helped launch the Vegetarian Society's magazine. And he shared head-table honors at one great vegetarian feast at which were present all the figureheads of reform—Metcalfe, Amelia Bloomer, Susan B. Anthony, Horace Greeley, and many others. Probably, Harriet Beecher Stowe was also present.

The toast of the evening was drunk in the purest of water. It was, "Total Abstinence, Women's Rights and Vegetarianism!"

The honor of proposing the toast was accorded to Dr. James Caleb Jackson, founder of the Glen Haven Water Cure. And thereby hangs a significant tale.

5

Water, Water, Everywhere

Any time after 1858, if you were looking for a little excitement in Dansville, in upstate New York, you could always check to see if the flag was up over Liberty Hall. The flag was a big triangle emblazoned with the letter "J," and it could be seen from the edge of town by looking down Health Street to the famed Glen Haven Water Cure.

In fact, some days it was worth just standing at the end of Health Street to see who was in the carriages that rolled down to the Cure. For most of the big names in reform went there sooner or later. You might catch Amelia Bloomer, William Alcott, or even Clara Barton coming back from the rigors of starting the Red Cross.

Indeed the Cure was the scene for many a fateful meeting of the opinion makers of the time, who shaped many of our own ideas about health and food. But probably none of the meetings had more consequences than that of James Caleb Jackson with Ellen Harmon White.

It was Dr. Jackson for whose initial the "J" flag flew, denoting that he had something new to tell the world. His doctorate was a casual affair, mainly earned by helping out healers; Jackson had been a farmer by trade, in Manlius, New York, until 1847 when he was 36 years old. Then his health had failed. The diagnoses had ranged from heart disease to kidney trouble to dyspepsia. Worried, he had gone to Cuba, New York, for intensive care at Greenwood Spring.

There was no real clinic or hospital at Greenwood Spring. There was mainly water, for in the mid-19th century, water represented a primary method of treatment.

Although the idea can be traced to early Greek, Roman and Chinese practices, the great water resurgence in the western world probably began with Vincent Preissnitz. Preissnitz was one of the philosopher-healers who emerged from the school of *Naturphilosophie.* In Grafenburg, Germany, he squirted his patients with water on the outside, made them drink up to 40 glasses a day for their insides, and denied them any food at all until they conceded that they were well again. No doubt the denial of food helped persuade patients that they were much better. It was through the Preissnitz method, modified by a "natural" vegetarian diet, that Jackson recovered.

Probably no one gave more impetus to water-curing than a little man in Worishofen, Bavaria. In the photographs which were taken late in his life, Father Sebastian Kneipp appears a stout, rosy-cheeked, white-haired cleric in monk's robes. He might have resembled one of those elfin winemakers or brewmasters one sees on German labels, except that he insisted on being photographed with his regular medical instrument—his watering can.

Born in 1821, Father Kneipp was a frail child, and he very nearly found himself dismissed from theology school because of his constant ill health. Prayer and medical study were unavailing. Fearing for his vocation, Sebastian Kneipp began to read about Preissnitz' water cures.

At first he tested the power of water gingerly. One rainy day he decided to remove his shoes and go for a walk. He felt better. So he again doffed his shoes and tried walking in an icy stream and felt still better. Finally he began to plunge his whole body into cold water, and he became well enough to be accepted into the priesthood.

It is not surprising that, once he had his own little parish in the mountains, he recommended water to the sick in his flock. Word spread that he was a healer. (There is an obvious extra impact, one suspects, for a simple country people of great faith, in the aqueous anointing by a priest. But it should be made clear, to Father Kneipp's credit, that he carefully divided his lay and clerical roles, never exploiting the Church.)

In his book, *My Water Cure,* Father Kneipp suggests three key reasons why water heals:

1. Taken inside or out, water dissolves poisonous elements in the blood.
2. Water withdraws all unhealthful matter from the body, other than the blood poisons.
3. Water strengthens and braces the constitution. It is a primary stimulant (especially at the temperature of Bavarian streams).

How much value is there in such ideas? Were they convincing only to our forefathers? Let us consider Father Kneipp's frequent prescription for walking barefoot in wet grass, preferably dawn dew, and a modern opinion about it.

We turn to one of the most popular food authors of our own time, the late Jerome I. Rodale, founder of the modern "organic" movement and of the foremost journal of "natural" eating, *Prevention.* In one of his basic works, *Health Builder,* Rodale discusses how to prevent and cure cancer. He gives much attention to a visit which he made to Oxford, England, and the laboratory of George Delawarr and his family.

Writing of the Delawarrs, Rodale establishes their scientific prowess by noting that, "With their specially developed camera which costs in the thousands of dollars, they were able to diagnose a person's disease from a tiny specimen of blood taken by pricking the finger."

Rodale uses the Delawarrs' work to corroborate some of his own theories about the electrical qualities of cancer and other diseases. He cites a letter from George Delawarr, in which he says: "It was originally supposed that by walking barefoot on dewy ground one's body was 'earthed' in some way, but it is now known that more than this goes on—there is a contact with the basic life force that is being evoked in the living soil." That force, Delawarr says, is electricity. "Yes," he concludes to Rodale, "put your hands in the soil as much as you can; handle living plants and drain their health-giving electrical charges into your body."

Rodale concurs. In fact, he explains that this is one reason why weeding is so healthful. "In pulling out an undesired plant," Rodale says, the gardener, ". . . touches it while it is alive, and thus he drains its health-giving electrical charges into his own body. He, therefore, gets electricity both from placing his hands in the soil and also from the plant. Mr. Delawarr in his letter, touches upon another aspect of how one can absorb earth electricity and that is by walking barefoot on dewy ground."

Mr. Rodale is often said to have made up for his lack of formal training in medicine by extensive reading. He demonstrates his acquaintance with medical literature by recalling Father Kneipp, and cites a long passage from *My Water Cure:*

"I knew a priest," writes Father Kneipp in the quotation, "who went every year to stay for a few days with a friend . . . and there his morning walk was always taken barefooted in the wet grass. He has many times spoken in glowing terms of the excellent effects . . ."

Father Kneipp gives examples of "a number of persons of the highest ranks of society," who do this and benefit. And he adds:

"The wetter the grass, the longer one perseveres . . . and the oftener it is repeated, the more perfect will be the success . . . After the promenade all the improper adherents, such as leaves, or sand, must be quickly wiped off the feet; yet the feet are not to be dried, but must be left wet . . . Dry stockings and shoes have to be put on, however, without delay. The walking in the grass has to be followed by walking with covered feet on a dry path . . ."

Comments Rodale: "Father Kneipp's work should be re-evaluated based on the possibility that in walking on the dewy grass one absorbs liberal charges of earth electricity. . . . Man . . . should live where he can take his shoes off occasionally and walk barefoot."

Father Kneipp healed for some three decades, drawing thousands to little Worishofen, which is said thereby to have grown from a village of 500 to a little city of 15,000. For the curing became an industry. Townsfolk took in patients as boarders, fed them, sold them warm woolens and guided them toward the best cold streams. Only Father Kneipp's advice was free. How was it obtained?

The believers lined up in long queues at the parish house and the church. The Father admitted them to his presence in groups of five and ten, a well-filled watering can in his hand and his faithful little white Pomeranian at his feet, the sleeves of his simple cassock somewhat drawn up.

Quickly he walked from one to the other, asking, "Where does it hurt?" Answered, he often gave treatment on the spot. An arthritic hand? Slosh, the cold spring water spilled from the can.

Eventually the Father was in such demand that he saw only the problem cases himself, leaving the bulk of the watering to his parishioners. They built their own watering rooms, bought watering cans and sloshed for a fee.

Special tubs and basins were constructed, on the premise that only the affected part should be sloshed. For some unexplained reason, merely having everyone bathe would not work.

Take the heart patient. He removed his shirt, put on special coverings for his shoes and trousers and bent backward over an upper-body tub, while an attendant was sent running down to a frigid mountain stream with a watering can. The room was warm, and the shock must have been considerable.

There were other special treatments. In his later years Father Kneipp added steam-treating under a blanket, wet-straw walking, icy-stream walking and snow-walking. He warned, however, of the hazards of walking in old, dirty snow; the snow had to be newfallen. Special walks were matched to special ailments. Bowel, bladder or kidney trouble, for example, called for stream walking, just knee-deep. The lung victim was bent over a tub while the chill water was administered, just one frigid drop at a time onto his warm and trembling skin.

One of the few personal reports of Father Kneipp's therapy stems from his last years, toward the close of the 19th century. It is from the pen of Dr. Henry Lindlahr. Dr. Lindlahr eventually took this Bavarian medicine to Chicago, became licensed as a "drugless practitioner," and taught his art to his son, Victor Lindlahr, a 1930's radio foodist.

Henry had been making a lot of money buying land ahead of the railroads in Montana. In fact, by 1893, he was the banker and mayor of Kalispell. Then suddenly this rotund little man (five feet six and 250 pounds) was stricken with diabetes and told he was incurable. He sought help in Vienna, but was merely told to prepare for death.

As a last resort, Henry turned to Bavaria and the priestly watering can. Severely ill as he was, he had to wait several days to see the Father. As his son Victor tells us, the interview was short. "The priest smelled his breath, surveyed his 250 pounds, and said bluntly: 'You are a pig. You will take sitz baths, live on fruits and greens and vegetables alone.' " Soon Henry Lindlahr was indeed a much healthier man.*

Henry Lindlahr, we may estimate, was some 50 percent over medically desirable weight, yet he considered his figure "not unbecoming," according to the fashion of the time. In a few months of restricting his diet to fruits and vegetables, he lost 43 pounds and then kept losing. These facts suggest the origin in Henry Lindlahr's case, and in many others of his time, of a good many of the "cures" effected by water and food reform.

By the time he wrote his book, Father Kneipp's usual practice was to have the Sisters of his church give dietary advice, once he had made some basic determinations, such as where and how the water should go. These early dietitians prescribed diets which were vegetarian and sparse, and also featured drinking much water and a little of the local beer.

The tales of Preissnitz and Kneipp were not slow to reach American shores. Of course, many healers began to feel that if the water looked and smelled bad, it was even better. Thus the mineral-spring spas, in all their sulphurous glory, appeared.

*The chief factor in the modern management of most diabetes is no longer insulin or the severe restriction of dietary carbohydrates; it is weight control. The typical diabetic is, before treatment, likely to be obese—if his case, like the vast majority, is *diabetes mellitus,* with its onset in mature years. Weight reduction usually has considerable value in managing the diabetic's illness, as it does in heart disease, high blood pressure, arthritis and other ills.

But whether the waters at the "cures" were mineral or plain, they became the social and medical centers of the day. By 1850, the *American Water Cure Journal and Health Reform* magazine had 20,000 subscribers. Any issue would have half a hundred ads for water cures. By the Civil War, it is estimated that there were some 2,000 spas and cures in business in the U.S. We have reminders of them still in many of the names of eminent and ancient resorts which end in the word "Springs." So wet was American life that the *Knickerbocker Magazine* of that era printed this poem:

> It's water, water everywhere,
> And quarts to drink if you can bear;
> 'Tis well that we are made of clay
> For common dust would wash away!

Meanwhile, back in New York, Dr. James Caleb Jackson, having been impressed not only by the health magic of water, but also by its economic potential, had acquired the title of *Doctor*. It wasn't hard in those days. By 1850, a flood of new medical schools had opened up. In many places, one could start a medical school just by declaring one. Degrees might be handed out after a few months' study in some, which advertised their speedy teaching, or even offered degrees without any actual attendance.

At first Jackson set up a cure at Skaneateles Lake, with a Dr. Gleason. Realizing that reform and success in the health field went hand in hand, Jackson began attending meetings such as those of the Vegetarian Society, adopted food treatment, broke with his partner and opened his own place at Dansville in 1858.

Dr. Jackson's following was assured after he achieved a "brain cure" with water and diet counseling. He held a kind of press conference to advertise it. Over 100 of the thinkers and the press of reform, including Amelia Bloomer in her noteworthy pants, showed up for the party, and Jackson's name was made.

For treating women, he had the assistance of Dr. Harriet Austin. Where she got *her* doctorate, we do not know. She was said to be Jackson's adopted daughter. Her early education had been under the aegis of Mary "Free Love" Gove. She got her patients out of their false hair and tight corsets, and into the standard reform bloomers. Both she and Jackson prescribed diets of fruits and Graham crackers and bread, waters, naps and walks.

Meanwhile, Dr. Jackson began issuing pamphlets about the value of whole wheat. (He was merely repeating what Sylvester Graham had said, but the mark of the successful health-fooder is that he or she can plagiarize without conscience and recite old fallacies as if they were new discoveries.)

Jackson began to sell foods such as a coffee made of cereals, which he called *Somo*. Also, there was a baked concoction of Graham flour and water, which he broke into bits. These two products were marketed so that people who could not come to *Our Home*, as his spa became known, could buy them and use them at home. They were widely bought, especially the baked crumbs, which Dr. Jackson named *Granula*. In all probability, these were the first commercial health-food products in the U.S.

In 1863, *Our Home, Somo* and *Granula* were famous among food reformers. It was in that year that Ellen Harmon White appeared in Dansville, worn out by her labors and seeking physical restoration.

Born in 1828, Ellen Harmon's church was that of William Miller, who was to fail in predicting Christ's coming to New England. Indeed, on that October day in 1844 when the Millerites waited on the hills with their laundry baskets, sixteen-year-old Ellen waited on a hill in Maine.

Hers was not a family belief. At 14, she heard Miller preach the Second Coming and joined what was beginning to be called the Adventist congregation in Portland, Maine.

When the Coming did not materialize, Ellen was profoundly disappointed, but not, like so many, wholly disenchanted. She brooded over the failure. And two months later, she had a vision.

Ellen saw 144,000 saints entering heaven, each with a harp and each instantly able to play it. The Lord invited then to supper, showing them a solid silver table laden with fruits, nuts and manna. Seated on a throne of jasper, He held a book with seven seals. The throne was set on a glass dais, and it was rimmed with a rainbow. The Lord was attended by 24 elders in white robes, and He was hailed by four ugly monsters who recited, "Holy, Holy, Holy."

The vision gave Ellen much attention, especially from

Adventist Elder James White, who married her when she was 18. Together they journeyed across the country, exhorting and organizing new congregations.

Sister White, as she was now known, began to have more and more visions. "I present the Word of the Lord God of Israel," she always began. And she would offer the revelations which had been granted to her. Some of her revelations began to deal with problems of administering the Church and setting matters of policy.

As a religious entity, the Adventists were loosely organized. The members believed in and waited for an imminent Second Coming; indeed, this belief was the main source of their unity. The Whites' effort became the strengthening and formalizing of the fabric of the Church. Poor but dedicated, they moved from one meeting to the next, going by whatever conveyance they could find. And their fame spread, in part because to so many congregations, they represented the only real contact with the Church as a whole.

By 1863, they had reached Otsego, Michigan. Sister White was now 35, a little heavy in the manner of the time, face strong, hair pulled tight, dress plain and dark. In the kitchen of the Otsego home where they stayed, Ellen White knelt to lead prayers. Suddenly she began to speak in a strange tone. "Glory, glory, glory," she said. Her eyes were open, yet she seemed unaware of the others. She appeared not even to breathe, but her hands moved as she described her vision.

Sister White was being given a Divine injunction to health reform. No meat. Only two meals a day. No whiskey or tobacco. The faithful were to eat fruits, vegetables and Graham bread, because meat stirred animal passions. They were to disdain salt and other condiments, use no lard or cake and drink only water.

Sister Ellen spoke for nearly an hour and then collapsed. In that time, she set forth many of the basic practical tenets of what we now know as the Seventh Day Adventist Church. She wrote them out the next day.

The living pattern embodied in the revelation was strikingly like that of Cowherd and Metcalfe and the Bible Christians. It was an emphasis on a Christian duty to care for the body as for the soul, not only of oneself, but of others. Whatever the psychology or the theology of the revelation, it is—for all its reflection of the health reform of the time—the foundation stone of a caring tradition of medical education and service. Nevertheless, as we shall see, the development of that tradition took some curious turns.

The vision and its central concept had an electrifying effect on the Adventists. They were eager to obey.

From that time, Sister White skipped dinner. She traveled with apples and Graham bread as her basic provender.

It was a time of trial for Adventists. For since they did not believe in war or killing, they refused to participate in the Civil War and were persecuted as cowards or traitors in many areas. The new emphasis seemed to give them a rallying point.

But a problem remained. The Lord had called for care of the body. It was important to learn how best to do this. Recognizing that the new health principles paralleled those of Graham and reform, the Elders of Adventism gathered up the money to send observers to a fine medical center. Thus did the Whites start eastward to *Our Home,* to Dr. James Caleb Jackson and the doctrines of water and wheat.

6

Snap! Crackle!
Enter Dr. Kellogg!

It was an eager team of Adventists that James and Ellen White led to *Our Home*. Their sense of urgency was born partly of zeal at fulfilling the Lord's commands and partly of a shortage of cash, which would permit them to stay only a short time. *Our Home* was not cheap.

Such was their eagerness and hurry that they apparently shut their eyes to some of the sinfulness which unfolded. For at Glen Haven the elders were confronted by a world that tolerated theater-going, card-playing and even social dancing.

Sister White's control was such that she steeled herself to conversations with Dr. Harriet Austin, admired her bloomers, and borrowed a pattern for them. She bought a supply of irons for baking Graham Gems and scavenged the library for the books and pamphlets which were to become the nucleus of Adventist learning on health. She and the others scrupulously studied all the secrets of water and diet cures. Occasionally, she disagreed with Dr. Jackson on medical theory; after all, she had received her medical knowledge from an unquestionable Source. Soon the Adventists agreed that they had mastered all that the healers of Glen Haven knew. After all, three weeks had passed. They were ready to turn west again.

Because the new era of Adventism had begun there, Sister White felt that her mission lay in southern Michigan. But for a year she received no further instructions for using what she had learned at Glen Haven. Then the Lord spoke to her. She was to build a health center, a cure, at Battle Creek, some 30 miles east of Otsego.

It was 1865 before the Adventists were ready to begin. But in the meantime, a number of other tasks had been laid before Sister White.

For example, in one vision, she was shown three costumes for Adventist women, from which she selected one. Included was a bloomer pattern for the faithful, which she said were The Lord's bloomers. She drew a pattern from the vision and offered it for a dollar. She was also instructed to begin a health magazine, called *The Health Reformer.*

The Western Health Reform Institute at Battle Creek opened its doors in 1866. It had no doctors of medicine, though few cures did. Its staff was composed of those who had shared the three weeks at Dr. Jackson's. It was agreed that some of the men should pursue a doctoral degree. They chose degrees in naturopathic medicine; they bought them for $25 each. They really needed no further training. For their main medical armamentarium was to be a severe Graham diet, much like that of Dove Cottage, along with a lot of water.

Even the faithful, however, were a little skeptical about putting themselves in the hands of the Institute, knowing the backgrounds of its staff. Sister White was a realist. She began to look for a real doctor of medicine.

She tried Adventists with all manner of training. But it would be ten years before she had made the final choice. His name was John Harvey Kellogg. And if you are beginning to connect the name of Kellogg, the town of Battle Creek and an awesome flow of breakfast cereal, you are absolutely right.

John Harvey was the son of a Michigan broom-maker who had become an Adventist convert. His father could afford the largest contribution—$500—to the building of the Institute. But John and his younger brother Will (better known to the world in later years as W.K. Kellogg) grew up hard. From childhood, they helped to make the brooms.

True, John Harvey was given the money to study medicine in New York, at famed Bellevue Medical College. But his budget was so tight that he had to skimp on meals. His education was another donation to the Adventist cause, a kind of faithful offering. The elder Kellogg and John Harvey both knew from the beginning where the new physician was to use that education. It had already been discussed with the Whites.

This foreknowledge imposed some limitations on what Bellevue could teach young Kellogg. He knew as well as any other Adventist what sort of practice the Lord wanted at Battle Creek. Grain, water and vegetables were to be his only medicament; except for the requirements for his degree, he could ignore the rest.

John Harvey graduated in 1874, and in the same year he became editor of *The Health Reformer*. Then he wrote two short works in which he attempted to sum up modern medical knowledge. One was *The Use of Water in Health and Disease*. The other was *Proper Diet for Man*. No one could ever say that John Harvey Kellogg, M.D. did not know on which side his Graham cracker was buttered.

The two books made certain what was already assumed. In 1876, John Harvey took over the direction of the Western Health Reform Institute, and almost at once he changed the name to the Battle Creek Sanitarium.

Brother Will was one of the first employees John hired, to be chief clerk and to fill orders for copies of John Harvey's books. Will, ten years junior to his brother, had always been bossed around by him. And John Harvey continued to treat Will as a flunky until the younger Kellogg was into his forties.

John was 25 when he took over "The San" and was both clean and efficient. For example, one refinement of water-curing which he introduced at Battle Creek was the enema. He liked to start every day with an inner cleansing, and to make the time count, he dictated to Will during the purge. He was also a passionate admirer of the bicycle. After his enema, he liked to take a little bicycle exercise in the Sanitarium yard. And it seemed sensible to continue his dictation, while Will ran behind him with a notebook. It should be said, of course, that John Harvey rode slowly, and in circles, out of consideration for his brother.

Dr. Kellogg soon added a new dimension to health reform, and one which foreshadowed our own day. For until his entry upon the scene, wearing medical white—his suit, shirt, tie, shoes, hat, etc., were all white—foodism had been based upon religious and philosophic intuition. Vegetarianism and whole grain advocacies had been born of inspiration. But John Harvey now set out to give these ideas scientific support.

At once, he began to write furiously, asserting a scientific basis for The San and its regimens. His works were full of threats. "The oyster," he wrote, "is a scavenger. He dines on germs. His body is covered and filled with bacteria . . . and his slimy juice . . . is simply alive with wriggly germs."

"Bouillon," he asserted, "is a veritable solution of poisons." According to "the world's greatest authority"—John Harvey was seldom specific about his sources—"a quart of beef tea contains enough creatin to kill nine guinea pigs."

John Harvey had a way of using such scientific words as *creatin*. Chances are that scarcely anyone among his lay readers understood the word. But the way the Doctor used it, there was no mistaking that this was bad stuff indeed.

Every Adventist principle was so substantiated. "Coffee," he wrote, "cripples the liver." (In fact, it probably caused diabetes.) And of course anyone who combined drinking coffee and smoking was in deep trouble, since ". . . the liver is the only thing which stands between the smoker and death."

Tea? He quoted an antique opinion given by the Irish Commissioners for Lunacy, which held that tea was a main cause of insanity. Cola drinks, he wrote, "are an insidious poison."

Meanwhile, in a businesslike way, John Harvey poured every nickel of income back into The San. One after another, he built new buildings. The grounds were landscaped with broad lawns and masses of shrubs. The walks and drives were graveled. Fountains were added, along with spacious glassed-in verandas. Tame deer and other animals were installed on the grounds, to entertain the visitor and waken his sympathy for abstention from meat. He put string orchestras into the dining room and offered evening marches and entertainments. And he bought the newest and most scientific-looking machines for watering and rubbing his patients. He got hold of an enema machine that could put 15 gallons of water through the bowels in a matter of minutes.

But perhaps more than any other factor which built the good name of The San, there was John Harvey's tight control over who was admitted as a patient. He refused contagious diseases. He admitted no one on a stretcher. He accepted no new patient whose appearance was unsightly.

What he looked for above all were tired businessmen, sufferers from dyspepsia and victims of *neurasthenia,* a catch-all phrase of the time for neuroses. These he could cope with. Kellogg wanted no one dying under his care at Battle Creek. He did not want to disturb the cheery atmosphere which he had spent so much to create.

The only repugnances allowed at The San were those which justified the therapy. Following Dr. James Caleb Jackson's technique, Kellogg gave evening lectures, replete with shocking lantern slides, mainly aimed at meat eating. He liked to recall for his audiences how, in his student days at Bellevue, some patients were sent to nearby slaughterhouses, so that they could "drink the hot blood of the slain as it gushed from the throat." And he used slides to demonstrate that "fresh meat is usually swarming with putrefactive bacteria." (He did not bother to mention what every medical student knew—that even water could be used to reveal the prevalence of swarming life throughout the micro-world.)

Eventually, John Harvey's strategies filled The San with America's rich and famous. Henry Ford, John D. Rockefeller and Harvey Firestone became his patients. In all, well over 200,000 people, most of them well to do, were to experience the regimes of The San.

Dr. Kellogg thought that the Adventist elders would be delighted by his success. He even evolved a plan to promote gradual conversion to Adventist eating. Each group of tables in the dining room was progressively more abstemious. At The Radical Table, the food was mainly water, Graham crackers and vegetables.

But Sister White was critical. The place did not belong to the Adventists. If they were really sick, they were not the sort of patients Kellogg wanted. If they were only mildly ill, chances were that they could not afford the prices or feel comfortable in the flossy company.

Moreover, Battle Creek had been envisioned as a training center for the Adventist young, a teaching hospital from which they might go out into the world, serve the sick and spread the Word. John Harvey found this idea useful from a business point of view. The training was free, but the work was largely unpaid. Thus John Harvey got ample free help. Nurses, clerks and dietitians got room and board but no money, at first. And as their skills developed, they were given only token sums. Even W.K. Kellogg, the real administrator of The San, for some time earned only six dollars a week. John Harvey liked the system. It made both sense and money.

But to Sister White, Kellogg's cultivation of the rich was providing an atmosphere of luxury which did not square with the vision of life she wanted the Adventist youngsters to have. She and the other elders also saw evidence that Kellogg was exploiting both the faithful and a basic article of their faith.

For the Adventists were convinced that the Biblical injunction to rest on the Seventh Day should be interpreted in the Judaic manner, so that the Sabbath fell on Saturday. This made it difficult for Adventists to find work, for in those times there were no 40-hour weeks. Saturday was a workday, and people who refused to work on Saturday were likely to go without work. Sister White had seen her Institute as a source of jobs without this prejudice. But Kellogg's substandard wages exploited the need of Adventists for work that allowed a Saturday Sabbath.

Overall, Sister Ellen felt that The San was rapidly becoming John Harvey's, not hers or the Church's. "The great display you are making," she warned him, "is not after God's order."

For years, John Harvey staved off these incursions with a fine defense: "After all," he would say to the elders, "I'm not taking a penny of salary for myself. The money is all for The San, and thus, the advancement of the Church. The least you can do is to leave the administration of this medical institution in my hands."

It was a nice ploy, and it worked quite well for 13 years. But there was a gimmick. As head of The San, Dr. Kellogg was selling books, and with them he was marketing some other products, all of which fattened his personal bank account.

In his third year at The San, 1879, however, he married Miss Ella Eaton, of Alfred Center, New York. Eventually, it was through this curious marriage that his own take from The San was to become apparent and cause real trouble.

Ella brought something new into Dr. Kellogg's celibate and rather lonely life—imaginative cooking. She soon had an experimental kitchen at The San, in which she concocted things that stayed within the narrow range of the Adventist diet, yet tasted good. For example, she invented a number of vegetarian products with flavors rather like beef or pork or veal, which helped non-Adventist patients to accept The San's herbivorous constraints.

Partly as a reward for this good work—which was Ella's main function in the marriage—after ten years, Dr. Kellogg built his bride a home just outside The San grounds. It was a Queen Anne mansion of 20 rooms, lavish, with a fireplace copied from Anne Hathaway's home in England. On the sprawling estate were great gardens and vegetable patches, orchards, greenhouses, a swimming pool and a deer park. It was not what Sister White thought of as the model Adventist home.

In fairness, it should be said that Kellogg's new house did have some redeeming moral features. For example, it had separate bedrooms. There were no children of Ella and John Harvey's marriage. He had stated publicly, and repeatedly, that sex bred evil diseases, especially in men. (One recalls Sylvester Graham's finding that lewdness contributed to the onset of cholera.) Thus John Harvey was determined to live without sex, to prove that it could be done. He and his bride were, however, always good friends. And in the end they adopted 42 children, who helped provide a sense of family.

Since Ella had neither children nor housework for some years—servants being plentifully supplied from the Adventist

youngsters in training at The San—she was free to join John
Harvey in what may have been the greatest food invention of them
all. The Doctor tells us how the multi-billion-dollar idea came
about:

"The writer," he records, ". . . early became convinced that
indigestions and decay of teeth were encouraged to a marked
degree by failure to use the teeth sufficiently in a thorough
mastication of the food. He accordingly made it a practice to
require his patients to begin each meal by chewing slowly a small
slice of dry *zweibach* (the hard German twice-baked bread). One
day a patient came into the office with a complaint that the
prescription had broken her teeth, for which she jokingly demanded compensation."

Whether or not she had actually spoken "jokingly," Dr.
Kellogg preferred to consider her complaint to be jocular, his
frugality being legend. It was one of the Doctor's few excursions
into humor.

"The impracticability of *zweibach* was at once apparent," he
writes. "Patients with artificial teeth, with sore teeth or diseased
gums needed something they could chew . . . without running
the risk of injury . . . Experiments were begun to produce toasted
or dextrinized cereals [those in which the carbohydrate was
partially broken down] in a form which, while dry and crisp, could
be properly offered to such persons and eaten by them *without the
addition of milk or cream, which would destroy their value as a dry
food.*" (Italics added.)

The doctor is speaking of the cereal flake. And he adds some
historical notes. "The first flakes were wheat flakes and were
known as *Granose* and later as *Toasted Wheat Flakes.*" But, he
laments, "various imitations" were soon made, such as "Malta
Vita, Force, Vim, Egg-O-See, etc."

Dr. Kellogg also came up with a product which consisted of
broken bits of baked wheat. They were indeed reminiscent of Dr.
James Caleb Jackson's *Granula.* And when John Harvey made a
similar product, and called it *Granola,* he was sued. He changed the
name reluctantly.

Such products as the cereal flake paid for most of the Queen

Anne mansion. But soon other cereal inventors took the field, and with it some of Kellogg's market and profit.

A dyspeptic inventor named Henry D. Perky baked whole wheat into mattress-shaped molds and called it *Shredded Wheat*. Eventually, he took out 47 patents to protect it and established a factory at Niagara Falls, which accounts for the cascade on the package. It was intended to be consumed in soup and sold rather slowly. Kellogg had a chance to buy the rights. But he haggled over the price ($100,000) and finally lost the deal.

Still without salary at The San, John Harvey was making his wheat flakes at a new $50,000 Battle Creek building, under the name of the Sanitarium Health Food Company—perhaps the first commercial use of the term "health food." Even though he still pushed the flakes for chewing exercise, and cautioned against getting them soggy with milk, he sold over 100,000 pounds in the first year. And cereal flakes weigh very little.

Kellogg had opened up a gold mine. And he found another with his coffee substitute, *Caramel Coffee*. To help sell it, he adduced antique medical advice, such as that of the 18th century French gastronome Brillat-Savarin: "Every mother and father should forbid their children to take any coffee, unless they wish to see them shriveled up, bony and withered little things before they are twenty years old."

But, as the money poured in, both to The San and to Kellogg's pocket, Sister White lost patience. The two fought for the support of the Church elders. When John Harvey quietly slipped meat onto the menu for the wealthy guests who might want it, Ellen White insisted on a total ban and won. Then she invoked the Adventist two-meal-a-day rule, and Kellogg became infuriated.

He managed, however, by resorting to one of his stock gambits with guests—making a medical discovery. In this case he announced that excessive eating produced stress on the cerebrum, the major portion of the brain. To remove this stress, he said, he was forced to remove supper. (However, he would permit a snack of a few dates or raisins with "a few nuts added, if well chewed.")

To understand how Kellogg could convince his high-paying

patients to do without food, we must keep in mind that his essential treatment was an "Anti-Toxic Diet," with which he promised to remove poisons from their bodies. And even before Sister Ellen tightened the screws, this diet had not been Lucullan. It looked like this:

Breakfast
Cantaloupe and Stewed Raisins
Graham gems, Malt honey   Brose (A wheat invention)
Cereal Coffee
Bran

Dinner (at noon)
Vegetable Soup with Noodles
Baked Sweet Potato   Buttered Asparagus
Swiss Chard
Cabbage salad   Bran bread
Yogurt and Buttermilk
Watermelon
Bran

Supper
Okra Soup
2 oz. shredded carrot (with lemon)   Graham bread
3 oz. Baked Cornlet (A Kellogg invention)
Blackberries
Bran

Gradually Dr. Kellogg became bolder. In addition to his regular fees, he would ask the steel magnate or the coal baron for an extra $10,000 to $100,000 for The San. And often he would get it.

Sister White heard of these donations, and kept visiting Kellogg's study to ask for a share for other projects of the Church—a new organ or hospital or school. The San and the food enterprises (in which John Harvey usually held a major stock interest) were the only big sources of cash which the Church could tap. To Kellogg, it seemed that the Church's appetite for *his* money was insatiable. At first he evaded Sister White. Finally, angry, he flatly refused her.

Sister had visions to clarify the situation. The Lord, she said, had changed his mind about Battle Creek. The schools must be moved, along with the Church and its offices. If they left, John Harvey knew, his cheap labor would be gone with them. But still he resisted. He asked for a new charter for The San, on the grounds of protecting it from taxation. To avoid taxes, The San would have to be nondenominational. He won this point, and with it some protection from the Church's cash raids.

Among the Adventist people, there was division. Half sympathized with Sister White and went to the church in town; half went on Saturday to the chapel at The San, signifying support for John Harvey.

"Dr. Kellogg," said an elder who stood with Sister White, "has an imperious will which needs to be broken."

And then Sister White had a new vision. She saw a Sword of Fire poised over The San and Battle Creek. And whenever Sister White had a vision, you had better look out.

7

The Battles of Battle Creek

More than money was involved in the mounting conflict between Dr. Kellogg and the Church. The Adventist elders were disturbed by what many felt was a commercializing of a spiritual enterprise. And among other areas of conflict, there was a running battle along the alimentary canal, particularly in the large intestine.

To gain insight into this important battle, which still influences American health thinking, we might look at a recorded exchange between the Doctor and an elder who charged John Harvey with "waywardness." The elder doubted that Kellogg was adhering to the revealed Word on medicine. Repeatedly, he challenged the Doctor's medical opinions, invoking rules derived from Sister White's visions. Finally Kellogg turned on his questioner vehemently:

"Is God a man with two arms and legs like me?" he asked.

"Does He have eyes, a head?"

The elder hesitated, thinking about these questions. And John Harvey seized the chance to loose what he felt was a master stroke: "Does He have bowels?"

"No!" the elder shot back at once, deeply offended.

"Well I do," cried Kellogg. "And that makes me more wonderful than He is!"

The fact was that John Harvey's medical thinking had changed. While he still put great emphasis on the "naturalness" of diet, more and more he was preoccupied with poisoned intestines as the real cause of disease.

Remember that the Adventist diet did not begin as the product of nutrition research. Sister White got her dietary rules from spiritual, not scientific revelations. And like the vegetarianism of the Bible Christians or the Grahamism of so many intellectuals of an earlier day, the Adventist diet was also a fundamental expression of philosophy.

Kellogg had initially intrigued the Adventists, and gained the interest of outsiders as well, by substantiating this ordinance of spirit and philosophy with evidence which he gleaned from science. But to the faithful Adventist, this "scientific" confirmation, though useful, was not really necessary. The Word of God did not need Dr. Kellogg's endorsement, and certainly not his improvements.

At first Kellogg's stream of books—which were often over 1,000 pages long, and rarely shorter than 500—were seen as missionary instruments. It was comforting to have John Harvey write, for example, that, "The writer has met many cases in which a single meal of cold storage game, long dead and neglected to be buried, has been the cause of many years of misery."

It was useful to Adventist evangelism to be able to quote the famous physician to the effect that he knew of many terrible deaths from, "eating a sausage, a sturgeon or a codfish."

It was nice to be able to show that violating the food ordinances of the Lord had specific biological consequences. For example, to support the revelation that food should be eaten cold, Dr. Kellogg wrote: "The art of cookery has been used not only to render food more digestible, but more often to lessen its digestibility and transform the simple wholesome products of Nature into noxious, disease-producing mixtures." Hot food, he added, could cause cancer.

It was helpful that the Doctor, whose books became the staple home medical references of families across the nation, said that salt and condiments were risky. As an instance, he warned of the use of vinegar and pickling spices. "Vinegar," he said, "is a chemical compound of use only as a reagent in the laboratory . . . It is a poison, not a food."

But soon a combination of genuine curiosity and medical ego led Kellogg to ask *why* bad foods were bad. To those of faith, this was a pointless exercise. But John Harvey was mindful both of his medical reputation and of his hardheaded business clientele. The latter came to him mainly because they thought they were not as healthy as they might be. After all, *sanitaria* were commonly known as "cures." It was not enough for Kellogg to teach his patients the "natural" ways of eating and living. He was expected to repair the damage of a former "unnatural" pattern of life and make people feel better.

In 1878, in a reputable scientific journal, one Dr. Brieger propounded a theory that much disease originated with the putrefaction of proteins in the intestines. (The chemistry of proteins was then only vaguely understood, as was the knowledge of human protein need.) By 1880, Dr. Brieger had refined a principle that meat was full of germs, blood and perspiration, all of which would rot in the intestines to form poisons, thus causing illness and early death.

Kellogg, of course, was quick to seize upon this idea. And he was not alone. Scientists began experiments to assess the dietary value of protein versus that of carbohydrate. (The fact that almost *all* food is a mixture of protein, fat and carbohydrate was obscure to most researchers.) At the University of Michigan, Dr. L.H. Newburgh proved the "deadliness" of meat by feeding pure meat diets to rabbits, who had been quite healthy while they ate only vegetables. "The larger the amount of protein they got," Dr. Kellogg explained, "the worse it was."

(Of course, it was not to be known for some time that herbivorous animals and omnivorous animals such as man have very different enzyme systems, with the result that they may use very different food sources. Humans, to take an extreme situation, would not do well if turned out to graze in a pasture or kept on hay in the winter.)

Dr. Kellogg was fond of citing a study by the German scientist, Liebig, in which, as he tells us: "A bear kept at the Anatomical Museum at Gressen showed a quiet gentle nature as long as he was fed on bread, but a few days . . . on meat made him vicious." It did not seem to occur to either Liebig or Kellogg that a bear sustained only on bread might be too malnourished to be combative.

Putting such data together, John Harvey concluded that meat did its evil work by rotting in the intestines and making poison. The meat-eaters and those on other "unnatural" diets must thus be in toxic states. The key to therapy was to clean out the poisons and purify the patient. Cleaning up the bowel became an obsession for Kellogg—and eventually for millions of Americans. For the Doctor rhapsodized about the potential beauty and vitality of the bowel. He wrote whole books about it.

The interest was then a common medical one. Some physicians offered bread diets; others fed sterilized foods. Kellogg soon became the leader of the movement (no pun intended). At The San, he assaulted the bowel with sterilized bran and paraffin oil from above at every meal—and daily hosed it out with torrents of water from below.

For Dr. Kellogg, there were some clear signs of bacterially compromised bowel. One was a coated tongue. Such a tongue, he believed, was the signal of an "acid stomach." Soon he had much of America looking at its own and its children's tongues.

A sure sign of trouble, of course, was "irregularity." Dependable daily bowel movements, Dr. Kellogg convinced much of the nation, and many of us still believe, were essential to healthful life.

The patient with a coated tongue became not only a target for the enema crews, but the recipient of a standard purifying diet of lettuce, celery, cucumbers, green corn, cabbage, turnips and bran. It was a veritable fodder bag of "roughage"; Dr. Kellogg even insisted that patients eat lettuce for breakfast.

For long periods, carrots were served at every San meal, often with sauerkraut. The coarse Graham bread helped, too. But Kellogg insisted that it not be eaten fresh. Its proper state for human consumption, he decided, was when it had stood for some days, drying out until even the very core crumbled when rubbed between the fingers.

"Bran does not irritate," asserted Dr. Kellogg. "It titillates!"

(We shall see more of the function of food fiber later on. But Kellogg's idea that it worked by a kind of tickling of the intestines—because of its rough texture—is not quite right. Even though he liked to refer to "roughage" as "nature's broom," a natural image for a broom-maker's son, we now know that fiber provides bulk by passing through the intestine undigested and holding quantities of water. Fiber need not be readily apparent to us through coarseness. For example, mashed potatoes, though they are smooth to the taste, still contain useful fiber.)

The purifying rituals grew more and more severe—and more and more remote from Adventist revelations—until each patient with a "toxic" bowel got nothing to eat for two weeks but fruit, four times a day—followed by several days more on nothing but milk. "This," said Kellogg, "changes the intestinal flora and restores health."

If a patient showed increased blood pressure, he might get a meal of ten ounces of strawberries with copious draughts of water. If the pressure was really high, Kellogg fed the victim ten to fourteen pounds of grapes a day, with the seeds and skins painstakingly removed by the young Adventist trainees.

Milk was another favorite of the Doctor's. Some patients who paid full board got an exact seven ounces of milk four times a day, and nothing else. Others were drenched with milk, for reasons that remained obscure. Many were given half a pint every half hour, 26 feedings in all per day between awakening and soggy sleep. The only supplements were fruit at 10 A.M. and 4 P.M. and three tablespoons of paraffin oil four times a day. Their nights, one may speculate, were probably not restful.

Often, Dr. Kellogg decided patients were underweight. Such a patient was put to bed for absolute rest. Immobility was assured by wedging 20-pound sacks of sand under the buttocks from either side. "To increase food absorption," another sandbag, often heavier, was placed on the abdomen during each meal, to remain until digestion was thought to be well under way.

With those on the 26-milk-feedings-a-day plan, there was a lot of sandbagging. Moreover, the Doctor liked things nice and clean. But since he did not want the patient to exert himself, after each meal an attendant would swab the patient's mouth, brush the teeth and then polish each tooth with a special paper polisher. This regime usually lasted for from 40 days to three months.

Dr. Kellogg called all these regimens "biological eating," a phrase which annoyed the elders. Biology was not their objective. The elders could certainly find no trace of Adventism in Kellogg's even stranger ideas, such as giving a patient a goat to follow about the countryside, with instructions to take nourishment, kid-like, directly from the source.

Odd treatments were standard at The San. In the bath houses, patients held onto iron hooks while attendants rubbed their nude bodies with a mushy paste of salt and water. Then followed a forced, high-speed enema from a machine, or some electrical stinging and tickling of the skin.

Once The San got rolling, some 3,000 men and women were subjected to such rituals every day. Among them were some of the richest, best educated and most politically influential people of the day. Hundreds of thousands of other Americans practiced the methods at home from the instructions in John Harvey's books. And the royalties poured in, financing the Queen Anne mansion, the wide travels throughout both Europe and America (which served nicely as publicity tours), and such personal accoutrements as the closets of white clothes, with the white now encompassing even the frames of his spectacles. But perhaps more important than anything else, the money built the Doctor's factories.

The Sanitarium Health Food Company, in which neither Church nor San had any financial interest, was booming. It had begun small, making the special San menu items—such as Caramel Coffee—so that patients and guests could continue to get them after they returned home. But Dr. Kellogg was building steadily, and gradually Battle Creek became another kind of battleground.

Perhaps the most impressive of the wars developed between Kellogg and a Sanitarium guest named Charles W. Post, who arrived at the San in 1891. Born in Springfield, Illinois, in 1854, Post had wandered in search of success until, at age 37, he had become a well-to-do real estate salesman and blanket manufacturer in Fort Worth, Texas. He had also become a sick man, though we do not know the nature of his illness.

We do know that Dr. Kellogg promptly put Post in a wheelchair, and that after a few months the Texas blanket maker hadn't enough cash left to remain a San resident; he had to become an outpatient. So he and his wife and daughter lived in a rented room in town, while Mrs. Post sewed suspenders to pay her husband's medical bills. In his white Stetson hat, Post wheeled about town spieling from his stock of salesman's stories and was soon well known in Battle Creek.

But by the end of nine months, Post was getting desperate. He still felt sick, and now he was destitute to boot. He pleaded with the Doctor to keep him on as a patient. He had spent quite a little time around Mrs. Kellogg's experimental kitchen. He knew that Kellogg had a new cereal coffee, called *Minute Brew,* and begged to help promote and sell the coffee in exchange for treatment and a little share of the profits.

Post was coldly refused. John Harvey was not a loose man with money. And he did not believe in sharing profits with anyone. He had refused Sister White and the Church any part of his health-food take. Why let Post in?

So Post studied the powers of the mind, took up Christian Science, determinedly repeated to himself, "I am well," got out of his wheelchair and went to work. He had studied the economics of The San and liked what he saw. So with his gift of persuasion, he raised some money and by 1892 established his small La Vita Inn on a plot of 10 acres. Here diet and mental healing were combined, and at prices much lower than those of The San. Meat was allowed to lure those who wanted it. But despite these and other inducements, Mrs. Post still had to go on sewing suspenders.

Post got some of Kellogg's overflow, some of his malcontent clients and some of his employees. He talked up his own powers to heal with faith and hypnosis. But things were still so slow that he went back to Kellogg and offered to pray for San patients for only $50 a week. The answer was the usual *no*.

So now Post began writing a book—*I Am Well! The Modern Practice of Natural Suggestion as Distinct from Hypnotic or Unnatural Influence. Scientiae Vitae*. It was signed, "By C.W. Post, worded for Plain People."

The book featured amazing stories of instant cures—no waiting around for months and taking all those enemas. In some cases of bad teeth, dyspepsia or troubled bladder, one could hope for same-day service. He also knocked out a pamphlet, *The Road to Wellville*, which he gave away. In both the book and the pamphlet he criticized Kellogg, making the Doctor his certain enemy.

Later on, the San magazine, *Good Health*, would say that Post had spent a lot of time around the San kitchen. The clear implication was that Post had borrowed some of the formulas for his products. *Good Health* quoted Kellogg as saying, "Let him see everything that we are doing. I shall be delighted if he makes a cereal coffee and wish him every success. The more he sells of it the less coffee will be consumed, and this will be of great benefit to the American people."

In January of 1895, the year Dr. Kellogg discovered and launched the cereal flake, C.W. Post put out *Postum Cereal Food Coffee*. The original marketing tool was a handcart which was pushed through the town of Battle Creek.

Soon Post took samples to Grand Rapids, Michigan. Almost without capital, he told wholesale grocers they could pay him if and when they sold their Postum. He talked newspapers into ad credit on the strength of the line, "It Makes Red Blood." By the end of the year, his sales amounted to over $250,000. In three years, they tripled.

Steadily Post opened wider and wider markets, using ads for which he invented such ailments as "coffee neuralgia" and "coffee heart." Postum could cure them, he said. "Lost Eyesight Through Coffee Drinking" was another of his gambits. And they worked; 50 years later Postum was still being sold as the answer to "coffee nerves."

He ploughed a fortune into advertising, using every cent of profit and borrowing more. He began to take ads in the *New York Magazine of Mysteries,* offering spot cash to get testimonials of cures.

Largely because sales of Postum fell off in summer, Post came up with a cereal to try and take up the warm-weather slack. Remarkably like Dr. James Caleb Jackson's *Granula,* it was broken into rock-hard bits crumbled from sheets of baked wheat. He called it *Grape Nuts,* and he pulled out all the stops to announce its curative properties. According to ads which first ran in 1898, it was almost a specific for appendicitis. It tightened up loose teeth, fed the brain through what was implied to be almost a direct pipeline and quickly disposed of tuberculosis and malaria. Of course, it worked better when consumed with a certain amount of faith; so Post put a copy of *The Road to Wellville* in each package.

By 1901, C.W. Post was *netting* a million dollars a year. Tales of his and Kellogg's success were turning Battle Creek into a new kind of boom town.

The little city became synonymous with health in a package. New companies blossomed like desert weeds after a rain. Literally scores of cereal firms, each with bolder advertising claims than the last, took the field. The population mushroomed so rapidly that many employees lived in tents around the uncompleted (but producing) factories in which they worked. Post and Kellogg remained the fountainheads, however.

Malta Vita, started with the help of a Kellogg's foreman, soon garnered five million dollars and led to the birth of *Vim Wheat Flakes.* Another Kellogg defector helped Duke Ellsworth to launch *Force. Mapl-Flakes* made the Hygienic Food Company rich—with the help of college football players' testimonials. John Linihan built *Cero-Fruito* into a fortune.

Workers and ad copy were pirated. Partners broke up and formed rival companies. *Monk's Brew, Golden Manna, Food of Eden, Norka Oats, Tryabita*—a thousand get-well-quick schemes bloomed—with most foundering, a few building empires.

The cereals and cereal coffees offered little of nutritive value, really. Postum, for example, was made of bran and molasses, neither with any great food value. And one or two ounces of grain made into cereal, with some sugar, is no more nutritive than one or two ounces of bread.

Yet whatever came from Battle Creek was deemed healthful. Diamonds and fine carriages appeared in the town. At least 44 companies were in production at one time, and stock issues were as numerous as oil-well shares in Oklahoma's early days. Everyone in Battle Creek owned a bit of the dream of cereal riches.

This was the corrupted Battle Creek which Sister White deplored. And beginning in 1901, she began to show true exasperation. This cereal Sodom was what John Harvey Kellogg had produced from Divine vision.

Then the worst sort of fears among the elders were realized in 1904, when C.W. Post divorced his suspender-sewing wife and married his typist. He was in his fifties; she was in her twenties. The grains which had symbolized the Lord's Word had been made the instruments of Satan. From the holy seed kernels had come a crop of cupidity, vanity and venality.

Dr. Kellogg was no less disturbed, but for different reasons. These people were taking business away from the Battle Creek Sanitarium Food Company. And he blamed one man. As he had written, early in the boom:

"More than a score of these food enterprises have been launched in Battle Creek . . . and as many more elsewhere in the country. By ingenious advertising, much after the method of the medical quacks, some of these concerns have built up large business interests and have waxed rich by their ill-gotten gains. *One party in particular has made some millions by the sale of a cheap mixture of bran and molasses."* (Italics added.)

Kellogg repeatedly disavowed any connection between The San and the Battle Creek companies. "The prestige of Battle Creek as a health center," he said, "has made this an attractive place for the operations of various charlatans, and not the least pretentious and predatory of these are the numerous food charlatans."

Sister White and the elders blamed Kellogg for the situation. She had seen a Sword of Fire. In 1901, it materialized; there was a bad fire at The San, and then still another.

Commented the *Detroit News*: "While the idea that the fire was a fulfillment of the 'flaming-sword' prophecy of Mrs. Ellen White, founder of the denomination, is flouted to some extent, it is pointed out that this was the thirteenth big fire in Battle Creek's West End, and every building save one that was part of the Adventist group at the time Mrs. White gave what was purported to be a vision, has fallen victim of the fire god."

While the fires threatened Kellogg's structural space, The San always had cash, and generous donors. Building after building was rebuilt, grander than before. But Sister White persuaded the elders to move the headquarters of Adventism to Washington, D.C., to clarify the fact that Kellogg had been cut off from the Church.

And almost at once, Kellogg suffered another defection. Little brother Will, now in his forties and the real director of the gradual rebuilding and refinancing of The San, still abused as in the days when he had taken notes during John Harvey's morning enemas, began still another battle. W.K. Kellogg now wanted to expand the sales of The San's cornflakes along Post's lines. John Harvey demurred. The medical community was beginning to look askance at his methods and his products; and he had enough money. He wanted to go slow.

Quietly, Will found some money and proceeded to acquire control of the cornflakes. For while the Doctor had kept all rights and patents in his own name, he had made a mistake. To save salary money, he had persuaded San staffers to accept cornflake stock in lieu of some of their pay. Now Will used funds from a St. Louis insurance man to buy up these bits and pieces. By 1906, he had control of the Kellogg Toasted Corn Flake Company.

Thus challenged on all sides, by his church, his brother, and the free-enterprise system, John Harvey struck out at his tormentors. He called his competitors thieves and frauds, his brother a traitor—and finally, his co-religionists fools.

In 1907, an anonymous pamphlet appeared. Attributed to Dr. Kellogg's coterie, it was called *Responses to an Urgent Testimony from Mrs. Ellen H. White Concerning Contradictions, Inconsistencies and Other Errors in Her Writings.*

Sister White had invited anyone to question her visions or

their infallibility. A copy of the pamphlet went to her first. After a month with no reply, it was published. In general, it intimated broadly that Sister White was a fraud.

Dr. Charles Stewart, a close friend of the Doctor's was said to have done the writing. "I believe she is a victim of auto-hypnotism," he said. "She has actually hypnotised herself into believing that these visions are genuine. I don't think she willingly sets out to deceive—she's gotten into the visionary habit—but I do blame those who foist upon the people a scheme which is nothing more or less than a gross fraud."

The elders of Adventism seemed to have little doubt about the presence of Dr. Kellogg's hand in the *Responses,* which they assessed and rejected. They held eighteen hours of inquiry into Dr. Kellogg's religious demeanor and beliefs. Learning of the inquiry, the Doctor clarified his position bluntly: "I do not believe in Mrs. White's infallibility and never did."

A month later, John Harvey Kellogg was summarily expelled from the Seventh Day Adventist Church.

Neither in public nor in private did Dr. Kellogg ever record the smallest regret or dismay. He had separated the Church from The San for tax reasons. Adventism had no hand in his books. He felt that he had given the Church far more than it had given to him. He did not deem himself wounded, but freed.

Besides, the Church had never been his real interest. He had much to do. He was 56 years old. He was fit; his intestines were immaculate. And the world of medicine seemed to have more and more to gain from joining him in his militant vigil along the alimentary canal.

8

Life along
the Alimentary Canal

In 1907, when John Harvey Kellogg was expelled from the Adventist Church, the bowel was just coming into its own, both in America and in Europe. And while many influences led to this new prominence, none were more profound than the writings of Russian-born biologist Élie Metchnikoff.

Metchnikoff (really Ilya Ilyich Mechnikov) first came to fame as a professor at the University of Odessa. But his most important work was conducted in Paris, where he became Louis Pasteur's right hand and, after Pasteur's death, deputy director of the Pasteur Institute.

An orthodox scientist of immaculate credentials, he was the author of the brilliant book, *Infectious Diseases* (1901). He also developed the landmark theory of *phagocytosis*—explaining the basic defense against infection, in which the white blood cells engulf and destroy foreign substances entering the body, especially harmful bacteria.

Then Metchnikoff began to worry about his age. He started to search the world for examples of long life with the hope of learning the secrets of survival. The result was that in 1907, at the age of 62, he published *The Prolongation of Life*. It became a bestseller, a diet revolution of its day. For it revealed a simple recipe for the forestalling of death—yogurt.

Metchnikoff first discovered that Bulgarians seemed to live longer than most peoples of Europe. Why? Ilya Ilyitch looked at the special characteristics of Bulgarian life. Influenced by the 19th century vision of food as medicine, he paid special attention to eating habits and noted that Bulgarians ate a lot of yogurt, a kind of soured milk. Finding nothing else remarkable on the Bulgarian table, he assumed that yogurt must be the reason for the national longevity.

Why should this be? Looking to medicine, Ilya Ilyich soon found an answer. Some of the best known physicians of the time, such as Dr. John Harvey Kellogg, said that much disease was caused by putrefying protein in the intestines.

Recall that Metchnikoff's greatest triumph was his theory of how good cells overcame bad ones. And note that yogurt is full of bacteria, as is any soured milk product. (Metchnikoff dubbed the little fellows in yogurt *Lactobacillus Bulgaricus*—literally, "Bulgarian milk bacteria"—and assumed that when lots of them were resident in the intestines, the putrefying proteins were attacked as foreign substances and neutralized.

Odds are that *The Prolongation of Life* would not have received so much attention, except for one thing. In 1908, shortly after the book's publication, Metchnikoff was awarded the Nobel Prize in Physiology and Medicine. Of course the Nobel did not go to him for his work with yogurt. It was for his theory of phagocytosis. But the public does not delineate these matters well. Metchnikoff was a Nobelist, and Metchnikoff said that yogurt would make you healthy and long-lived. Never mind that he was not a physician or nutritionist; he was a brilliant scientist, was he not? In the public mind, "science" tends to be a single entity, which the "scientist" understands.

Interestingly, yogurt seemed to cause more excitement in England than in France. But some physicians were skeptical. *Lancet,* the most distinguished British medical journal, felt obliged to editorialize:

MacCauley says, "We know of no spectacle as ridiculous as the British public in one of its periodic fits of morality. The same public in a fit of new-found panaceal therapy affords a spectacle only slightly less ridiculous." Metchnikoff was the innocent cause of one of these . . . One heard of nothing but the Bulgarian bacillus. The bacillus shared with Mr. Lloyd George's budget the honor of monopolizing the conversation at the dinner tables of the great. He dominated Belgravia, frolicked in Fulham, and bestrode Birmingham and the whole of the British Isles. . . . That he himself, or a colorable imitation of him which was put upon the market by the unscrupulous, did a great deal of harm is quite certain."

Metchnikoff also popularized a catchword which neatly summed up the supposed effect of poisons in the bowel. It was *auto-intoxication.*

Ironically, today yogurt is once again the fastest-growing product in the dairy industry. Why?

Says health-food author Cathryn Elwood, "Eli Metchnikoff . . . who discovered the white blood corpuscles, was the first to call our attention to the longevity of the Bulgarians. At the same time he propounded the scientific truth as to their exuberant health and youthful appearance . . . that these people are so unusually healthy because they have used such large quantities of a cultured milk called 'yogurt.' Modern nutritional scientists have corroborated his investigation and shown that 'yogurt milk' plays an important role in the health of the intestinal tract . . . Yogurt bacteria . . . produce lactic acid . . . Lactic acid inhibits growth of the germs of putrefaction."

Says the late founder of *Prevention,* Jerome Rodale, "Yogurt's therapeutic effects lie in its reducing putrefaction of the bowel."

Says Adelle Davis, "Yogurt . . . has long been the principal food for the Bulgarians and is considered responsible for their unusual health."

Says Linda Clark, columnist for the magazine *Let's Live:*

"Although yogurt is looked upon by the uninformed as a 'fad,' nothing could be further from the truth . . . Actually, yogurt has been used since Biblical times . . . to eradicate . . . auto-intoxication."

Unfortunately, nutritionists do not support these views. The handbooks of food composition show us that yogurt is scarcely different from ordinary milk in nutritive value. It is, after all, just milk in which some extra organisms happen to be living.

With or without yogurt in the diet, the bacterial flora of normal people does not change much. In general, the opinion of science is summed up by the authors of two standard nutrition textbooks:

Says S.R. Williams, former president of the Society for Nutrition Education: "Yogurt is merely a fermented, culture form of milk; it has no mysterious additional properties."

Comment Drs. Bogert, Briggs and Calloway, all professors at the University of California: "Yogurt is a very nutritious food, but offers no magical promise of good health or longevity beyond milk itself."

When the word about yogurt and the bowel reached Battle Creek, Dr. Kellogg was greatly excited. Here was real support for his life's work. He rushed to England.

In addition to spending time with the Metchnikoff-minded physicians of Britain, Kellogg also visited his surgeon friend, Sir Arbuthnot Lane. At about the time of Metchnikoff's yogurt discovery, Lane, who had long worried about the colon as a "common sink," decided to do something bold about this supposed problem. He believed that he had identified one particular part of the bowel as the main site for such intoxication, and he began to cut it out. Diagnosing *auto-intoxication* in literally hundreds of patients, Lane promptly relieved them of that section of bowel where he thought that wastes slowed down. His skeptical colleagues soon referred to the section as "Lane's Kink."

Thus did Kellogg return to Battle Creek armed with a new confidence in the villainy of the bowel, and some bold new weapons to combat it. He had a new three point program:

First, no "putrescible" foods would be allowed at The San. And all fruit would be disinfected with chemicals, operating-room style, before patients were allowed to consume it.

Second, Kellogg would drive toxin-making cells out of the intestine by making his patients drink half-pint doses of whey culture, made from milk. Then, as though to trap the poor little bacteria in a crossfire, after each daily cleansing enema, the patient got a second enema—with another half pint of whey culture.

Finally, on the way home Kellogg had thought a lot about Lane's brisk surgical traffic. And he decided that Lane had really missed the colon's kinkiest part. John Harvey selected a new twist of bowel as the target, and soon he was cutting it out of as many as twenty patients a day, at fees appropriate to his international stature.

In explaining what had been learned, the Doctor often used constipation as proof of the perils of auto-intoxication. When one's elimination was slowed down, the putrescence and its poisons had longer to do their dirty work. This accounted for the symptoms of constipation. Not until 1916 was this idea disproven experimentally. In that year Dr. A.N. Donaldson merely packed some cotton into the colon and got the effects of constipation.

As time passed, Dr. Kellogg took the principles of putrefaction more and more to heart, modifying the San diet even more to deal with it. For example, he said that "a luxurious bill of fare" could be composed of only "bananas, figs, dates, raisins, prunes and a few nuts." In fact, he decided that the only safe foods for humans were nuts, fruits, grains, juicy roots, eggs and milk.

Nuts figured larger and larger in Kellogg's dietary scheme. "There is no danger of a food shortage," he wrote, "if we give the noble nut a chance." At one point he was deeply involved in a plot to plant 400 square miles of nut trees, to revolutionize American eating.

Actually, John Harvey had always liked nuts. Rather early in his career, for example, he had worried about those patients whose teeth were in no condition to manage nuts. In 1893 he had found a solution to the problem by inventing peanut butter.

Kellogg now began to worry about the intestinal intoxication of children, too. He set out three rules for child health. The first was to feed them his simple, narrow diet. The second was to make them chew everything to a liquid pulp before swallowing. And third, he dictated, "Prompt and regular evacuation of the bowels at least three times a day." Many an American household sought to comply, confronting countless hapless children with an unending stream of enemas and castor oil.

By 1920, the Doctor went so far as to lay out the dictum: "It is of far more consequence for a teacher to know whether a child's colon is evacuated regularly and frequently than to know that he is acquiring proficiency in mathematics."

One might think that the increasing stringency of life at The San would have driven away all but the most earnest or desperate enthusiasts. Yet Kellogg was still so swamped with rich patients that he built a 15-story luxury tower to accommodate the most baronial tastes. Around the spectacular "Acidophilus Milk Bar," the showpiece of his new Palm Garden, gathered the biggest names of the day.

There you could see comedian Eddie Cantor and Johnny Weissmuller, greatest of the Tarzans. Amelia Earhart came in her plane and flew the Doctor around for his first air view of The San. "I like Dr. Kellogg's philosophy," said Henry Ford, who returned frequently to The San, always wearing a buckwheat blossom in his lapel. And Joel Cheek, the founder of Maxwell House, listened attentively to Kellogg's evening lectures on the toxicity of coffee.

Explorers liked to come to The San to be restored. There were Admiral Byrd, Roald Amundsen, Wilfred Grenfell and adventurer-author Richard Halliburton.

There was Mrs. Knox, whose gelatin was repudiated by John Harvey, and the Gerbers, whose baby food he disdained. There were tycoons, from John D. Rockefeller to Messrs. Kress and Kresge. There were bigtime politicians from the Congress and the Cabinet.

And all of them, at the end of the day, listened to the new Sanitarium Philharmonic Orchestra, sitting restlessly on their half pints of whey culture, full of nuts and berries. Here and there, as the bran and the paraffin oil did their work, members of the audience would rise and hurry toward their rooms. But everyone understood and discreetly pretended not to notice.

Why were so many people so susceptible to the odd diets of the 19th century, to the rigors and rituals of The San? The questions are worth trying to answer, because such susceptibility is with us still.

Let us look again at the state of medicine, say, in 1876, when Kellogg took charge of the Western Health Reform Institute. The age of science had begun. Darwin had published his theory. Balloons were taking men into the air. The steam engine had brought new power and speed. The telegraph had opened new rapid communication. Machines, then as now the primary evidence to the public of scientific achievement, were taking over more and more of life—machines to farm, to sew, to roll cigarettes, to shape hard steel, to tunnel into the earth.

But while people had begun to believe in what science could do, medicine had achieved little to meet the popular expectation. At John Harvey Kellogg's medical alma mater, Bellevue, when doctors were faced with a case of typhus, they still gave whiskey and milk and told the family to pray for the best.

Actually strides were being made in basic knowledge. Insights into the functions of circulation, of breathing, body energy, and microbial life were laying a groundwork for later accomplishments. But the physician, having read or heard of these things, had to go back to the bedside with little of practical value save the old, inadequate nostrums.

In 1858, the *Medical and Surgical Journal* ran an article with the depressing title, "To What Cause Are We To Attribute the Diminished Respectability of the Medical Profession in the Estimation of the American Public?" And the physicians' lack of confidence made it hard for even some well-trained doctors to make a living. So often medicine did not attract the best minds. In 1870 the dean of Harvard's Medical School was asked why his students did not take written examinations. He replied that too few of the graduates could write well enough to make the test fair.

As Kellogg took over at Battle Creek, some physicians were still trying to prove that bleeding or leeching did not cure fevers. Pasteur's microbial theories were still doubted by many. Many physicians were still scoffing at Semmelweiss for saying that they should wash their hands between deliveries of babies. And despite the development of vaccines, until about 1900 efforts to require immunizations were frustrated by public distrust.

In brief, medicine could make few promises, compared to those made by less scrupulous healers. As late as 1900, a study showed that 75 of every 100 American medical school graduates turned to other work within five years of taking the Hippocratic oath.

The failures of medicine in the 19th century left the way clear to those with much imagination and little conscience, or for the well-meaning but ignorant. Most began with antique ideas of "natural" cures. For example, Adolph Just's *Return to Nature* became a big seller. It laid down precepts about walking on wet lawns and sand, and stressed the importance of sleeping on the ground. Louis Kuhne's *New Science of Healing* opposed all drugs. It offered a Grahamite "natural" diet, moved on to water therapy in the form of steam baths, and added exposure to sunlight. Heinrich Lahman discovered that the real cause of illness was eating salt and drinking water with meals.

As the knowledge of the role of bacteria in disease began to emerge, but with few means other than ordinary cleanliness to control those bacteria, Antoine Bechamp came up with another popular theory: the presence of bacteria in sick people indicated only that *disease produced bacteria.*

This latter idea of Bechamp's is still quite popular in some foodist circles today. One of the bestsellers in our health-food stores is Dr. Henry G. Bieler's *Food Is Your Best Medicine.* As Bieler wrote in 1965: "Germs are merely a concomitant of disease . . . able to multiply in a sick person because of disturbed function . . . Discarding the germ theory of disease opened the way for me to explore new methods of eliminating the stagnating waste products from the body. Briefly stated, my position is: improper foods cause disease; proper foods cure disease." Hundreds of thousands of copies of the book have been sold. But Bieler's unusual ideas—such as his belief that eating ice cream is the real cause of polio—have also been spread by his patients, among whom were some of Hollywood's most famous people. They have carried his concepts both into the media and into our law.*

---

*Similar popular thinking about non-microbial origins of what medicine knows to be contagious disease is found in *The Mucusless Diet.* This concept centers about unfounded hypotheses that certain foods cause excess mucus to be formed by various organs, leading to illness. It is commonly believed among some counter-culture groups.

Healing such as Bieler's, without drugs or surgery, is often dignified with the name "naturopathy." And one person who popularized naturopathic ideas in America was Andrew Taylor Still, the inventor of *osteopathy*. It all began in 1874, the year Dr. Kellogg graduated from Bellevue.

Son of a Methodist missionary to the Indians, Still got his medical education from watching his father attend an occasional Shawnee. Shortly before 1874, Still saw his two daughters die of unknown causes, which may have led to his bitterness toward orthodox medicine. Whatever the reason, Still was soon writing that "Osteopathy" [a word he made up, meaning illness of the bones] "is the greatest scientific gift of God to man."

He put it this way because the theory was given to him in a revelatory vision. It may be worth noting that for a time Still had been an Adventist convert and, of course, a vegetarian. As he explains his system: "God has placed the remedy for every disease within the material house in which the spirit of life dwells . . . They [the remedies] can be administered by adjusting the body in such a manner that the remedies may naturally associate themselves together."

The bodily maladjustments, he says, rejecting germ theory, are of the nerves or blood circulation. They are brought about by tiny dislocations of bones in the spine. For these displacements he invented the term "subluxations of the vertebrae." At first he said that when "subluxations" were "adjusted" relief should be instantaneous, but he soon modified this position. *Adjustment* of the spine was to be accomplished by twisting and wrenching the patient. *Snap! Crackle! Pop!* might apply to osteopathy as nicely as it does to breakfast food.

Not until 1910 did Still get his thoughts on paper. (In the meantime, he had practiced extensively and had opened the first school of osteopathy at Kirksville, Missouri.) His book certifies that, with proper osteopathic manipulation of the skeleton one can cure yellow fever, baldness, piles, rickets, dandruff, obesity, diabetes, malaria, cancer and kidney trouble.

Today's osteopathy still manipulates the spine, but also uses conventional drugs and surgery. The training of something less than 10,000 practitioners varies in quality, but in a few states is compared to that of orthodox medicine. Nevertheless, many osteopaths still claim that adjusting a couple of bones in the neck can cure *schizophrenia,* and some 40 of our states give them about as much license to practice as they give to M.D.s.

The acceptance of Still and his followers helped to open the way for another group of "healers," the chiropractors. And it is worth knowing a little about the origins of their beliefs, because they are perhaps the largest group of licensed health practitioners who use foods as "cures."

Twelve years after Still invented osteopathy, a Canadian-born fish peddler and grocer named Daniel Palmer left What Cheer, Iowa—and also the first of his six wives—and moved to the town of Davenport. There he turned to curing people with "animal magnetism." Soon he met a janitor named Harvey Lillard, who had become stone deaf 17 years before, after he heard something go "pop" in his back. The rest of the story is told by Daniel's son, B.J. Palmer, who became the popularizer of chiropractic:

"Harvey Lillard came in thoroughly deaf. Father looked him over, and there was a great subluxation of the back. Harvey said he became deaf within two minutes after that popping . . . Father thought of this thing, which was that if something went wrong in the back and caused deafness, then reduction of this subluxation should cure it. The bump was adjusted, and within ten minutes Harvey regained his hearing."

Ignoring Andrew Still's then 20-year-old discovery, Palmer called himself a medical inventor. Later, he wrote his textbook on chiropractic, *The Science, Art, and Philosophy of Chiropractic,* in 1910, the same year that Still finally published *his* book.

As Palmer explained, "A subluxated vertebra . . . is the cause of 95 percent of all diseases." As for the other five percent, they are caused by displaced bones . . . "more especially those of the tarsus, metatarsus and phalanges (of the foot and toes) which, by their displacement, are the cause of bunions and corns."

Daniel Palmer set up a school of chiropractic, which taught this amazing new science in three months for between $300 and $500. But very possibly, his invention would have received little notice, except for the efforts of his son, B.J. (Bartlett Joshua) Palmer. B.J. said he started practicing chiropractic at the age of eleven.

As one dean of the Palmer School reports B.J. Palmer's early life: "The first twenty years of this boy's life were spent in being educated to hate people and everything they did or were connected with.

"His mother died when he was one-and-a-half years old. From then on, he was at the mercy of five cruel stepmothers . . . forced to sleep in dry-goods boxes in alleys, often with the weather below zero . . ."

In 1906, the year before Metchnikoff discovered yogurt, Daniel Palmer was sent to jail for practicing medicine without a license. So son B.J. bought out his interest in the school. Seven years later, Daniel, who had left town and then returned to set up his own school, tried to lead a Homecoming parade of alumni through Davenport. Daniel charged that B.J. responded by running into him with his car. Daniel died three months later. His executors filed suit, claiming the automotive assault, and the district attorney sought a murder indictment. But B.J. avoided trial—as always, showing great skill in adjustment.

One can hardly accuse B.J. of concealing his real interests. "Our school," he said, "is on a business, not a professional basis. We manufacture chiropractors . . . In regard to educational qualifications, do not allow this to annoy you. We hold no entrance examinations."

These basic principles have been followed steadfastly since Today, Ralph Lee Smith, author of the authoritative book on chiropractic, estimates that there are perhaps 20,000 chiropractors, although the American Chiropractic Association claims there are 25,000. However many there are, a basic aspect of their approach to the healing art is perhaps best suggested by one small segment of B.J. Palmer's book, *Answers:*
"Q. What are the principal functions of the spine?
A. To support the head
   To support the ribs
   To support the chiropractor."
Osteopathy and chiropractic were not the only concepts

developed to fill the gaps in medicine. For instance, there were the *heliotherapists,* or sun healers, who prescribed vegetarian diets, had their patients run barefoot in the snow and took their pictures lying naked (but decent) on their stomachs in the sunny wards and balconies of their "cures."

Typical of the turn-of-the-century new therapies was Movement Therapy. This held that the body need merely be jiggled to run right again, much as one deals with a recalcitrant wristwatch.

What we might call the Movement movement began in Germany, but quickly spread to the U.S. It used many new techniques. One was a pair of ropes, fastened both to floor and ceiling. The patient held the ropes. Two attendants then, at a signal from the doctor, whipped his legs over his head, to stimulate blood vessels of the head and thus cure disorders of the ears, eyes or nose.

The greatest success of Movement Therapy, however, appears to have been with women. For example, breast therapy, using movement by the hands, seemed to help many. Even more effective was manipulation of the womb, including prolonged movement of the female genitalia. The German theorists of Movement found this very helpful in cases of headache and indigestion. But they were never able to explain why.

Such was the spectrum of medicine in the latter part of the 19th century and the earliest part of the 20th. It was in this context that Kellogg offered his diets, his enemas and all the rest.

Now consider Dr. Kellogg's promises of diets to "cure cancer of the stomach, ulcers, diabetes, schizophrenia, manic depression, acne . . . asthenia, migraine and premature age." And remember that the most ethical practitioners of medicine had to say that they had no answer for these ills. Wouldn't almost anyone have *wanted* to believe Kellogg? And what was the risk of trying his way?

Indeed, even in our own time no one can honestly guarantee to spare us from heart disease, stroke, cancer, even from the common cold. Shall we simply submit to our fate? It is not really in most human hearts to concede mortality—or even the inevitability of a stuffy nose—without a fight. What if the answer just might be only a change of dinner or a few dollars worth of vitamin E? Once we begin to fear for our existence, what price will we not pay for even the smallest better chance?

The problem is not just one of the last century. The dilemma is still with us.

Thus could Kellogg draw the nation's best and wisest people. Thus could he still, in 1927, float a $3 million bond to keep building facilities. Thus, as late as 1931, could he persuade aircraft tycoon Glenn Curtiss to give him an estate in Miami Springs, Florida, which was to become Miami-Battle Creek. Thus could Kellogg scarcely be turned aside in the 1930's, when the Dionne Quintuplets, then of world fame, developed a digestive problem and John Harvey flew unbidden to their aid.

But the Depression dried up the incomes that San patients needed to pay Kellogg's bills. In 1933, The San was more than $3 million in debt. By 1938, Kellogg had to order it closed.

C.W. Post was long gone. In 1914, having tried to build his own city in Texas, and having failed to make it flourish by setting off explosions to bring rain, he had been depressed. In his Santa Barbara, California, home, he fired one of his own fine rifles into his head.

John Harvey Kellogg hung on until 1942, when pneumonia finally took his life at the age of 91. Only one of the old Battle Creek crowd survived him.

W.K. Kellogg ("The original bears this signature") survived until 1951, when he died at 92. But his spirit, and those of all the veterans of the old Battle Creek wars, is still with us.

Let us look back again to the turn of the century to see how and why.

9

The Jungle, the Sausage
and the Law

Many a history student knows that in 1906 a young writer named
Upton Sinclair published a book called *The Jungle,* and that the
public outcry at his revelations about the food industry ended with
the formation of the U.S. Food and Drug Administration. Students
have also learned that the effort toward food-industry reform was
led by President Theodore Roosevelt, who was supposedly
shocked by Sinclair's tale of chicanery among Chicago's meat-
packers, and grateful to young Sinclair and his fellow "Muck-
rakers." The end of the story is thought to be the triumph of
Sinclair's crusade for pure food.

It makes a memorable yarn this way. But the truth is a little
different.

To begin with, Sinclair was always angered by the belief that
he sought improvements in the food supply. His story is about a

95

Lithuanian emigrant who becomes an underpaid worker in Chicago's packing houses and who, with family and friends, is cruelly used by a rapacious economic system. His hero, Jurgis (pronounced *Yoorgis*) Rudkus, was supposed to be seen as a victim of capitalism, not of bad meat. The critic Clarence Andrews tells us that Sinclair, "became discouraged when he discovered that his readers were more alarmed by his disclosures of . . . the production of food supplies."

Some packinghouse scenes in *The Jungle* were indeed startling. For example: "As for the other men, who worked in tank rooms full of steam, and in some of which there were open vats near the level of the floor, their particular trouble was that they fell into the vats; and when they were fished out, there was never enough of them left to be worth exhibiting—sometimes they would be overlooked for days, till all but the bones of them had gone out into the world as Durham's Pure Leaf Lard!"

Or: "And then there was 'potted game' and 'potted grouse,' 'potted ham' and 'deviled ham' . . . made out of the waste ends of smoked beef . . . and also tripe, dyed with chemicals so that it would not show white . . . and potatoes, skins and all, and finally the hard, cartillaginous gullets of beef . . . All this ingenious mixture was ground up and flavored with spices to make it taste like something . . . It was hard to think of anything new in a place where . . . men welcomed tuberculosis in cattle . . . because it made them fatten more quickly. . . ."

While *The Jungle* was actually a plea for socialism, ironically, Sinclair did indeed end by becoming a food crusader. Unfortunately, his concepts of food and health were not much more realistic than his ideas of socialism. His two main socialistic schemes failed—a community in Englewood, New Jersey, and a western program called EPIC (End Poverty In California). To suggest the realism of his socio-economic thinking, he ends *The Jungle* with a complaint that, "the competitive wage system compels a man to work all the time to live." And he pleads for a new system in which, "anyone would be able to support himself by an hour's work a day."

If we recall that Teddy Roosevelt was a Republican of the old school, who believed in the virtue of individual enterprise without question, we can see why, when Teddy used the term "Muck-rakers," he hissed it through his large clenched teeth.

The novel would probably not have been taken seriously by the President if a great deal more had not happened to set the stage for reform. There was then urgent reason to worry about harmful and exploitative food processing—though foodist writers today give us the impression that the time of *The Jungle* was a kind of golden era of wholesomeness, now lost and lamented. As Adelle Davis commented in an interview shortly before her death:

"Up to 50 years ago, organic food was the only kind anybody knew of. Now we use hundreds of thousands of pounds of chemicals that destroy nutrients. Time was in this country that when you opened your mouth, you put in good food. That was when real brains got developed—Washington, Jefferson, people like that. These days we don't grow enough skulls to put a brain in anymore."

But the adulteration of food is as old as trade. For example, Pliny writes: "The dealers have set up regular factories where they give a dark hue to their wine by means of smoke, and . . . employ noxious herbs." Early Sanskrit law set fines for those who adulterated grains, oils and other products. By the second century B.C. in China there was a "Supervisor of Markets" whose agents spot-checked to catch adulterated foods. The code of China's T'ang Dynasty provided that when, ". . . meats cause men to become ill . . . the violator will be flogged 90 strokes. He who deliberately . . . sells it to another will be banished for a year, and if the person to whom it has been . . . sold dies, the offender will be hanged."

The more food was processed, as in the selling of flour instead of grain, the greater the opportunities grew for fraud. By medieval days, laws to prevent and punish such offenses were on every nation's books, and the tradesmen's guilds were trying to police their members. Bread was the prime target for many such laws. In England, some of these were codified by King John, in 1202; penalties for bakers included hanging false loaves about their necks, the pillory or having their ovens pulled down. French law in the 13th century dealt with bread, butter and harmful additives, such as resins, in beer.

So commonplace were offenses, however, that the punishments had to be stepped up. The Turks would simply nail the ear of an errant baker to his doorpost. In Germany of 1482, a vintner who had used forbidden additives in wine was forced to drink six quarts of it and died. At Nuremberg, an adulterator of costly saffron was burned at the stake, over a fire of his own spices.

More and more inspectors were appointed, and tests of purity became increasingly ingenious. For example, His Majesty's "ale tasters" in England would not only sip the brew to taste for adulterants, they also poured some on a bench and sat on it in leather trousers. If they stuck to the bench, it was deduced that sugar had been added to the beer.

By the 18th century that Adelle Davis so reveres, when she says that big brains were made by "organic foods," Smollett describes the food supply in London (and the situation was then much the same in the U.S.) in this way: "The wine . . . is balderdashed with cider, corn spirit and the juice of aloes." Bread was a "deleterious paste, mixed up with chalk, alum and bone-ash, insipid to the taste and destructive to the constitution." Cream was "the worst milk, thickened with the worst flour into a bad likeness of cream."

Tea in the 18th century was costly, so it was tempting to sellers to adulterate it. Iron filings, clay, and gypsum were added to make it weigh more. Old tea leaves were bought from inns and used to stretch out the new. The tea was sometimes thinned with whatever leaves came to hand, which were then colored with everything from molasses, clay, logwood, dyes and paints to sheep dung.

At the end of the century, Frederick Accum set up the first food-testing lab in England, and his revelations were shocking. He reported that many poisonous substances were used in food, as in the greening of pickles with copper sulphate. He tells of a woman who ate such pickles whenever she went to her hairdresser, and finally died. He tells of red lead being used in cheese, of additives such as oil of vitriol, turpentine and arsenic to give foods pungency. Accum's writings generated such an outcry that embarrassed officials procured his indictment on a criminal charge—failing to return books taken from a library. Faced with jail, he skipped bail and left England.

In the U.S., Massachusetts had the first pure-food law, passed in 1784. New York, New Jersey, Rhode Island and other states soon followed suit. But few of these laws were well enforced. By 1853, more than half the New York City milk supply was "swill milk." It was produced by cows fed on the exhausted grains which had been used to make beer and whiskey. It was commonly watered, then doctored with chalk or plaster of Paris to change its suspicious, thin blue look.

Not until 1859 did Massachusetts ban swill milk. In Buffalo, New York, in 1880, 73 percent of milk was found to be watered; 71 percent of the olive oil produced in Massachusetts was adulterated; 69 of 171 samples of ground coffee in New York were faked; 46 percent of candy samples in Boston had mineral coloring, chiefly lead chromate. In New Hampshire, the state found that only 21 of 41 "maple syrup" samples were real.

Again turning to England, where the food industry was much better policed, a physician named A.H. Hassall began to do some food checking, largely physical inspections with a microscope. In the 1850's, Hassall, working with a special sanitary commission appointed by the journal *Lancet,* published the following results:

In brown sugar, 40 of 72 samples showed such dilution as potato flour, starch, grit and tapioca. All of 74 bread samples had alum. Four of eight flour samples held alum. 48 of 56 cocoa samples had cocoanut shell, colored earth, etc. 16 of 30 oatmeal samples had barley meal and husks. All of 42 mustard samples had been colored. Cayenne pepper had been colored with such as cinnabar, ochre and red lead in 24 of 28 samples. 32 of 61 vinegar samples held sulfuric acid.

Some of the adulterants were quite imaginative. For example, Hassall found coffee which had been stretched out with the roasted livers of horses and oxen.

Medicine was so poor in this time, moreover, that most of the illness which resulted from adulterated foods was misdiagnosed. But in 1900 a dangerous beer was sold in the Manchester-Sheffield area; it had been made from a brewer's sugar, which in turn had been made by breaking apart starch with sulfuric acid. The ore from which the acid had been made contained arsenic. Seventy people died. Six thousand were poisoned.

With the rotting of food such a key health and economic problem, the manufacturers took steps to solve it. They began to dump preservatives into the cooking and preserving kettles. They merely found what was roughly the smallest amount needed to prevent decay and then tossed it in. It was hardly their responsibility to find out what their customers' bodies would tolerate. They used boric acid, borax, benzoic acid, and benzoates, and the deadly caustic, carbolic acid.

They soon found that these chemicals had still another use. If you sloshed them on foods which were already somewhat decayed, sometimes it stopped the decay and often made the stuff look good enough to sell.

In many cases it was difficult to tell foods from drugs. The two were often used interchangeably, and there were no controls on claims or content.

The patterns in British and American industry were similar, although the U.S. had no such patent-medicine villain as the British "Soothing Syrup," remarkably effective at quieting youngsters, but so loaded with then-cheap narcotics that it was estimated to kill 15,000 children a year. Anything could legally be used in such "cures," in either nation.

By the end of the century, there was Sears' *White Star Liquor Cure.* In the Sears-Roebuck catalog, the wife was instructed simply to slip this into her drinking husband's coffee after dinner; he would go right to sleep instead of slipping off to the neighborhood saloon. And the cure apparently had enough narcotic in it to fulfill the claim. (Not to worry; on the same page was an ad for *Sears' Narcotic Cure.*)

There was *Dr. Rupert Welk's Radiated Fluid for Cancer.* ("It will cure you at home without pain, plaster or operation.") One such medicine did indeed contain radioactive material, and led to some deaths before it left the market.

Dr. Kilmer's Swamp Root was claimed to cure "Bright's Disease or Dropsy" (dangerous kidney ailments). These and many similar medicines, as for coughs and tonics, often did make the patient feel better, for the moment, because they were largely alcohol.

"Female remedies" were legion. A group called the Thompsonians paved the way for many of these, by heralding a system of vegetable cures. Thus did *Lydia Pinkham's Vegetable Compound* make a fortune.

Many patent-medicine ads offered free consultation by mail. The women were offered advice from wise old ladies; men were counselled by "Viennese doctors," most often on "male weakness." Almost all the advice proved to have been written by imaginative young men, who often sat around a large table in the advertising office. The advice was always the same: use more of the product.

Tent shows went on the road with nostrums and wild promises. At one point, Healey and Bigelow had 20 companies out, rivalling the vaudeville circuits as they sold *Kickapoo Indian Sagwa*.

Sidewalk displays were set up to lure innocents into "examinations" and "consultations" which ended with the sale of magic foods or concoctions. The business became so big that newspapers depended on it for revenue. So no questions were asked when ad copy read: "In any woman's breast, any lump is Cancer," as it did for *Dr. and Mrs. Chandless' Cure.* And of course they got many testimonials of cancer survival, since most lumps found in women's breasts are *not* malignant but are harmless cysts.

All this chicanery did not go unnoticed. A counterattack began on two fronts about the turn of the century. One wing of this assault originated with an Indiana chemist named Harvey Washington Wiley who in 1883 became chief of the Chemistry Division of the U.S. Department of Agriculture.

As a chemist, Dr. Wiley was no slouch, within the limits of his time. In 1884 he founded the Association of Official Analytical Chemists (whose methods are today the standards for determining the nutrient content of foods). And in 1893 he became president of the American Chemical Society. He also was an M.D., and thus had the interests and knowledge of the physician.

To check out his concerns about food adulteration, Wiley chose a daring method, one which would not be permitted today. He formed a squad of 12 volunteers, who ate their meals under his eye at the Agriculture Department. Wiley put various materials into their food to see what happened to them, and he often ate with them.

In 1902, Wiley began to issue reports on these studies, which caught the attention of Congress. Thus, in part, was the stage set for Upton Sinclair. For Wiley's reports began to scare people.

But clever as Wiley was, he had made a basic error. And that error is today compounded in much of our popular thinking about food safety. In essence, the mistake centers about the scientific fact that there is really no such thing as a poison.

If this seems to contravert the great danger of, say, arsenic in the making of beer, look again. For there is arsenic (and also its more toxic chemical cousin, selenium) in our soil. And both are taken up by the plants we eat. But both these elements have roles in nutrition—healthful roles.

Or recall Frederick Accum's account of the lady who died of eating pickles which contained copper sulphate. Both copper and sulphur are essential nutrients for the human body, found in many every-day foods.

How can such substances be "toxic" and yet also be necessary to life? Toxicity is a question of *amount*. There is no nutrient which is not toxic if we consume enough of it. Excess table salt or even water can kill. Conversely, there is no substance so deadly that small amounts of it are not safe.

Thus Dr. Wiley's error. For example, having added sizable amounts of benzoic acid to the food of the "poison squad," he wrote in one of his pamphlets:

"The administration of benzoic acid either as such or in the form of benzoate of soda, is highly objectionable and produces a very serious disturbance of the metabolic functions, attended with injury to digestion and health."

Scientifically, this statement cannot be made accurately without specifying the *amount* of benzoic acid of which one speaks, and making some estimate of *how frequently* it will be used. To many non-scientists, this seems like a quibble. The attitude is often, "If this stuff can be toxic in any amount, why use it at all? Why not get rid of it?"

The answer is, if we were to apply this thinking, *we literally could not eat anything*. Indeed, the legal limitations on the permissible amount of a number of chemicals are often far below the levels which are found in such everyday foods as spinach, rhubarb or potatoes.

Yet in 1970, a well-meaning Ralph Nader study group issued a book, *The Chemical Feast*, by James Turner. The group and Turner are properly admiring of Dr. Wiley's work. But they miss a key point. "Four of the chief major struggles that Dr. Wiley directed," writes Turner, ". . . were against bleached flour, Coca-Cola, saccharin and benzoate of soda." In each case, Wiley was disturbed by the presence of chemicals such as caffeine which, in *large* amounts, could be harmful. But we know today that in the small amounts in which they are useful in food, they do no harm. If there were knowledge to the contrary, the products would *have* to be taken from the market. The law demands it.

Despite his error, however, Dr. Wiley had suggested a vital principle, that the government has a duty to protect the public health by controlling the adulteration of food with any chemical which might be injurious to the consumer. The principle has an important corollary—that use of any additive should not be permitted until testing has assayed its effect on the body and certified its harmlessness in the quantity to be used.

In 1905 another important blow was struck, this time by author and editor Samuel Hopkins Adams. Adams had investigated the patent-medicine business. In a series of articles called, "The Great American Fraud," he discussed some of the factors we have considered in the making and selling of nostrums.

Perhaps the most important principle he set down was that "On every dollar out of which you are cozened by a fraudulently advertised article, the publication which carries the advertising gets a percentage . . . As a partner in the enterprise the (publication) cannot share the profit without also sharing the responsibility."

At this, several publications, such as *The Ladies' Home Journal*, dumped all the questionable drug advertising they had carried for years. It was a noble thing to do, for the patent-medicine pitchmen were probably the biggest group of national advertisers at the time. However, it seems significant that a good deal of highly questionable food advertising continued.

When Post advertised for Grape Nuts, "Makes Sturdy

Legs!" no one complained. Nor did anyone question him when he published a Postum ad showing coffee dripping. "Constant dripping," read the copy, "wears away the stone. Perhaps a hole has been started in you. . . . Try leaving off coffee for ten days and use Postum Food Coffee."

In 1904, the California State Journal of Medicine said, "Prominent among the deceptions practiced . . . may be noted several proprietary foods: infant foods, cereal breakfast foods and coffee substitutes. (These deceptions are) not in the foods themselves, but in the labels. They convey to the minds of the laity decidedly wrong impressions."

And there were always a few sound laymen who chuckled at the claims of the overenthusiastic scientists about foods. A German physiologist named Moleschott had discovered that there was considerable phosphorus in the human brain. He laid down a law: *"Ohne Phosphor, kein Gedanke,"* which was widely quoted and meant, "Without phosphorus, no thought."

Jumping at this, Professor Louis Agassiz of Harvard quickly reminded himself that fish possessed a great deal of phosphorus. So when he was making a speech on behalf of the Fish Commission in Massachusetts, he made the statement that one nice thing about eating fish was that it would make you think better.

This was a rash assumption, scientifically speaking; it required little scientific training to examine the evidence and draw common-sense conclusions about it. Mark Twain suggested his feeling about the idea, in writing in the magazine *Galaxy* an answer to the question of a "Young Author."

"Yes, Agassiz does recommend authors to eat fish, because phosphorus in it makes brains. So far you are correct. But I cannot help you to a decision about the amount you need to eat—at least, with certainty. If the specimen composition you send is about your fair, usual average, I should judge that perhaps a couple of whales would be all you would want for the present. Not the largest kind, but simply good middling-sized whales."

On January 1, 1907 the Food and Drug Law went into effect. It subjected foods and drugs to restrictions with regard to the danger they entailed for the user. It banned interstate shipment of such items, and it provided mild penalties. Dr. Harvey Wiley was given charge.

But disappointment lay ahead. As originally passed in 1906, the law had seemed to both legislators and doctors to promise a bar to rash statements about curative effects. Almost at once the Food and Drug people cracked down on Dr. Johnson's Cancer Cure ("Available Everywhere").

The case went to the Supreme Court before it was over, and the Court ruled that the Food and Drug Law referred only to statements on composition or identity. Dr. Johnson's Cancer Cure could go right back to its old ways.

Wiley became bitter. He had encountered not only legal limitations, but also administrative ones. In a biography of Wiley, a meeting in Teddy Roosevelt's office is described, a meeting of the President, representatives of the food industry, cabinet-rank officials and Wiley. Roosevelt listened a bit to both sides on the matter of benzoate of soda and snapped, "Gentlemen, if this drug is injurious you shall not put it in foods."

Then came saccharin. Said Congressman Sherman, representing industry, "My firm saved $4,000 last year using saccharin instead of sugar."

Said Wiley, "Everyone who eats these products is deceived, believing he is eating sugar, and moreover the health is threatened by this drug."

"Anybody," Roosevelt interposed, "who says saccharin is injurious is an idiot. Dr. Rixby gives it to me every day."

Dr. Wiley had discovered how whimsical can be the rationale by which government applies rules, and the perennial complication that everyone believes himself an expert on the relationship between foods and health. He had patience with neither. In 1912, he resigned, thereafter to attack government food policy and to write *The History of a Crime Against the Food Law*, published in 1929. He also went to work for *Good Housekeeping*.

Soon after Wiley's resignation, Congress added the Sherley Amendment (1912) to the Food and Drug Law. The Amendment made violators liable, ". . . if the package shall bear or contain . . . any statement . . . which is false or fraudulent."

However, this referred only to the package label. C.W. Post and W.K. Kellogg could say what they pleased in ads. The most ethical magazines still accepted their hucksterism. No one complained when Post advertised that Grape Nuts "Makes Sturdy Legs!"

The makers of *Eckman's Alterative* challenged the new label restrictions and lost. But an ad was not a label. And not for another quarter of a century could ads be challenged. Yet the lead and arsenic came out of baking powder and gelatin. Copper was no longer used to color peas green. Fewer decomposed beans and polluted oysters were sold.

As for Upton Sinclair, he was still unhappy because he thought the point of his book had been missed. At the same time, he now considered himself an authority on food. He espoused one food cause after another.

In 1908, for example, one Hereward Carrington wrote a book called *Fasting and Nutrition,* which maintained that most human ills could be cured if only the patient would stop eating. Sinclair championed Carrington's cause. In fact, by 1911 he had issued his own book on the subject, *The Fasting Cure.*

In another of his books, *The Book of Life,* Sinclair opines, "I would not like to guess just what percentage of dying people in our hospitals might be saved if the doctors would withdraw all food from them . . ."*

Later he went on into other medical explorations. He took up the cause, among others, of Gaylord Wilshire, who was promoting I-On-A-Co, an electric collar which, it was claimed, when worn around the neck for fifteen minutes a day could cure almost everything.

Sinclair was also smitten with Albert Abrams, whom the American Medical Association has stated simply, "easily ranked as the dean of all 20th Century charlatans."

Claiming that vibrations were the cause of all disease, Abrams came up with a series of outrageous concepts. At first he

---

*Fasting is unknown as a valuable cure for any problem except obesity. Even when normal eating is impossible or ill-advised (as in certain surgical patients) nutrient intake is continued through the circulatory system (*parenteral* nutrition).

said he could diagnose any illness by tapping the patient's stomach, listening to the vibrations, and getting the special sound each disease carried. But this method was slow, and it limited his customers to those who could see him personally. So Abrams invented the *oscilloclast*, into which he could put a single drop of blood and get a complete diagnosis.

Thus Abrams could collect fees from all over the United States, from people who sent him a drop of blood. Later he found the machine would also determine the patient's sex and religion. And then he discovered how to make diagnoses from handwriting samples.

But how to cure the people in far-off places—Abrams worked from California—was the problem. He found he could direct radio waves at them with the right vibratory rates. For desperate cases he made the diagnosis and sent the cure over the telephone.

It is estimated that Abrams sold some four thousand oscilloclasts, most of them to osteopaths and chiropractors, at a price of $450, which included a course on how to use them. The AMA sent Abrams the blood specimen of a healthy guinea pig, under the name of "Miss Bell." Abrams reported quickly that Miss Bell had an infected sinus, a streptococcic infection of the left Fallopian tube, and cancer.

One private physician sent a drop of blood from a rooster. The diagnosis was diabetes, cancer, malaria and two venereal diseases.

What did Upton Sinclair say about this? "He (Abrams) has made the most revolutionary discovery of this or any other age. I venture to stake whatever reputation I ever hope to have that he has discovered the great secret of the diagnosis and cure of all major diseases."

Later he counseled his readers, "So is opened to our eyes a wonderful vision of a new race, purified and made fit for life . . . Find out about this new work and help make it known to the world."

Of course Sinclair was not the only important writer to become interested in odd medical ideas. To mention only two more of the period, George Bernard Shaw was a militant vegetarian. And as late as 1944 he was an ardent defender of naturopathy. He believed that drugs were useless and that epidemics were caused by the intermingling of handkerchiefs in laundries. He did not like vaccination, either, and he spoke up on most of these subjects in Bernarr Macfadden's naturopathic magazine, *Physical Culture.*

Philosopher John Dewey attributed his longevity to the theories of an Australian named Frederick Matthias Alexander, a reciter who lost his voice, then retrieved it by a weird system of subtle muscular exercises. He not only taught these exercises to Dewey, but in a school he established in 1904 in London he trained to his method Aldous Huxley and Sir Stafford Cripps.

The interest of famous men in odd or absurd ideas is not really surprising, however. What is surprising is that readers will turn to an Upton Sinclair, a Bernard Shaw or an Aldous Huxley for medical advice. It is a little like finding the best possible plumber, to service your car. Yet medicine seems to be the only field in which personal prejudice is deemed sufficient qualification not only to defy informed opinion, but to spread misinformation to the world at large with impunity.

Soon after *The Jungle* appeared, the newly made authority on health, Mr. Sinclair, realized that he needed more training in these matters. He had found a career, and he wanted to enter it without reservation. He boarded a train for Battle Creek. There he found a new and marvelous diet—a regimen of milk and honey.

Things were still churning along at The San; you could always count on finding the latest ideas there. Dr. Kellogg had discovered the litchi nut and concluded that its sugar should be substituted for cane sugar in America. He never realized his plan for planting 800 acres of litchi nuts, but patients at The San could get litchi-nut sugar. It was as standard a San menu item as *Malted Nuts*—which John Harvey said Post had stolen from him and called *Grape Nuts*—or *Protose,* a blend of peanut meal and flour to substitute for meat.

Reindeer moss was catching Kellogg's fancy at the time. So was a weed known as Abyssinian rumex. Upton Sinclair felt right at home. He was especially interested in Dr. Kellogg's new sign. After all, there were not many signs at The San, except for such traditional ones as that which hung over a live turkey each Thanksgiving: "A Thankful Turkey."

But Dr. Kellogg was so enthusiastic about a new idea that he had raised a ten-foot banner across the Grand Dining Room. It was emblazoned with a single, powerful word—"Fletcherize!"

In fact, Horace Fletcher, from whose name the word came, was actually there. Sinclair sat with him at the Radical Table (perhaps because he mistook the label to be political rather than nutritional), and the two became friends and mutual supporters.

At the very least, the new association provided Upton with some good copy. The magazines were hungry for new stories about food and health. A new era of health communications had begun.

Sinclair listened carefully as Horace Fletcher confided to him the simple code of health which he had devised. Then Upton wrote it down. It was all summed up in a little poem:

> "Nature will castigate
> Those who don't masticate."

10

Chew, Chew, Horace

In 1909, *The Ladies' Home Journal*—having disdained the big money of patent-medicine advertising which misled the public or risked its health—fell into a new journalistic trap. It has not fully emerged since.

The fall was heralded by the publication of an article by Horace Fletcher. The *Journal* had waited some years after the launching of Fletcher's chewing theories. Today, it is quicker off the mark.

Wags of the time were fond of saying that, whatever the scientific value of Horace Fletcher's ideas, they certainly had teeth in them. The *Journal* brooked no such levity. Instead, it introduced Horace's work in a convincingly pretentious manner. Said the editors, in their September issue for that year:

"Fletcherism has become a fact. Ten years ago it was laughed at. Today the most famous men of science indorse it and teach its principles. Scientific leaders at Cambridge University; University of Turin, Italy; University of Berne, Switzerland; Université de là Sorbonne, France; the Universities of Berlin, Brussels, St. Petersburg . . . as well as Harvard, Yale and Johns Hopkins . . . all indorse Fletcherism and its principles. The honorary degree of M.A. has been conferred on him at Dartmouth. Professor William James of Harvard and Professors Fisher and Chittenden, of Yale, have endorsed his principles. Chautauqua made him its lecturer on Vital Economics. It has been established that more than 200,000 families in America are living according to Fletcherism. It is no longer a question of doubt that of all the many current movements for sane eating and living, Mr. Fletcher and his principles have emerged at the very front."

The *Journal* was not alone in its support. Virtually every important magazine of the time took note of Horace and ended by conceding that he had something.

But let us double-check the magazine sources before we too accept this new idea. Let us attend to the words of pioneer Harvard psychologist William James.

"I tried Fletcherism for three months," he writes. "It nearly killed me." He was not alone in his feeling. And he was guilty of little exaggeration.

In 1889, Horace, then a wealthy businessman, had been ready to retire. His family wanted to live in Japan, and Horace had felt spent, sick and old.

"At 40 years of age," he later wrote, " ny hair was white. I weighed 217 pounds . . . I was afflicted with that 'tired feeling.' "

Horace's waist was some 15 inches bigger around than it should have been. Today, 20 percent obesity is considered a medical concern. Horace was about 40 percent overweight.

But he had been strong. In *McClure's* magazine, popular at that time, we read that he had begun as an apprentice clerk in Shanghai. "He surpassed all his associates in running, jumping and wrestling and could lift dead weights of pig iron that the strongest sailor could not move."

At 40, his hair already white, his face and body round and cherubic, he was the picture of physical incompetence. He applied for life insurance and was refused. He later made much of this rejection, but the truth seems to be that it was due to only one problem—he was fat.

The rejection frightened Horace. He went to Venice to regain his health, saying that exercise made his breath short and his heart pound. He never seems to have known that his excess weight could have accounted for these and other symptoms.

In 1898, thinking himself moribund, Horace went to Chicago, to close some business affairs. Having to wait, he read. And what he read was literature about health.

Here he followed a common lay pattern of making medical inquiry. Laymen may read either medical books, dull and hard to understand, or lucid simplifications, more often than not based on half-truths and fantasies. Horace chose the popular literature. Having done so, he became convinced that Nature had the answers. "I determined," he writes, "to consult Mother Nature herself for direction."

Somewhere, Horace read that Gladstone, the British statesman, felt there must be a reason why humans had 32 teeth. As Gladstone saw it, there was one possible explanation; Nature intended that each bite of food should be chewed 32 times. (It may be that Gladstone assumed a kind of British fair play among teeth, each taking its turn, in gentlemanly rotation.)

Mulling this over, Horace was sure that Nature had given us clues to what she expected. That secret, he writes, "was not hidden away in the dark folds and coils of the alimentary canal." It was in the mouth.

Testing, Horace took a bite of food. He chewed thoroughly and slowly. After 50 or 60 chews, the food became so much thick liquid. And then came the miracle. The flavor extracted, the food suddenly disappeared. What Horace called the "food gate" opened, of its own volition, and the mouthful was gone.

The observation has some accuracy. The reader might like to Fletcherize just one bite of food to test it. Remember Horace's advice, however, to "Hold the face down so that the tongue hangs perpendicular in the mouth." Then keep chewing until Nature does the swallowing.

One can draw many conclusions from the results. Elbert

Hubbard—self-styled philosopher, moralist and psychologist—explained in his *Cosmopolitan* article of 1908, "The Gentle Art of Fletcherizing": "Try to sip your Martini. Fletcherize it, hold it in your mouth and taste, taste, taste it, and you are a hero if you can empty the glass. Nature rebels after two or three very little sips, and it tastes like kerosene."

"Nature knows," asserted Hubbard. "Trust her!"

When Horace Fletcher found his idea, he went back to Venice to think and write about it. Here his works, *The ABZ of Human Nutrition* and *How I Became Young at 60,* took shape. And in the city of canals, Fletcher met a sick physician, a Dr. Van Someren.

By now Horace felt like a new man. He was 65 pounds lighter. (If the reader wonders why, he need only try Fletcherizing a few meals. He will see how soon oral exhaustion comes.) Moreover, many obese people do bolt their meals. And one of the objects of modern *behavior modification* therapy in obesity is to slow down the process of eating, so that the eater realizes that he has satisfied his appetite, before bolting excess food.

Van Someren was no lightweight. He tried the idea, lost weight, liked the whole concept and presented it to the British Medical Society.

Among the audience was Sir Michael Foster of the University of Cambridge, Julian Huxley's successor as secretary of the Royal Society. He was impressed. This British acceptance led to Fletcher's being invited to address the American Physiological Association in Washington, D.C.

Horace concluded that, because people ate little when they Fletcherized, that man must need very little food. For two weeks in Venice, he tried eating milk alone. Fletcherizing, he found that he wanted no more than a quart a day.

Back in Battle Creek, Dr. Kellogg was asked about Fletcherizing. He said that the principle was correct; in fact, he had discovered it some 20 to 30 years before.

If a man would know what foods were best, Kellogg wrote, he must be "willing to listen attentively. And to *listen,* one must take care to chew each morsel of food . . . until the main part of its flavor has been set free and appreciated. Anyone who will take his food in this manner will have little occasion to consult diet specialists or call for professional aid of any sort; *for there is no one thing which comes so near to being a panacea for all gastric ills and nutritional disorders as thorough mastication of food and careful attention to the natural promptings of a disciplined and intelligently studied sense of taste.*"

This thinking had great appeal. It was accepted, among others, by Professor Russell Chittenden of Yale, a noted physiologist who was not feeling well at the time. He, with his colleague Irving Fisher, conducted experiments that became the main scientific arguments for Fletcherism.

The 1909 *Journal* contains a photo of one of the tests. It shows a chubby little man with eyeglasses and a benign expression. He is sitting by some apparatus, looking something like a cherubic plumber working with some steam pipes. The caption: "Mr. Fletcher Making a World's Record on the Dynamometer Without Training."

On this contrivance, using leg muscles only, Fletcher lifted a 300-pound weight 350 times. Athletes had crumpled after only 125 lifts. How Fletcher did it, no one knows. From his youth, this little barrel of a man had shown great strength. The only thing we know certainly is that his performance was an anomaly.

Fletcher was certain that chewing did it. And he set out after further proofs. He took off his shirt and exercised in his underwear with young football players. He had himself photographed in the high dive and doing push-ups, and boasted, "It's all in the mouth."

Reactions came in a steady stream. General Leonard Wood told reporters that he had seen the benefits of chewing and little food. "I noticed this," he said, "while chasing Indians."

Yale's Chittenden now had groups of vegetarians from Battle Creek's Sanitarium staff compete with Yale meat-eaters. He reported that the vegetarians could hold out their arms longer, without quivering, than could the New Haven carnivores.

This, Chittenden considered, was a major finding. For all agreed that when one Fletcherized, meat became a bore; it took so long to chew it to a pulp. Thus, meat was "unnatural" food. When Yale men Fletcherized and were given free food choice, they soon disdained steaks for mashed potatoes.

Scientifically, we might say that there were two genuine conclusions. First, Battle Creek staffers, who had engaged in Grahamish setting-up exercises for years, could do more of them than could Yale faculty members. Second, beef is harder to chew into a liquid state than are mashed potatoes. But Chittenden and *The Ladies' Home Journal* were awed.

But science went further. Hubert Higgins, demonstrator of anatomy at Cambridge, studied the palates of the horse and dog, to identify the secret automatic-swallowing reflex. Then he wrote (in 1907) *Human Culture,* which described in unprecedented detail the chewing of a currant cake. *Current Literature,* then an important magazine, was so fascinated that it reviewed the book in a lengthy article called *Poltophagic Protest.* The contention was that man was intended to chew things in this manner; only lower animals were meant to swallow lumps.

As the data built up, the War Department joined in. West Point was Fletcherizing, to strengthen future officers. So 30 soldiers were assigned to Chittenden for a definitive study. When the project was explained to them, six deserted.

One worry of the soldiers was that their total food intake was to be slashed to 3,000 calories a day—a goodly amount, but food intake was larger than it is today.

When a researcher named Mendel took up Fletcherism, his dietary was cut to: a small breakfast of a few hundred calories; a lunch of lima beans, mashed potatoes, bread, fried hominy, syrup and coffee; a dinner of consommé, string beans, mashed potatoes, rice croquettes, syrup, cranberry jam, bread and coffee with cream and sugar. Mendel announced that this was less than a *third* of his previous dietary.

The soldiers who took part in the Yale test were more vigorous as the weeks passed, and they thinned. Also, as the War Department was pleased to learn, deprived of meat and other things they liked to eat, "they developed a marked readiness to kill."

By 1907, Elbert Hubbard reported that West Point was firmly entrenched in Fletcherism. "At the present time," he wrote, "it amounts to quite a tidal wave of reform."

Hubbard's belief that "food poisoning" accounted for most disease was by now a common press view, much like today's false belief that eating protein prevents or cures obesity. "Eczema," wrote Hubbard, "gout, headache, pimples, boils, bad breath, that foggy feeling, these are all symptoms of food-poisoning." (Remember, only a year before Metchnikoff had started the yogurt fad and confirmed the illusion of "auto-intoxication.")

Hubbard could not say enough about Fletcher's genius. He wrote: "As a biologist he has very few living peers. His statements are safe, conservative and the fruit of long study, careful observation and patient experiment. The excellence of his philosophy is so apparent that no one can argue it down."

Hubbard and others said Americans could save at least 20 percent of their food by Fletcherizing, with great benefit to health. "Epileptics," he said, "are gormands [the spelling is Hubbard's] who through disease have lost the sense of taste." And in a final maelstrom of semantics, in the best tradition of foodist rhetoric:

"Much insanity can be traced directly to the well of . . . manhood undefiled. The engine works, the wheels revolve, but the screw is befouled with a hawser and the pilot is drunk at his post. Ruin in high heels laughs a hysterical cry like the wail of a keener drunk on pepper sauce. And pardi, your soul is awash on a sea of bilge."

Fletcher kept going further. He ate even less, banning spices, stringy vegetables and tobacco. And his influence increased. *Current Literature* said that through his work, "scientists of the greatest distinction" were convinced, "that the dietetic ideas upon which . . . the standard theory is based will have to be revised." *McClure's* agreed, saying: "The first man to stir wide popular interest in nutrition was not a scientific man but a layman . . . Mr. Horace Fletcher."

Encouraged, Horace confined his diet to potatoes, cornbread, beans—and sometimes eggs, milk, cream and "fish balls composed mainly of potato." Then he tried living on two quarts of milk for 17 days and decided that his earlier diet was too liberal. He found that breakfast was unnatural, and finally ate only one meal a day.

Two years later he concluded that one must begin to

Fletcherize by fasting for several days, so that "unnatural" appetite disappears. One should wait for the true call of the stomach, feed it a Fletcherized cracker, then wait again.

In a later *Ladies' Home Journal* Fletcher noted that such eating "simplified woman's work." And it was economical. "Two hundred thousand families," he wrote, "save as much as one dollar a day on food." The Christian Endeavor Society adopted his plan and hoped thus to have its members save "hundreds of thousands of dollars a day" for good works.

Horace now discovered that what were usually thought of as the signs of hunger were really symptoms of overeating. "A person should brave discomfort for a week and even go without food entirely to . . . 'clean house.' Then the real sensation of hunger will be expressed . . . True hunger is never a discomfort."

In 1914, *The Ladies' Home Journal* was still militantly Fletcherite. It announced that John D. Rockefeller was one of many thousands of converts. "Don't gobble your food," the *Journal* warned. " 'Fletcherize' . . . Thus will demon indigestion be encompassed."

A poet at San Francisco's Bohemian Club commented:

> "Troubles in gobble and guzzle lurk;
> They give the stomach hard, needless work;
> They poison the blood and make it sour . . ."

Of Rockefeller's Fletcherite efforts, the poet added:

> "Eight years of health with golf to burn
> While saving the cost of a funeral urn
> Are some of the dividends John did earn."

Fletcher Clinics began to pop up around the world. The New York Academy of Medicine admitted that some of its members were practicing the method. And to much fanfare, Thomas A. Edison joined the movement, railing against "food drunks."

But as the first World War began, Horace was not feeling

well. Quietly, he sought medical help—at Battle Creek, where each day he could look up at the huge dining-room banner which commanded patients to "FLETCHERIZE!"

Kellogg had written, "This discovery of Mr. Fletcher's was one of priceless value." But John Harvey was sure that Horace had gone too far. He reports, for example, that Horace had begun to spit out anything left over after the flavor was gone. Where, John Harvey wanted to know, was Horace to get roughage?

And because Horace would now accept nothing but liquids and purees, Kellogg said, his patient showed "rapid decay of his teeth." Far worse, Kellogg noted that the Great Masticator suffered from "a most obstinate constipation." He adds, "Mr. Fletcher told me on several occasions that his bowels moved only once or twice a week."

(As a technical note, while daily elimination is hardly considered necessary by modern medicine, it is likely that Mr. Fletcher's record would have been of concern to the gastroenterologist as well, though not such horrified concern. But to Horace, this was an achievement. He told Kellogg that it was a sign of near "perfect absorption of food," so that no residue remained to be expelled or for germs to live on. He called this a "natural sterilizing process," and even proudly sent a sample of what he considered perfect elimination to a Federal laboratory, as a gift, by first class mail.)

Horace and John Harvey argued for weeks, but Fletcher continued to weaken. Finally, to Kellogg's great relief, Horace accepted a laxative. The Doctor reports that it "gave rise to a stool which greatly astonished him by its loathsomeness."

"But it was too late," mourns Kellogg. "His vital stamina and resistance to disease had been exhausted by many years' struggle against colon poisons, and he died of chronic bronchitis."

(It should be noted that there is not really a direct medical connection between chronic bronchitis and constipation. One suspects that Horace may have developed pneumonia or expired from the effects of *cardiopulmonary failure*. John Harvey always did have a little trouble with diagnosis.)

From that time on, however, Kellogg cites Fletcher's death as the tragic monument to the folly of insufficient roughage. In one of his books, he devotes an entire chapter to "Horace Fletcher's Fatal Mistake."

Characteristically, we have no way of knowing what was the real health impact of Fletcherism as practiced at hundreds of thousands of American dining tables. Certainly, teaching so many children to choose foods according to how nicely they liquefied and slipped down the gullet was undesirable. But as Horace passed, so did his ideas begin to slip away.

Surely, some nonsense remained of the fad. But it left one positive legacy. It generated a suspicion that gluttony might exact a price in health. During this era, the nation's pioneer traditions of eating also passed. There were certainly other factors that influenced the dietary changes—the shift of populations to the cities, less physical work, new wealth and the introduction of labor-saving machines, to name a few.

But somehow, looking again at Horace Fletcher's earnest, cherubic face, full of quiet pride beside the Yale dynamometer, it is nice to believe that his life work accomplished something more than helping to make America's magazines a fountainhead of foodism.

11

The Bare Torso King
Goes Public

Bernarr Macfadden, the man who made physical culture a household word both in America and Europe, was a man of many parts, and he aggressively exposed virtually all of them to the public.

The mere sight of a camera was enough to send him flinging off his rumpled clothes; often, only the photographer's air brush stood between Bernarr and complete self-revelation. In his myriad portraits, he is largely nude, with chin and stomach tensed, biceps, triceps and quadriceps straining, wiry hair flying out toward the planets, a picture of manly strength; it is hard to believe he is only five feet six inches tall.

He built a fortune from misinforming the public about nutrition and health. He was the first to use modern mass-media techniques in the process, setting a pattern which has endured.

Macfadden's history is dramatic. Horatio Alger would have been awed by his rise from penniless orphan to tycoon. Dickens might have felt that his childhood was too pathetic to record. "The Bare Torso King," as a Detroit newspaper called him—the editor of the *Journal of the American Medical Association* preferred the title "Body-Love Macfadden"—had bleak beginnings.

Macfadden was born in 1868 on a farm near Mill Springs, Missouri. His father was a devotee of cheap whiskey and fast horses, and often lay in a ditch outside the rundown farmhouse, shouting threats and obscenities. The father died in *delirium tremens* when Bernarr was only four.

The boy was sent first to a cheap boarding school. There his only food was often a dinner of peanuts, then thought useless except as livestock feed. The headmaster thought it might save peanuts if pupils ate the shells too. The peanut diet did little for the weakling child, but at last he was sent to live with an uncle and aunt outside Chicago.

They ran a sleazy boardinghouse. They quickly put their six-year-old nephew to boot-blacking, emptying spittoons and slops, and running midnight errands. Macfadden says that his workday was 18 hours.

Far away, struggling to earn Bernarr's keep, his mother was finally stricken with tuberculosis and died. The boy was told, roughly. He overheard his uncle say that Bernarr also looked consumptive and would probably be gone in a year or so.

Little Bernarr was terrified. He had become so sickly that he could work little. When an Illinois farmer named Hunter offered to take him, the uncle quickly agreed.

Now eleven, Bernarr strengthened with farm life. Later, he was to say that he had cured himself of tuberculosis by diet and exercise. But the diagnosis made by his uncle is questionable.

That winter, the boy stole a cigar and a jug of cider, tried them and found that they did not agree with him. Ever after, he liked to say that he had tried smoking and drinking and that either would kill.

At twelve, Bernarr was laughed at in town because he had no shoes. When he asked for some, Farmer Hunter refused, and the boy immediately ran away to begin a search for relatives with money. But his relations proved to be as poor as he, and Bernarr began to cough again. He decided that the tuberculosis had returned.

At this point, Macfadden tried scientific medicine. That is, he took some patent-medicine made by an uncle. In fact, to give a number of medicines a chance, he stirred them together, tasted, gagged, and decided that both drugs and doctors were useless to humankind.

Then, at fifteen, the boy discovered the magic of the gymnasium. He began hard workouts and carried a ten-pound lump of lead with him wherever he went. In his spare time, he worked with a wrestler, who got him a few inconsequential bouts.

For three years, Bernarr devoted all his energies to his muscles. At 18, bulging nicely, he rented a store and hung out a sign:

BERNARR MACFADDEN—KINISTHERAPIST
TEACHER OF HIGHER PHYSICAL CULTURE

Bernarr was never sure where he had got that word, *kinistherapist*. Nor could he say what it meant. But it attracted few customers. He soon closed his store and took a job in a school at Bunker Hill, Illinois. It was here that he received his only education.

He spent his spare time, mainly, wrestling and reading melodramatic novels. Soon he determined to write a novel of his own, *The Athlete's Conquest*. A Chicago publisher turned him down. So, yearning for bright lights and big money, he set out for New York.

On that city's 18th Street, he used his last $50 to rent a bare, second-story space and have a sign painted:

WEAKNESS A CRIME. DON'T BE A CRIMINAL.

Keenly aware of the value of publicity, Bernarr had his first semi-nude photos taken and presented them to the New York newspapers, along with 50 articles which he had written on the joy of muscle. Nothing happened. He was ready to throw in his loin cloth, when suddenly a businessman came in to be rejuvenated. Bernarr recalls that he would have been glad to get 20 cents for supper as his fee, but impulsively, he asked for $50. "Done," said the man, and Macfadden was on his way.

The King still had to take side jobs to survive. At the Chicago Fair, he demonstrated a muscle-building gadget and sold 300 of them. At once, he designed a gadget of his own, took it to England and began to sell it at public gatherings. He drew small crowds by standing in a box lined with black velvet, almost naked, and striking poses such as "Atlas Supporting the World," and "Achilles Disposing of Hector." He sold exercisers by the dozen, but found that he could make more by just posing.

The English sortie gave Bernarr capital. He returned to New York and in 1896 founded a magazine, *Physical Culture* ("Weakness a Crime!"). By 1898 he had 100,000 subscribers.

Bernarr guaranteed low overhead by his choice of staff. It consisted for some time of Bernarr Macfadden, the editor, who used the reporting of Bernarr Macfadden, along with such fine works of fiction as *The Athlete's Conquest,* by Bernarr Macfadden, serialized for months.

In the next few years, *Physical Culture* reached a circulation of a million—with such articles as "Is Muscle Bad for Brain?" "Marriage of the Unfit," "Some Practical Suggestions in Voice Culture," and "Paderewski on Strong Muscles in Piano Playing." Soon he began to realize, however, that women were also buying his photos of undraped males. He started, and soon closed, a magazine called *Women's Physical Development,* for which he wrote on female complaints under the sobriquet "Emma M. Harbottle." He ended by merging the failing journal (by then called *Beauty and Health*) with *Physical Culture.*

Physical Culture outlined a pattern of success for a whole skein of "natural health" magazines which were to follow, right up to the *Prevention* of our own day. Looking at its principles, we see a disdain for modern medical and nutritional science. *Physical Culture* instead depended upon the "natural" health ideas of the past century.

Two themes ran through almost every story. One was that drugs and even vaccinations were to be rejected, in favor of "natural" methods gleaned from Grahamism, Father Kneipp and

Battle Creek. And the other, of course, was a special health-giving nutrition regimen.

As his chief biographer, Fulton Oursler, wrote for *The Reader's Digest* in 1929: "At the foundation of the whole problem he places food. The keystone is diet and fasting. Energies of the body are largely concentrated on digesting unnecessary food . . . If one eats less, the body will have more time to take care of its repairs."

Oursler was sure that this worked. As an example, he wrote, "When something goes wrong, go on a fast. If you have a cold . . . a fast will cure it in a few days."

Macfadden said that fasting would make students stronger and keener-minded in a week. Cancer? He told the victims to fast for a few days and then go on a diet of all the grapes they could eat.

"Is it any wonder the doctors felt outraged?" asks Oursler, in discussing Macfadden's prescriptions for cancer and syphilis. "To them such statements sound simply idiotic. Yet I can find no record where they have actually experimented along Macfadden's lines."

More and more Macfadden dared to apply his simple solutions to all disease. When the subject was really controversial, he would write two opposing articles, each under a different pseudonym. Finally, he was so sure that no human ill could resist his "natural" methods that he wrote his *Encyclopedia of Physical Culture*—five fat volumes in which every ailment was listed, and along with each, "complete instructions for the cure of all diseases through physcultopathy."

There were no hedges, no disclaimers. As long as the reader followed directions and used no drug, he would get well. Macfadden even offered $10,000 to anyone who could prove that grapes would not cure cancer. In addition to the encyclopedia, he spun out 20 books on especially vexing problems of health, from *Foot Troubles* to *Hair Culture*. By 1905, he had the support of the natural-healing world of the time—naturopaths, chiropractors, osteopaths, water-curists and all the rest. He had created a potent medium of communication, and they were all eager to use it. Even George Bernard Shaw contributed articles on the merits of the vegetarian life.

There was no way to stop Macfadden, though many medical

men were outraged. They had no cures for heart disease, for cancer, for defective eyes—above all, none for aging. But Macfadden offered to deal with them all. The Law? There is no legal way, in America, to stop anyone from circulating an idea, no matter how ridiculous. Personal opinions are free from any control under the First Amendment of the Constitution.

In 1904, Macfadden proved the worth of his ideas by taking a handful of the infirm to a life of fasting and deep breathing in the country north of New York City. They all wrote testimonials to their cures—Macfadden, of course, diagnosed the illnesses—and an idea was born

From this experiment came Physical Culture City, a place where people could fast, build muscles and eat without meat. Its chief ornament was to be Physical Culture University, in which anyone could enroll. The students got special exercises to do, which Bernarr incorporated into all the labor of building the City. They were even paid, 15 cents a day. After only five and a half years, each student would receive a certificate of graduation which testified that he was physically superior and qualified to teach Physical Culture.

By summer of 1905, 125 tents had blossomed in Physical Culture City. A reporter for the *New York World* revealed that each tent usually housed one male and one female student, one way of engendering school loyalty. Macfadden sued the *World* for $50,000. But he lost. The judge ruled that the reporter had merely written what he saw.

Other New York reporters had fun with Physical Culture City. They found out how cheaply Bernarr had bought the property. Then they speculated about what it would be worth after a few hundred students had worked on it for some years. They called it a swindle. And having learned a little about legal rights, this time Bernarr did not sue.

Physical Culture City was soon in condition to accept paying guests for the warm weather. Among the first of these was a young writer who was hard at work on a novel which was to be a plea for reform. The author was Upton Sinclair, and the book was *The Jungle*. Upton helped to pay his way by writing praises of The City.

Also in residence was another young writer, named John

Coryell. Few people today remember his name, but many remember his hero, *Nick Carter, Detective.* Coryell believed in Macfadden because of the fasting. Both he and Bernarr were believers in Horace Fletcher's health ideas. And while Macfadden did not take Sinclair seriously, he believed that Coryell was a man of destiny, and offered him a deal. Macfadden envisioned a moral novel which he "did not have time to write." To be called *Wild Oats,* it would limn intimately not only the horrors of syphilis, but the exact conditions under which it was contracted. The novel would be serialized in *Physical Culture.*

Coryell assented. But famed blue-nose Anthony Comstock was waiting. He had been waiting ever since Bernarr's magazine had offered a book on sex as a premium to new subscribers. By our standards, it was a moral book. It showed in great detail the pitfalls of young men who were lured to "indiscretions." It pleaded not only for loyalty to wives, but also for restraint in overly-frequent marital connections as merciful and morally right. But despite the moral tone, Comstock knew the exploitation of sensuality when he saw it. (*Wild Oats* seemed to him to lack what today's Supreme Court would call "redeeming social values.")

Comstock hurried down to a New York auditorium where Macfadden was holding physical-culture exhibitions. Sure enough, there was lewdness. Women were exercising in tights. And *Wild Oats* was being offered. Comstock took his private police to Macfadden's office and discovered "filthy pictures" of women exercising, together with Coryell's "lewd" book. He made a citizen's arrest. Macfadden was fined $2,000 and sentenced to two years in jail (suspended). Physical Culture City was condemned to ruin, in the public mind, as a fleshpot.

With this, Macfadden decided that nutrition was safer than sex. He opened first a one-cent, and then a five-cent, restaurant. The food was the same in each (the basic price bought a plate of soup or beans), but the more expensive eatery drew more traffic. Soon Bernarr had 20 Physical Culture restaurants.

"Their menus were extraordinary," writes biographer Oursler. "One could buy a hamburger steak, made of chopped nuts and vegetables, and have all the illusion of eating good bloody beef, without the danger of high blood pressure afterward."

By 1911, with the magazine and restaurants coining money

and apostles going out regularly from the Physical Culture Training School, with the *Encyclopedia* streaming from the presses, Macfadden approached his finest hours. Once again, he set sail for England, though physical culture did not remedy his tendency to seasickness.

This time the posing box did not draw crowds. So Bernarr launched a contest, for "the most perfect woman in England." Victorious was Miss Mary Williamson, a lady runner and swimmer of impressively bulging thighs. Bernarr gave her not only the promised 100 pounds, but himself. Of his four marriages this was the best. This muscular 19-year-old was to be the love of his life.

Macfadden took Miss Mary to France for their honeymoon. There they shared the dreams that overflowed Bernarr's 44-year-old heart, with mile runs before breakfast and barefoot walks in the grass to draw vitality from the earth. And in the privacy of their bedroom there were many deep-breathing exercises, tooth-straightening (by biting a towel and pulling on the other end) and quiet meals of honey and water.

Finally there was an ultimate ecstasy. In the course of their nightly lectures, Miss Mary joined in by jumping barefoot from a table to land on the exposed belly of Macfadden.

Returning to America, Bernarr began to narrow the focus of his teaching. He now believed, for example, that fasting would cure some 30 diseases, from rectal ills to eye trouble. "While a patient is getting thinner during the fast," he wrote, "what he is really losing is not good flesh but the disease from which he is suffering." And he espoused Fletcherism with all his heart.

A typical Macfadden follower rose at 6 A.M., drank a cup of hot water (for his bowels), did neck exercises for his thyroid gland, and exercised his spine, while sipping two quarts of hot water to cleanse away his bodily poisons.

Finally, the Macfaddenite (or Macfaddist, as some called them) was ready for a "dry friction bath," with the aid of a coarse towel, and for the first of daily "air baths." "The air," Bernarr wrote, "coming in contact with the skin is of value at all times, but is especially required in important parts of the body organism." (Macfadden does not say precisely what these parts are. However, the implication is plain enough. Not only did he disdain all confining clothing, such as collars, corsets and even tight hats, but he especially lamented the practice of wearing trousers. He praised kilts and never wore underwear. His private seeking of air for vital organs caused a recurring servant problem. "Many weaknesses are brought about," he wrote, "through the unhealthful covering and restriction of these parts.")

Macfadden also had his followers bathe in cold water. Then, before breakfast, they had a good laugh, and sang to set a good mood and exercise the lungs. Anyone who wishes to try this remedy, as practiced in the Macfadden "health hotels," need only use the tune of *Jingle Bells* to sing:

> "Day by day in every way,
> I am getting well (Ha!)
> I am filled with health and strength
> More than I can tell (Ho!)
> Now I know, I can go
> All along the way (Ha!)
> Growing better all the time
> And singing every day! (Ho!)"

The most devout Macfaddenites followed the song, as he did himself, with a long, thoughtful chew on a lump of mahogany, to strengthen the teeth. Then, after one more lusty laugh—laughing was a ritual of bending, slapping the thighs, throwing up the hands and howling—Bernarr was ready to skip breakfast.

Less assiduous followers were allowed a breakfast of two foods. One was acid fruit. The other was milk, permissible only when following Bernarr's special technique of drinking and swallowing, which he had developed after long study of the "natural" way, emulating the sucking and swallowing of babies at the breast.

To help the health routine, Macfadden designed a Physical Culture watch. At 8 A.M. it pointed to "No breakfast. Take glass cool water."

After skipping breakfast, the follower went to work, barefoot, so as to absorb magnetic forces from the earth, his chin out to show his "fighting spirits." At the office, he braced himself erect at his desk and made quick decisions. Preferably, he stood on his head to decide faster. Macfadden commonly worked in this posture and advised, "Don't stand on your rights, stand on your head."

Bernarr always walked to work barefoot, even when, in his sixties, he had moved to Nyack, some 20 miles north of his city office. He arrived at his office by noon, after leaving at dawn, there to take his first "hearty meal of the day"—carrot strips, raw vegetables, nuts and berries. "Select only natural foods," he wrote. "A perfect diet is furnished by nuts and fruits."

He ate only when hungry, in the Fletcherite manner. He said that a half gallon of water drunk in the morning "not only strengthens the heart, it conquers constipation." He exercised his teeth and ate salads every day, seeing raw foods as the answer to many medical problems, and used fresh fruits to keep the intestines "antiseptic." He believed that in eating only "complete" foods— rather than processed white sugar and flour—one would eat less.

The rest of his day mirrored the first half—laughing, singing, showing the fighting heart, walking home to a dinner which was like lunch, air-bathing and then sleep, alone. He kept his blankets propped up tent-like, so that air could circulate over his body at night. Whether or not these personal habits had anything to do with his eventual total of four wives is not known.

Macfadden's ideas were not implanted by *Physical Culture* alone. During the First World War, he put out *True Story* magazine, and eventually took it to ten million readers. In 1919 *True Romances* was born, perhaps in answer to the editorial question, "Can anything be more syrupy than *True Story?*" And *True Experiences* was launched upon a similar sea of treacle. *True Detective* joined the pack soon after, and Macfadden Publications became a communications power.

There were failures, too: *Beautiful Womanhood, Midnight, Movie Weekly* and *National Brain Power Pictorial Monthly* all folded. But the losses were cut quickly, and by 1931 Bernarr admitted to a personal worth of $31 million.

All of these magazines were open to every eccentric health scheme. They were heavily editorialized, with as many as four editorials in an issue. They accepted any sort of advertising, from *Isham's California Waters of Life* to grass tea. Editorial matter supported these ads; for example, grass tea was recommended by that staunch female reformer, "Mother Teats," whose main theme was "Intercourse for procreation only!" And a number of foodist ideas were propounded by Eleanor Roosevelt, who for a time wrote a baby-care column for Bernarr. Whatever the main subject of the magazine, there was always in the background the scent of lettuce, the ripple of warm water and the clatter of dumbbells.

Early in the 1920's, Macfadden moved into the newspaper business, with the *New York Graphic,* which became a major New York City daily. As with the magazines, the reader's attention, and small change, were caught up by sensational headlines, as:

BEAT TWO NAKED GIRLS IN REFORM SCHOOL
WEED PARTIES IN SOLDIERS' LOVE NEST
RICH RED DROPS FREE LOVE

Bernarr had no scruples about snaring the buyer's interest. He used composite photos. For example, when a couple called Peaches and Daddy Browning were divorced, Macfadden's photo lab took a stock photo of a courtroom, superimposed a naked woman's torso and put Mrs. Browning's head on top of it.

Behind such attractions, the *Graphic* preached vegetarianism, air baths and tooth and hair exercise. Such articles usually came directly from Bernarr, who would sometimes dictate as many as 20 editorials and articles while standing on his head. Some of the sensation was provided by two new young columnists, Ed Sullivan and Walter Winchell.

In Macfadden's country house in Nyack, he led a simple family life, with nine children, to whom he taught physical culture, in the nude. As late as 1928, he lacked a son, however. Taking his readers into his confidence, he revealed his search for a natural method to spawn a male heir. In 1929, sure enough, Billy Macfadden was born. And Bernarr joyously began the training that was to make Billy the superbaby of physical culture. Then the one-year-old had a bad fall.

Macfadden permitted no ordinary physician to attend anyone on the Nyack estate. He took over Billy's care himself. Did he not know all that natural medicine could teach?

Three days after the fall, Billy began to have convulsions. Bernarr denied him food, to let the body heal itself. He devised special baths and water treatments. But soon Billy was dead.

For a time, the tragedy seemed to dampen some of Bernarr's naturopathic confidence. But soon he was back at the old stand. He attacked government for licensing some healers to do things that others were not permitted to do. "The government," he wrote, "has absolutely no right to allow any particular school of medicine any more privileges than those enjoyed by other schools of medicine." A man who trusted the free-enterprise system, he concluded that, "The healing art should be on a competitive basis . . ."

Macfadden's naturopathic methods were scarcely new—except for a few nuances, such as eating sand to relieve constipation, or dealing with this problem by pounding the abdomen with one's fist or rolling a baseball around on it. There was little new in his emphasis on baths, hot water, cold water, sun or air. But there was a certain courage in his promise that baths could cure not only colds, but also syphilis.

He developed and strengthened the writing style that attracts so many readers to popular health writers—an inflated statement of the obvious in the form of revelation. Concerning the heart, he exclaimed: "One cannot underestimate the functional importance of this organ." How much one learns from Macfadden, thinks the satisfied reader!

With the 1920's and 1930's, a new era was beginning in popular thinking about nutrition; there was a new awareness of the chemistry of nutrition, of the existence of vitamins and minerals. Macfadden acknowledged none of this. In fact he generally refused to admit science to a role in medicine. And with the 1930's, his physical-culture methods lost their old magic. A new style of foodism was coming into vogue. One by one, he lost his publications.

Physical culture was still accepted by many, but it now was given a scientific flavor. For instance, we might consider how a Californian named Jack La Lanne practices the art. He calls himself a physical culturist, but he adds the title of "nutritionist." With a string of conditioning parlors and a long career of television exercising, he is perhaps the best known modern of the physical-culture calling. And his thinking seems to typify that of The Great American Gymnasium.

La Lanne's history—as he reports it in a book called *The Jack La Lanne Way to Vibrant Good Health*—is in the best tradition. As a teenager, he says, he was "surely the most unattractive kid in California . . . For years I had an unsightly case of pimples . . . had to wear arch supports and special braces for my shoulders. I suffered from blinding headaches, from chronic constipation which drained all my energies, and from such violent tempers I actually tried three times to kill my brother Norman . . . every kid in the block beat up on me. (Even the girls.)"

La Lanne confesses that he spent his allowance on candy and milkshakes, pies, cakes and other desserts. He even admits that he stole from his mother's purse to feed his habit. Then as a little, sickly teenager, he heard a lecturer* speak of "natural laws and natural foods and how we disobey God's laws by our eating habits." With this, Jack prayed to be able to follow those laws.

So much of his story is not greatly different from those of Sylvester Graham or the Alcotts. Some of his exercises are reminiscent of Macfadden's. For example, La Lanne notes that, if he is dining out with people who order wine, he likes to chew on the cork ("as I listen to the table-talk") to exercise his gums and firm up his jaw line.

Much of La Lanne's nutrition is also in the old style. Take, for example, his recipes for "Clear-Eye Salad" or "Clear Skin Salad." He recommends brown rice, saying, "You could live your whole life, if need be, on rice and water." (Some *macrobiotic diet* enthusiasts have tried this and died of scurvy, or suffered from other serious nutritional deficiency disease.) He refers to ordinary garlic as "Russian penicillin," and says that, since pure garlic kills bacteria, he eats a lot of it. Like Macfadden, La Lanne believes that the head is best nurtured by being turned upside down, lower than the heart, which position gives "a wonderful beauty treatment to your hair and eyes." Like Macfadden, La Lanne is quite small (five feet seven inches) and is commonly photographed without shirt or trousers; he also performs various feats of strength.

*Paul Bragg, one of the earliest U.S. exponents of making juices from vegetables.

But there is a difference, the difference that made Bernarr go out of fashion. It is that La Lanne tries to be scientific. For example, he says that meat is a desirable food—though he was a vegetarian for seven years—because it is a source of, among other things, vitamins A, B, C, D and G. Of course, meat is actually a very poor source of vitamin C, and, except for a few organ meats, it is usually a meager provider of vitamins A and D. There is a rather large family of B vitamins, some of which are plentiful in meats and some of which are not. And nutrition science does not recognize a "vitamin G." But you can see that, except for some of these inaccuracies, La Lanne has the general idea that there are vitamins in foods, whereas Macfadden tended to ignore such newfangled ideas.

As an example of his food selection, La Lanne tells the story of Mrs. Housewife, who peels her potatoes and then "takes those wonderful peels—which contain nearly all the mineral salts and vitamins of the potato—and dumps them in the garbage can." Food-composition research has shown clearly that, while the peel of the potato does have nutritive values, only a small part of the nutrients of a potato are in the peel. In most cases, the peel holds perhaps a twentieth of the nutrients.

La Lanne's nutritional numbers are often a little askew.* As an instance, at the end of the Mrs. Housewife episode, she is said to put "3000 calories of butter or gravy" on the evening's potatoes. Three thousand calories of butter is just about a pound. Three thousand calories of brown meat gravy is better than a quart.

Bernarr Macfadden spent little time with the vagaries of biochemistry. He was preoccupied with more practical matters, such as a string of physical culture hotels. They ranged from

*In the television advertising for the La Lanne salons, "nutritional guidance" is said to be a part of the program. At a home economics meeting, the author happened to sit at lunch with a lady who identified herself as a "nutrition counsellor" with the La Lanne organization. She said that men who came to her were "terribly deficient" in protein. When the author expressed surprise, since most men in the U.S. consume fairly large amounts of meat, she replied that, "Some of these businessmen eat nothing but hamburgers, three times a day, especially the bachelors." Factually, the meat alone in three typical hamburgers would supply more than the whole daily protein requirement for an average male. The "nutrition counsellor" said she was recommending protein supplements for these patrons.

Danville, New York, to the big Macfadden Deauville in Florida. He also owned—and inculcated with physical culture—such institutions as the Castle Heights Military Academy in Tennessee and several summer camps along the eastern seaboard. In a nice touch, he acquired Charles Post's old La Vita Inn at Battle Creek, right across from Kellogg's Sanitarium.

To understand how seriously many Americans of the 1930's took Bernarr and his ideas, consider that he was nominated at the Republican National Convention for the presidency of the United States. (He lost out to Alf Landon.) As late as 1940, Bernarr won the nomination, but was defeated in the election, for United States Senator from Florida. He put everything he had into these campaigns, but his plans were too innovative for some. As an example, he proposed building a huge freezer to help deal with the depression. Into this he would put the unemployed. Later, he would "defrost them when good times return."

By World War II it seemed that Macfadden had outlived his time. The more America accepted science, the more it turned away from him. Control of his publications had gone to others, with the exception of a foundering *Physical Culture*, which he renamed *Health Review*. But he still kept in the public eye.

In 1950, he invited a reporter to join him in his barefoot walk home. It was his eighty-second birthday, and he carried a 40-pound sack of sand to celebrate. The reporter was surprised by the simplicity of the old man's lifestyle. The large, expensive apartment had no curtains, rugs or beds. Macfadden had slept on the floor for 67 years. A table and a few chairs were the main decoration. In the kitchen, Bernarr himself prepared a bowl of raw vegetables and some hamburger. He had accepted meat and now even took liver injections. He ate naturally, from the skillet and bowl, with his fingers. He was neither poor nor senile. But he was frugal. At the peak of his wealth and power, he had looked so shabby that his office staff had chipped in to buy him a suit.

On his next birthday, his eighty-third, Bernarr donned a business suit, tennis shoes, football knee guards and helmet and jumped out of an airplane over his Danville physical culture hotel. He and his guests enjoyed the stunt so much, and the papers made so much of it, that he did it again the following year.

The octogenarian Macfadden felt so good that he even

remarried. He was full of plans for the future, and had decided that man's proper lifespan was 120 years—especially now that he had recognized the power of meat. His main regret was that, despite his daily tooth exercises chewing on a lump of mahogany, he had only four teeth left and had to restrict himself to hamburger.

Then suddenly, in 1955, at the age of 87, Macfadden was ill. He decided that he had a liver problem, and he began a fast to rest the organ. In three days he was dead.

The attending physician—who was probably the first Bernarr had known—told reporters that the cause of death was "jaundice, aggravated by fasting." Surely, Macfadden would not have liked this.

Time's ordinarily astute obituary writers merely noted that he had, "Pioneered in popularizing bedboards, enriched flour, scanty swimsuits and sunbathing." Of course, they were wrong about these details. Macfadden did not think anything should be enriched—rather that food should be left in its "natural" state. Sleeping on the floor, he did not need a bedboard. He emphasized air, not sun, for bathing. And he believed that one could not properly air-bathe in pants of any kind, no matter how scanty.

The real point was that an American king was dead. And like so many of his European royal counterparts, he had lived a little too long, into an era in which he could no longer reign. New princes—who had learned to trade in the royal robes of purple for the new white smocks of science—had taken power.

12

How to Stop Your Cow from Drooling

Some years ago an advertisement appeared in the newspaper of a small California agricultural town. It read:

"SEND 10 CENTS IN COIN OR STAMPS
We will send you a method that will help
you to stop your cows from drooling."

There was nothing more, save the address.

For the benefit of those who have little conversance with either the social habits or the physiology of the cow, it should be emphasized that drooling is a normal, though messy, bovine trait. It symptomizes no disease, no deficiency, no fault of breeding. For centuries, cows have drooled but gone on growing, calving and giving milk. Drooling has simply not been an issue in cow husbandry.

Nevertheless, ten-cent pieces flooded in from the farm area. (We should note that in this time, letters cost only three cents to mail and postcards a penny; it was a time when a dime allowed for a profit margin.) The ad proved not to be a cheat. For once the dime was received, a postcard went at once to the sender. It said, simply:

"Teach your cow to spit."

This story tells us something about America's response to health offers. For the advertiser was brought to trial. (Later, California Food and Drug officials concluded that he was an honest fellow, but with a pranksterish sense of humor.) Victims were located and brought to court to testify. And testimony went something like this:

Q. You say you received a postcard in return?
A. Yep.
Q. But the information was useless, fraudulent?
A. I don't know if I'd say that.
Q. Well, do you feel you got fair value for your money?
A. Yep. Only cost 10 cents.
Q. Sir, the money is not the question. Legally, we want to know if the defendant defrauded you by means of false promises in an advertisement. Did he?
A. Nope.
Q. (With impatience.) Do you mean that this method of preventing a cow from drooling is workable?
A. Well—yes.
Q. (Exasperated.) You mean to say that you could teach your cow to spit?
A. Maybe—if I had the time.

The above is not an actual record, but a reconstruction. However, the fact remains that not one witness would admit to having been cheated by the drooling remedy, even to the extent of ten cents. And this is one of the factors which, from the time of George Washington and his tractors, has made it difficult to prosecute for fraudulent health claims. For it is a rare person who will admit to being gulled—unless perhaps he has lost a lot of money and hopes to recover it.

The drooling gambit also suggests how easily many people respond to almost any scheme that sounds exciting. In 1976, some of the wire services carried the story of an experimenter in human nature who took an ad which simply said, "Send one dollar . . ." and gave the address. Nothing was promised, and nothing was given. But enough dollars came in to pay for the ads.

If we remember the dearth of medical answers which were available during most of the 19th century, it is certainly easy to see why people might respond to advertising rather than fold their hands in resignation. Around the turn of the century, moreover, as science made enormous strides in every profession, the public began to believe in wonders on a wholly new basis. The promoters' claims did not really seem any more astonishing or implausible than the wonders which science was almost daily finding in the simplest aspects of the natural world.

Beginning at the end of the 19th century and continuing into the early years of the 20th, the changes were bewildering. Suddenly there were automobiles and airplanes. Suddenly the microscopic marvels of the body were being discovered. Suddenly many doors of basic science swung open, doors which led to the scientific triumphs of our own day.

We may get some insight into the change by looking at the first Nobel Prize winners. Remember that most of their work had begun in the 1880's and 1890's. The prizes for 1901 included Roentgen's discoveries of X-radiation and von Behring's elucidation of serums and antitoxins, which paved the way for the conquest of diphtheria and tetanus.

Thereafter, in rapid succession, prizes went to such people as Finsen (for harnessing ultraviolet light and using it in therapy), to Fischer (for penetrating the mysteries of sugars and proteins, and the comprehension of the linking of amino acids to make proteins), to the Curies for their work with radium, to Arrhenius (for his theories of ionization and *osmosis*), to von Baeyer (for opening up much of the basis of organic chemistry), to Cajal and Golgi (for explaining the workings of the nervous system), to Pavlov (for explaining the reflexes of psychological conditioning), to Koch (for so much of the understanding of contagion and immunity), to Buchner (for opening our insight into the body's enzymes and how they take our foods apart and put them together), and to Kocher (for revealing many mysteries of the cell and its making of proteins). All these awards came within 10 years.

And there were endless other discoveries of the era which did not receive the Nobel accolade. It was in these same years that Freud opened up the unconscious mind and laid the basis for modern psychiatry. It was in about 1900 that Mendel's work was rediscovered, to give us the basis for what we know of genetics. Speculation on the meaning of all these findings ran wild.

To both the scientist and layman of the time, it began to look as though anything were possible, so long as the person who tried it wore a lab coat.

It is scarcely surprising, in this milieu of excitement and amazement, that the layman might have trouble discriminating between real and bogus discoveries, between mind-boggling realities and outrageous fantasies. To add to the difficulty, all but the most educated had little background for understanding the new marvels.

Through the revelations of chemistry and physiology, the groundwork was now laid for opening up the mysteries of nutrition. It is really in the first decade of the 20th century that modern nutrition science begins. And it begins in a spectacular way. A young Polish chemist, Casimir Funk, is working in London with pigeons. With dietary insights gained in the preceding generation, he is able to afflict the pigeons with the Orient's dread nutritional deficiency disease, *beri-beri*. The word means, "I cannot." It describes the great physical lassitude and weakness, which precedes death, if treatment is not given.*

The pigeons are dying. Funk gives them an extract he has made from, of all things, sweepings from the floor of a grain mill, the "worthless" hulls of the grain. Within hours the pigeons are on their feet; they are pecking, moving about. In 1912, Casimir Funk announces the first vitamin.

*The Dutch scientist Eijkman actually performed the basic experiments which led to the vita-amine discovery, using chickens in Indonesia.

Actually, he made a number of errors. He called his magical food substance a *vita-amine,* a name derived from his belief that it was a compound of the group called *amines*—and said that it was *the* unknown lifegiving substance in food. Today, of course, we know that there are many vitamins, and that they are not amines, which is why the spelling was changed.

Within four years, Elmer McCollum, the famed nutritionist of the Wisconsin Agricultural Experiment Station, had identified a second "vita-amine." Unlike Funk's substance, which dissolved in water, McCollum's dissolved in fat. To differentiate them, he called the water-soluble chemical vitamin B and the fat-soluble one vitamin A.

Meanwhile, in 1915, Dr. Joseph Goldberger and his assistants had shown that *pellagra,* the painful killer of the American South, was also a deficiency disease—and that it could be cured quickly and dramatically by many foods rich in proteins.

It took a generation to unravel the real meaning and chemistry of these findings, to learn that Funk's substance was *thiamin* and that Goldberger's was another B vitamin, *niacin.* By this time, many more micronutrients had been identified. But long before the chemistry was untangled, long before World War I ended, all of the civilized world was aware of the magic of vitamins. There was great hope that many diseases which could not be prevented or cured before might yield to these potent chemicals, of which so little could mean the difference between life and death. (For example, less than one thirty-thousandth of an ounce daily of Funk's thiamin could save a person's life. One of Funk's errors, incidentally, was his belief that he had isolated his vita-amine; he had only made a preparation which contained a little of it.)

Almost at once, after Funk's announcement, the foodists began to explain the magic of their regimens and products by claiming that they provided life-giving minisubstances. And by the 1920's, the presence and absence of vitamins and minerals, real or imaginary, had become a standard of the food-and-health pitch.

Many an ad of this kind dressed things up dramatically. For example, August F. Glaive, former chief of the California State Food and Drug Laboratory, recalls, "The circular of one of the early ones pictured a dream building with white-robed scientists, weird contraptions . . . and a long line of people waiting their turn to enter. The come-on read as follows:

"All animals, man included, must get their nutrition directly or indirectly from the soil, from the vegetable kingdom, for there is to be found all of the fundamental substances or values which can be transformed readily into growth substances, into lifegiving, into health-producing matters; it is these last which permit us to avoid illness or overcome it. . . .

"Calcium, Iron, Potassium, Phosphorus are most essential to a normal healthy blood supply; and unless we have an abundant supply of these elements many forms of nerve disorder and infectious disease will be our lot . . . The anti-acid properties of minerals of vegetable origin, or vegetable salts, have been fully demonstrated by experiments in our laboratories . . .

"We obtain our magic vegetable salts by a new ultra scientific method of extraction. Under our process the vegetable salts remain vibrant and alive, not just masses of inert materials. Our salts are obtained from strong healthy and virile vegetation . . .

"For a modest sum we will send you a two-months supply of the results of our years of research and an additional supply of our detoxifiers."

"After investigation," writes Glaive, "the vegetable salts were found to come from industrial chemical factories, while the detoxifier consisted of tablets of phenolphthalein, a laxative . . . The so-called Research Institute was a barn, equipped with buckets, pans and shovels to mix 'scientifically' the 'vegetable salts.' "

Almost anything might serve as a carrier of magical micronutrients in the 1920's. An example is one clever source of minerals called *Cur-O-Sea*. Its distributor describes the supplement in these terms:

"This everlasting source of health has given a new health outlook to thousands . . . A never ending source of radiant energy. There is only one healer and that healer is Nature. *Cur-O-Sea* is one of the most glorious manifestations. Send $5 for the family size of one gallon."

Truly, *Cur-O-Sea* did prove to be one of the most glorious

manifestations of Nature on earth. It was the Pacific Ocean, bottled a gallon at a time.

Where was the protection of the law? Unfortunately, pre-posterous though the product might be, it was not unlawful to sell it. True, as early as 1905, two years before the initiation of the Federal Food and Drug Administration, California had passed a law which said that: "Any person, firm or corporation . . . who advertises or displays any brand of goods known to the general public . . . who shall make verbal or show written or printed false statements regarding the quality or merits of the goods advertised, is guilty of a misdemeanor."

But no false statement had been made for *Cur-O-Sea;* a preconditioned public had been appealed to on the basis of its belief in nutrition magic.

Would it be possible to sell people ocean water today? It not only would be legally possible, but it is evidently commercially acceptable. As this book is written, Sears, the giant retail chain, has begun to open health-food sections in its stores. One of the products for sale in the new department of a California Sears, less than 10 miles from the ocean, is water from the Pacific Ocean. It is filtered, of course. It sells for $1.95 for a pint bottle. But then, the price of everything has gone up.

The author has no doubt, furthermore, that Sears' ocean-by-the-pint is the real thing. This is important. For one water seller of the 1920's did not even want to take the trouble of going down to the beach. He merely sold "natural" water, which he got from his kitchen tap. Then on each bottle he put a label of a different color— blue for tuberculosis, red for heart disease, etc.

For the economy-minded there was *Zola, the Wonder Water.* To save shipping cost, the water was first dehydrated. (The reader may wish to take a moment to think this out.) What the buyer got was a little powder marked "concentrated water." It cost only a dollar. And from it, using 25 to 40 gallons of ordinary everyday water, the buyer could make "the best of life-giving beverages." (Actually, the powder proved to be five cents worth of Epsom salt.)

Another popular Pacific Ocean product of the 1920's was sea

weed—sold wet, dried, powdered, in bulk or capsule. There were *Sea-Wrack, Blad-Wrak, Min-Wrak* and the cleverly named *Al-G,* to name just a few. The prices were high.

Why would people buy sea weed? It had been found that some areas of the U.S. had soils which were low in iodine. The result of low iodine intake can be goiter, a swelling of the thyroid gland, in the neck. That is why salt is iodized. And since both the amount of iodine added to salt and the human need are very small (the U.S. RDA is 150 micrograms a day, or 150 millionths of a gram, a little more than five millionths of an ounce) iodized salt usually costs no more and is recommended by nutritionists.

However, J. I. Rodale, of *Prevention* fame, still recommends kelp to deal with goiter. "As always," he writes, "it is our belief that the body's nutritional needs should be met by natural food sources, not doctored-up drugs such as iodized salt." Adelle Davis concurs, urging her readers to take a teaspoon a day of "granulated kelp."

Not surprisingly, Sears offers *Nu Life* kelp for around a penny a tablet at this writing, selling for money what one could get free in one's daily salt. Indeed, Sears hands out a pamphlet in which "Norwegian kelp" is held to be one of 14 "basic products." It is, "harvested from the cold waters of Norway where the water is clean and uncontaminated . . . full of Iodine. . . ." (We might also observe that excessive iodine can be as harmful as a deficiency, but such an excess would be extremely unlikely from the levels of salt fortification.)

With impressive speed, industry moved to supply a food or supplement for every nutritional need, real or imagined. As an example, one manufacturer offered a product which contained "silicon for sparkling eyes." Nutritionally, the reasoning for this product is obscure. Silicon is one of the most plentiful elements on the surface of the earth, a principal component, for one thing, of sand. It is because of the silicon that sand is the main raw material of glass. Presumably, the sparkle was to be transferred from the sand to one's eyes.

The list of new products lengthened rapidly. There was *Globulation,* a "blend of choice Oriental fruits," which was "the real secret of the virility of a well-known and warlike tribe of headhunters in the South Pacific." As Food and Drug expert August Glaive notes, "The manufacturer confided . . . that these aborigines thought nothing of living to the age of 150. And twelve weeks of such virile eating cost only $39.50."

There were foods that carried radiation. There was *Aqua Miel,* the juice of the agave cactus, common to Mexico and the American southwest, ordinarily used for making *tequila.* It was said to cure Bright's disease, rheumatism, high blood pressure, stomach and kidney disorders. This product is noteworthy because, in 1928, it was one of the few items which was foreclosed from interstate shipment by the Food and Drug Administration. However, this did not bar its distribution *within* states.

In general, as Glaive says, "There was little we could do. Occasionally we brought into court one of these . . . merchants . . . But living testimonials flocked into the courtroom and succeeded in imparting their credulity to the judge or jury, and the case was lost. We continued our efforts, however, and when we found sufficient evidence of insect contamination or moldy food, often succeeded in getting a small fine imposed. But not infrequently, instead of punishment, this turned out to be a cheap way to advertise them, particularly if reporters could see a humorous feature of the case."

Toward the end of the twenties, herb teas became popular, as combinations of folk medicines and nutrient sources. One made by Chinese producers in San Francisco under such names as *Mexican Magic Tea, Kidney Herb, Desert Tea* and *Golden California Tea,* was made from the same herb but with different promises. Another tea maker used ginseng in his tea and advertised: "For three thousand years the wise men of the Orient have called Geng-Seng Fragrant Health. People do not like to see a sour-faced, sickly-looking man or woman. Would you not risk $1.00 to gain something worth millions to you? Send the amount in advance and we will guarantee joyful temper, plenty of pure red blood, and relief for your irritable bladder."

This has a certain charm. But let us consider the mood of the man who sends in his dollar. An old principle in advertising is that the customer must identify himself with the problem suggested in the ad. So we assume that the victim must have felt that he either

(a) did not have a joyful temper, (b) had too little red blood (or enough blood but of some other color) or (c) believed that his bladder was irritable. Of course he might simply have felt "sour-faced" or sickly looking, and ignored the other requirements.

Many aging people do have bladder problems. But even assuming this sort of identification, what motivates the dollar-sender? Does the language of the ad inspire confidence? Are any authorities cited for the claims made? Is any evidence given of a case in which Fragrant Health did the job? The mystifying factor in the health-food business is the ease with which certain people can be separated from their money; it requires almost no persuasion at all; just a muddled mumbling about "natural," "ancient remedy," and "quick relief" is usually sufficient. Sometimes the advertiser does not promise *what* the nostrum will relieve.

How much more sophisticated have we become? According to *New Times* magazine, which seems to know about such things, before each television show, John Denver has an infusion of *Mellow Mint*—a blend of mint, alfalfa, papaya and licorice. *Mellow Mint* is the product of a new firm which has received considerable publicity. Called Celestial Seasonings, its 27-year-old boss has, at this writing, taken its business to $3 million a year. It makes such products as *Red Zinger,* called by *New Times* the "ultimate organic refresher." *Red Zinger* is described as beginning with African hibiscus flowers, in the hands of young herb mixer Mo Siegel. "Because herb tea is an excellent preventative medicine," reports *New Times,* "he added vitamin C-rich Bulgarian rosehips . . . a little Spanish orange peel and Mexican lemon grass . . . Wisconsin peppermint . . . wild cherry bark." (Scientifically, we should note that the amount of vitamin C, or any other vitamin, which could be derived from the small amount of herb used to make a cup of tea, would be inconsequential.)

The 1920's saw the emergence of a rash of outlandish claims that dealt with various nutritional and health problems. For example, the truth about obesity is hard to take. It is that, to lose weight, we must eat less food than our bodies use as fuel. However, the threat of hunger is enough to lead millions to suspend their common sense.

In the 1920's, if you didn't want to eat less, you had a number of options. There were reducing baths which promised to remove body fat. (A couple proved to be nothing more than rock salt.) There was a cream called *Hollywood's Secret Formula 199*. The instructions told the buyer to rub it into her face and watch herself grow thin.

Similar remedies were widely sold into the 1930's, when *Helen's Liquid Reducer Compound* had a flurry of popularity. The ads read: "Gargle Your Fat Away!" When a California Food and Drug inspector went to the offices of *Helen's*, he found not only huge piles of mail from buyers, but a line of drop-ins three-quarters of a block long, waiting patiently for their gargle. The compound proved to be nothing more than a dilute solution of a cheap disinfectant, hydrogen peroxide, colored red and flavored peppermint.

Nutrition was part of almost every get-well-quick scheme; an example was *Spectro-Chrome Therapy*. This marvel was invented by Colonel Dinshah Pestanji Framji Ghadiali, a native of Bombay who was born there in 1873 and migrated to the U.S. in 1911. During the first World War, Ghadiali got his colonelcy in the New York Police Reserve Air Service. He was intrigued by diets and began to preach an unseasoned vegetarian regime pretty much like that of the Grahamites. But he was also fascinated by the recent triumphs of radiation, especially those of ultraviolet. And by 1920 he had invented the *Ghadiali Spectro-Chrome Machine*. This was a fancy box with an electric light in it. The light came through a lens, and the color of the light could be changed by slipping different gels into a frame, much as one changes the color of a spotlight, to play upon the body.

By 1924, the success of the machine had paid for the building of a Spectro-Chrome Institute in Malaga, New Jersey on a 50-acre estate, marked by big signs reading, "Our Aim: Spectro-Chrome in Every Home."

You could get a membership in the Institute by paying $90. This gave you use of a machine, plus that of a companion gadget called a *Favoroscope*, which told the best time of day for using the lights. In a few years, Ghadiali sold almost a million dollars worth of memberships. And since new members also had to pay $250 for a two-week course in healing, these fees produced another $2.5

million. He also sold copies of his two books, *Spectro-Chrome Metry Encyclopedia* and *Railroading a Citizen.*

The latter work explained his five-year penitentiary sentence for violating the Mann Act.* It told how the charge was trumped up by jealous physicians. Not until 1940, however, was Ghadiali prosecuted on the basis of his medical work. Then more than 100 witnesses came to testify that Spectro-Chrome had healed them—including one who first asserted that he had been cured of epilepsy and then collapsed in an epileptic seizure. Ghadiali lost, got a suspended jail sentence and a $20,000 fine. But in the 1960's his methods were still being used and his followers were still, in response to one of his basic injunctions, sleeping with their heads pointing north.

Almost every wonder cure had an accompanying diet. And this combination made it much harder for local and Federal authorities to prosecute. Such was the case with one of the most widely accepted cures of the time, *glyoxylide,* a cancer treatment developed in 1919 by a former professor of physiology at Detroit Medical College.

Perhaps no one has explained Dr. William F. Koch's methods better than Jerome Rodale, who refers to Koch as a healer of "honor and influence," and outlines his work like this:

"This Glyoxylide was a substance . . . to convert the poisons which he believed cause cancer into antitoxins . . . He used this substance in connection with a rigid diet. Dr. Koch insisted that . . . neither diet nor Glyoxylide would be effective separately."

This last factor was important, especially after Food and Drug analyzed *glyoxylide* and found it indistinguishable from water, for thousands were being injected with the "drug." Not for more than 20 years was Koch successfully prosecuted, and then only through an injunction, obtained by the Federal Trade Commission, to make Koch stop advertising his cure. This put a dent into what government officials estimated was a $100,000-a-year business.

*The Act is concerned with transporting persons across state lines for immoral purposes.

Other prosecutions, as late as 1943 and 1946, failed—the last when Koch fled to Brazil. But *glyoxylide* appears still to be in use by some who maintain that medical tests of it failed only because the prescribed diet was not properly included. Injections were recently shown to cost from $25 to $300 each.

The old naturopathic school was still in business. For example, Bernarr Macfadden and Elbert Hubbard (one of Horace Fletcher's leading apostles) both championed the work of Dr. E.R. Moras. Wrote Hubbard: "Dr. Moras has written a commonsense book on antology [a curious system which Moras invented] and by so doing placed the Standard Creed of Health farther to the front than any man who has lived for one thousand years."

Moras, however, steadily lost credibility. There were some police problems when he insulted a woman on a train, when he tried to blackmail a prominent man for a million dollars, and when he badgered the President to help him collect $50,000 from a drug company. They put him away.

In the 1930's, Wilbur Voliva stirred interest in living mainly on Brazil nuts and buttermilk. And he was able to form a colony of believers at Zion, Illinois, who shared not only his diet but his passionate espousal of the belief that the earth was flat.

As the states began, in those years, to establish more careful licensing for professions and to define the limits of practice for various healers, a legal tradition evolved. It was a kind of medical democracy, which still persists, and which holds that when a number of people believe in a mode of treatment, they have a right to receive it. This right to a treatment of choice is an interesting question, and one not easily resolved. Legislators have, however, tended to recognize such rights, and in so doing they have provided legal credibility for many a healer with curious ideas.

Typical of such laws is a Connecticut statute which was passed in the 1930's. It defines "naturopathy." And some legislators were persuaded to vote for this and similar legislation by the argument that licensing or definition would control such practitioners and clarify their work for the public. The Connecticut law reads:

"The practice of naturopathy shall be held to mean the practice of . . . psychological sciences such as psychotherapy, the mechanical sciences, such as mechanotherapy, articular manipulation, massage, correction and orthopedic adjustments, neurotherapy, physiotherapy, hypnotherapy, electrotherapy, thermotherapy, phototherapy . . . etc., and the material sciences such as dietetics . . ." It is a broad license—possibly, as the saying goes—to steal.

With such a statute, one can imagine, it is hard to prosecute a "naturopath" for going beyond the bounds of his profession. Making it even harder is the fact that some of the defining therapies have only the fuzziest definitions themselves. Yet one can easily understand how the legislator is persuaded that the use of light or heat, a backrub or a regimen of foods is really quite harmless. The politician is a practical man. Why, he reasons, antagonize a body of voters by taking from them some "harmless" thing they want?

In the 1920's and 1930's, that body of voters who sought food remedies for health was growing larger and more vocal than ever. Many of the old "natural-healing" movements had been resurrected and were reaching large new proportions. Ironically, new life had been breathed into them by scientific discovery, the very discovery which made the ideas logically preposterous.

In 1927, Meyer E. Jaffa, then chief of California's Bureau of Food and Drugs, wrote in the Bureau's *Bulletin:* "There is probably no science which has made greater progress in the last decade than nutrition; but at the same time no science has suffered as has nutrition in the hands of the faddists and those who market commercial food and vitamin preparations, the labels of which savor a repetition of the patent medicine propaganda."

In the 1920's, it was estimated that the American public was spending some 70 percent of its medical dollars on patent medicines, foods and dietary supplements. Food and Drug historian August Glaive writes of this twenties' trend:

"Eminent scientists and physicians were reporting their findings on nutrition in our scientific journals. This opened wonderful new vistas for the health fad boys. Vitamins in pill form and as yeast cake promised to cure most of the common ailments. The fact that many of the statements in their literature or on the label of their products were wild distortions of sober scientific findings did not seem to bother them at all.

"A few began to grow fat financially. These got out of the retail business and went into manufacturing . . . This proved so remunerative that they could afford tons of literature . . ."

Let us look at what was in that literature. For much of it is little changed today.

13

Eating for
the Hull of It

In 1898, the giant American Sugar Refining Company, which had been formed only the year before, began an ad campaign for its white sugar. The ad featured a photo of "A Disgusting Insect," which was said to have been found by an analyst in Dublin, in a package of brown sugar.

Magnified 220 times, the insect was not attractive. "It is a formidably organized, exceedingly lively and decidedly ugly little animal . . ." read the copy. "The number of these creatures found in raw sugar is exceedingly great and in no instance is raw sugar quite free from either the insects or their eggs. Brown sugar should never be used . . ."

The ad was convincing to many readers, but to foodists it appeared to be one more instance of robbing food of its value by processing. From the time Sylvester Graham had begun his cry of

"Put back the bran!" wheat had been the chief cause of such fears. But beginning shortly after the Civil War, white sugar also became an object of fear and suspicion. Many felt certain that the refiners were duping Americans into eating a less nutritive, as well as paler, product.

In truth, except for a brief period at the turn of the century, there was little promotion of white sugar. There seems to have been no need. In Civil War days, white sugar, because of refining expense, had cost 10 cents a pound extra, a great deal in those times. But by 1876, as processing methods improved, all sugar was cheaper, and the difference between brown and white dropped to three cents a pound. One might have expected the nation to take advantage of the bargain in brown sugar, but in fact, Americans began to buy less total sugar but more white. When American Sugar Refining reduced the price difference to a mere penny a pound, brown sugar began to go out of fashion.

Actually, consumers had long preferred white sugar. American plantation sugar, grown and refined in the south, was almost exclusively brown, and its quality and sweetness in cooking were undependable. So recipe books of America's early years always called for white sugar for more delicate dishes. It was imported and sold in 10-pound cones, and the best families all had sugar shears for cutting off what was needed.

There was certainly no health consideration in the making of different sugar grades. Essentially, sugar is made by boiling a crude extract from the cane (botanically, a grass, which was first cultivated in the State of Bihar, in India's Ganges Valley) and then letting this boiled extract crystallize. The first batch was the premium product, light brown. What was left was boiled and crystallized over and over again. The syrup left behind after the last boiling, the fourth or fifth, was blackstrap molasses, the least sweet and most impure product.

But as the 20th century dawned, suspicion arose about any refinement, whether of flour or sugar. As Gayelord Hauser still puts it: "The unprocessed, unrefined raw sugar, whether it is extracted from sugar cane or beets, is by far the most desirable to use . . ."

Despite scientific headshaking, one finds "raw" sugar—the somewhat less purified product—valued for health and sold at ironically high prices in health-food stores. This is despite the fact that, as the Council on Foods and Nutrition has pointed out, "The small quantity of vitamins and minerals available in partially refined sugar is of little, if any, nutritional significance."

In 1972, the myths of "raw" sugar were rejected by the government, when the Federal Trade Commission obtained a consent order in its case against Cumberland Packing Corporation, which made *Sugar in the Raw.* Among other things, the FTC had objected to representations that the product was a significant source of vitamins or minerals, or significantly superior in any nutritional way to ordinary white sugar.

Sales figures show that in 1898 most Americans were not put off by the efforts of American Refining to sell a whiter product. And indeed, the case was the same for flour. For while Sylvester Graham and his many followers caught the public attention, they did not seem to have great influence on most people's buying habits. Removing some bran made a more palatable bread for most tastes.

Until the Civil War, a great turning point for food processing, the American wheat was a soft winter wheat. It was easily ground between stones. Then it was "bolted" through a soft cloth to sieve out some of the bigger particles of bran—the process which Graham felt was against God's purpose.

But with the War between the States, there were many changes. A number of processes came into broader use, some of which had lain relatively dormant for generations. For example, early enough in the 1800's so that he could be decorated and rewarded by Napoleon, Nicholas Appert had discovered how to can foods with hermetical sealing. His theory was entirely wrong, but his process was right; putting food in jars, heating it to destroy bacteria, then sealing the jars to keep new bacteria out, Appert had created canning. By 1819 the process was being used in New York in a limited way. By 1825 there was a patent on a method for coating steel with tin to make cans for food preservation. By 1856, Gail Borden had perfected his process of condensing milk.

None of these processes was much used until the Civil War, with its long supply lines, brought new challenges for food preservation. Soon most of the fruit that went to the Union Army was being canned in California. Borden's condensation-and-canning process was being used not only for milk, but also for California blackberry juice.

Perhaps most important of all, the new lands of the Great Plains, with their harsh heat of summer and bitter freezes of winter, were becoming a new bread basket. Scandinavian and German emigrées moved into the virgin lands of Wisconsin, Minnesota, the Dakotas and Iowa. With them came a new, tough wheat, the hard spring wheat.

It was, and is, good wheat. But when the millers began to grind and bolt it, they found that much of the gluten, the primary food core of the wheat, stuck to the bran. When they followed their usual method of removing the hull of the wheat, a wasteful portion of the gluten went with it.

To leave the bran in the flour meant creating a product that only a Graham or an Alcott would buy: dark, coarse in texture, and hard to chew. Not surprisingly, the public rejected it.

The first solution to the problem was the "middlings purifier." *Middlings* is another term for the heart of the wheat—the gluten and the little kernel which is best known as wheat germ. In 1871, the Washburn Mill in Minneapolis installed a purifier in which a blast of air blew away the bran, so that the middlings were left for making flour.

In this process, quite a lot of the usable wheat was still lost, as it stuck to the bran. Moreover, since the germ was oily, flour made with it soon tended to develop an off flavor, for the oil soon became rancid. Bakers, who had no choice but to buy flour in quantity, ran the risk of waste.

The primary solution was the Hungarian Mill, or highmilling machine. It had six or seven sets of porcelain and chilled steel rollers, through which the wheat passed in turn. The first rollers cracked the kernel, releasing the germ and its oil. Other rollers took out the rest of the middlings. At once, the old war about wheat began anew.

Remember that Sylvester Graham, James Caleb Jackson and all the rest had never really known any reason to keep more bran in bread. They merely said it was "unnatural" to take any out. Dr. Kellogg's protests, which began about the time that the new wheat and the new milling methods arrived, were based on his belief in "auto-intoxication," which called for bran to "sweep out" the intestines and clear away their "toxins."

But as soon as Casimir Funk saved his pigeons from death with grain-mill sweepings, lights flashed and bands played in the minds of the worried. It had taken a century, but they were vindicated. The stuff they had feared to lose in whiter, more chewable bread was the *vita-amine*.

In the rush of vitamin and mineral discoveries which followed, the food extremists found a scientific argument, which they have pressed ever since. But along with the justification came an error of distortion,which also persists.

The reasoning goes something like this: Funk's pigeons—like other human and animal groups overly dependent on processed grain, such as Eijkman's beri-beri sufferers in Indonesia—sickened and died. When the hull of the grain, or an extract of it, was put into their diets, they were healed. Therefore, the hull was seen as the life-giving factor. The heart of the grain was seen as almost worthless. This reasoning is akin to thinking that, because a bad sparkplug is the cause of an auto breakdown, the rest of the car is useless, and one should use sparkplugs for transportation.

In a recent Federal study, some two-thirds of Americans believed that vitamins and minerals furnished energy to the body. This is not true. Our food energy comes from only four important sources—protein, carbohydrates, fat and alcohol. Yet *Prevention* magazine, not long ago, featured a letter from a reader who said she fed her child a breakfast of pure water and vitamins and minerals. The fact is that vitamins and minerals are important—they enable us to put the macronutrients (the sources of energy and building materials, such as protein) to work. But by themselves, without the macronutrients, they have little value.

We should keep in mind that foods vary in nutritional importance according to how much we consume and how often. If we eat cranberry sauce only once a year, on Thanksgiving, its nutritive value is not especially meaningful to our health. Our concern should be proportionate to the overall nutritional importance of the particular food.

For example, when the loss of nutrients from the milling of wheat first became a matter of interest, Americans were eating a great deal of bread. English sources estimate that in the middle of the 19th century, the typical Englishman ate perhaps a pound to a pound and a half of bread a day. So far as we know, these figures are probably true also for Americans of the time. Because it made up so large a part of the dietary, any major nutrient loss from wheat was critical.

Today Americans eat *per capita* only some one to four slices of bread a day, and consume just a little more than a third of a pound of cereal grains in *all* forms—bread, crackers, cakes, breakfast cereals, etc. When vitamins were first discovered, Americans were still eating somewhat more of cereal grains, but the trend toward lowered consumption was well under way. Our current dietary was taking shape, so the burden of supplying some vitamins and minerals was being transferred from wheat to other foods.

As one example, between 1952 and 1972, American *per capita* consumption of beef increased more than 80 percent. Chicken consumption increased even more. Both these meats supply some of the important vitamins and minerals found in wheat, though certainly not all.

The new "scientific" emphasis in foodism produced a boom in the selling of foods and supplements to provide the miraculous new vitamins and minerals. It brought a new breed of promoters to pave the way. Alfred Watterson McCann was typical.

Born in 1879, McCann was convinced that special diets had saved his life in childhood. The son of a Pennsylvania printer and engraver, he was fascinated by the printed word. At the College of the Holy Ghost, in Pittsburgh, his main interest was literature, and he showed a flair for journalism. Upon his graduation in 1899, he stayed on at the school, now known as Duquesne, as an English instructor.

Gradually, McCann began to supplement his income by writing ad copy for food companies, such as Francis Leggett and Company. It was the era when much food advertising was in the vein of the Battle Creek cereal kings. McCann refined the art, developing a style which combined short, punchy sentences and nutrition salesmanship.

The announcement of the vitamin discovery in 1912 fired McCann's imagination. He, like so many other foodists, suddenly had a vision of a depleted food supply from which nutrients were being stolen. When Harvey Wiley resigned from the Food and Drug Administration, McCann was suddenly fired into action. He wrote a hotly indignant article, "The Pure Food Movement," and the then-widely-read *New York Globe* gave it a full page on October 24, 1912.

The piece built readership, and soon McCann was in New York, writing series after series indicting various foods and the industry which produced them. In a day of wild, yellow journalism, McCann's work stood out for its sensationalism. His ability to snare readers is testified to by the fact that the *Globe* supplied him with a little lab and someone to perform tests of a crude sort. This let him refer to "work done in my laboratory." The *Globe* also retained a team of lawyers to defend the many libel and defamation suits which McCann brought to the paper. He spent much of the next 10 years in court. He also became the first important foodist to use the new medium of radio.

As one biographer characterizes his work: "He was able to arouse public interest by his bitter personalities, his unearthing of startling news, and by his torrent of catchy phrases."

In 1914, McCann summed up his thinking in the title of his first book, *Starving America*. Then he went on to the role, not merely of the food-consumerist, but of the dietetic expert.

In 1917, a revised edition of his book appeared under a new title, *The Science of Eating*. In this book, he asks the question, "Is there any evidence that God has prescribed a formula for the nourishment of the human family?" As old as this question is, the answer took on a new flavor. "The physician who follows these pages," he wrote in a nice ploy which suggested that he was the sort of authority whose work would be read by physicians, "will come into possession of facts not to be obtained in the medical schools of Europe or America. He will receive new information with regard to many of the causes of malnutrition, anemia, neurasthenia, edema, Bright's Disease, diabetes, cancer, hardening of the arteries, tuberculosis, and other preventable diseases . . ."

He advances two main premises. The first trades upon the new fascination with micronutrients. One can perceive the theme in such chapter titles as "Watery Tissues of the Hog," "Pasty Complexions of the Human," and "Rejected Food Minerals, a Mountain of Folly." He is saying that the food supply cannot support good health. He is saying that the path of Nature marks out methods of food choice and preparation for us, and that McCann knows her intent.

The second premise is a little hard to follow. But it is the forerunner of the current belief that industry turns food into disease-producing substances. For example, he says that when flour is bleached, it becomes a cause of cancer and heart disease.

To clarify McCann's style and thinking, and their effects upon his many successors, let us share a high point of his life. It is April 11, 1915. Big news in the U.S. is the docking of the *Kronprinz Wilhelm* at Newport News, Virginia. A German passenger vessel which had been converted into a cruiser with hidden guns, she has roamed the Atlantic, surprising and sinking 14 British and French merchantmen.

The U.S. then being neutral, the *Wilhelm* asked and got permission to come into port. 100 of her 500 men were seriously ill. The ship's doctor called the illness beri-beri. American doctors agreed that the men were ill, but disputed the diagnosis.

"I had been ordered to keep off," says the then 36-year-old McCann. "I had appealed to Washington in vain . . . I had tried all the prominent physicians of Newport News, the Collector of Customs, the politicians . . . Journalists were barred from that ship."

Having heard the symptoms, McCann is sure he knows how to cure the illness. But for some reason, the medical men are reluctant to ask for consultation from the famous copywriter and columnist. "Scientific bigotry and narrow ethics were keeping me out," he complains. "I was not a member of the inner circle . . . yet I had given more study to the cause of malnutrition and had addressed more physicians on that one subject than perhaps any man in America."

The latter claim is doubtful, since McCann had left Duquesne's English department less than three years before. Dauntless, he rushed to the scene anyway, bribed some people and tried to get on the ship disguised as a messenger for a local ship's chandler. They caught him and dumped him ashore.

Unrelenting, McCann now found in his wallet the calling card of a noted New York physician. He hired a power boat, stood up at the stern and ordered a course for the *Kronprinz Wilhelm.* McCann describes the short trip with great drama, as though at any moment the cruiser's guns might be brought to bear. (Odd, since they had not heard his theories.) Alongside, he sends his card to the ship's physician and is summoned aboard. But no sooner does he reach the officers' mess than one of eight doctors who are seated at a round table bursts out, "Why, here is McCann of the *New York Globe!*"

Talking fast, McCann says that the illness which troubles the crewmen is rampant in the U.S. "No man interrupted me," he reports. "I was as shocked at their silence as they were at my impertinence, so I kept on and reminded them of many of the neglected truths of the diseases of dietetic origin."

It is refined food which has laid low the seamen, explains McCann. They are poisoned. "After a diet of refined food," he tells them, "a mild chronic acidosis is set up which abstracts lime salts from the fibrous tissues, muscles, nerves, cartilages and bones . . . the loss of lime salts causes irritability and weakness of the muscles . . . continued loss of lime salts causes effusion into the joints . . . abstraction of lime salts is a cause of the rapid progress of tuberculosis."

This is utter physiologic nonsense—so confused and without foundation that it cannot even be explained as error. However, it is worth defining the term "acidosis," since it is used here as a popular faddist idea of the time and since many faddists (McCann included) used the term wrongly then and still do.

Acidosis refers to a disruption of the acid-base balance of the body. And while it denotes an excessively acid condition, as one medical dictionary explains, "The blood is never acid except in extreme pathological conditions."

Such extremity is not the result of eating things which taste acid, such as vinegar and lemonade. The body deals nicely and easily with the mild acids in foods. In fact, contrary to what many people believe, as Dr. Fredrick Stare points out, "Even such noticeably acidic fruits as lemons actually are base forming in the body because, after the metabolic breakdown . . . an alkaline residue of sodium and potassium remains."

As the reader may suspect, the acidity of the blood is a most subtle matter. And it is a condition that only a relative few need worry about. For example, acidosis is a threat to the diabetic. He cannot use carbohydrates efficiently. So he may use proteins and fats as his main energy sources. When he does this, there are certain acid waste products left, such as *ketones*. (These we shall see, help to make low-carbohydrate diets inadvisable.) The blood can become flooded with acid wastes, compromising normal body function and for example, causing the kidneys to labor hard to clear the blood.

Many foodists, however, have long imagined that the acidity or alkalinity of ordinary diets can make their bodies unusually acid or alkaline. They plan their food intake accordingly, but to no real purpose.

What really had happened to the sailors, we cannot say. However, it does appear that, cruising for months away from port, they may have been fed largely on bread and meat. That old enemy of the sea voyager, scurvy, caused by lack of vitamin C from fruits and vegetables, may have been at work here. On such a diet, the sailors may also have suffered some deficiency of certain B vitamins. McCann does note that such fruits and vegetables as there were went only to the officers' mess.

McCann proceeded to recommend an elaborate dietary pattern on the basis of a complex analysis of the problem. For example, he said that the sailors' fruit juices, "contaminated to some extent with salts of tin and sheet iron, acted possibly as an irritant to the kidneys, already taxed beyond their capacity with excess quantities of high protein and refined carbohydrate foods

. . . The condition of acidosis imposes a tremendous handicap upon pregnancy and lactation." (Never mind the odds against any of the *Wilhelm's* sailors being pregnant or nursing.)

McCann also believed that the stricken men might be suffering from other illness, since he maintained that, "Acidosis predisposes to measles, tuberculosis, pneumonia, appendicitis, meningitis, constipation and cancer." Fearing that all or any of these conditions might have taken hold, McCann gave the ship's doctor "a formula to replace lost salts."

"Soak one hundred pounds of bran in two hundred pounds of water for twelve hours, and give each man eight ounces in the morning. Give each man one teaspoon of wheat bran, morning and night, until contraindicated by loose stools.

Boil cabbage, carrots, parsnips, spinach, etc., and drain off the liquor. Feed with whole wheat bread. Wash and peel potatoes. Discard potatoes. Retain skins." (Jack La Lanne, we see, did not speak without precedent.) "Boil skins and give liquor to men, four ounces a day. Give them egg yolks and milk . . . one ounce fresh roast beef, for the psychological effect upon the men who have been taught to believe that without meat they cannot live."

McCann also added citrus juice, apples and apple sauce. As he saw it, on "April 16th, the men began to be saturated with soluble alkalines of vegetable origin to neutralise as quickly as possible the acidity . . . and the toxins poisoning them."

To the sickest of the sailors, McCann said, "You know you owe this to white bread and meat."

"Yes . . ." the poor man said, "we all owe it to white bread and meat, but there will be no more such food in the German Navy when they know what happened. . ."

McCann laments bitterly that neither Americans nor Germans learned from this incident the deadliness of refined food and meat. "God's laws," he says, "so easily discerned, remain ignored." In his books, he seeks solace from the fact that other great men of nutrition have not been heeded—above all "Sylvester Graham, M.D."

In truth, however, many were persuaded by McCann, including some who were not new to the theories. Typical of the pioneers was Dr. William Howard Hay, who graduated from the medical school of the University of the City of New York in 1891. In 1907, his health began to break down, and he sought to know why. He diagnosed himself as a victim of Bright's disease, high blood pressure and "dilated heart."

As Hay writes of himself in the third person, "He began to eat . . . only such things as he believed were intended by nature as foods for man, taking these in their natural form and in quantities no greater than seemed to be necessary." When he wrote his magnum opus, *How to Always . . . Be Well,* a book which on the surface can be criticized only for its split infinitive, he closed it with a chapter called *My Sacred Mission.*

What was this mission? It seems, like so much of what has gone before and what is advocated now, to be a hodge-podge of familiar ideas. For example, Dr. Hay points out that, "Cases fed à la Horace Fletcher, chewing all their carbohydrates till these disappeared and were swallowed involuntarily, developed more power and less fatigue on one-third or less of the intake of those who did not . . . and at the same time lived without the accompanying disease."

But above all, Hay believed that one must be terribly careful about how to *combine* one's foods. For example, he writes, "Any carbohydrate foods . . . require alkaline conditions for their complete digestion, so must not be combined with acids of any kind, as sour fruits, because the acid will neutralize . . . Neither should these be combined with a protein of concentrated sort . . . as these protein foods will excite too much hydrochloric acid during their stomach digestion." His most important principle was the idea that, "One can still wreck nutrition by . . . neglecting to observe . . . the correct chemical combination of the foods eaten." It is not hard to see where some of McCann's acid-alkaline notions came from.

Hay provides an elaborate system for combining foods. Typical of the system's science is the idea that "Milk is not good with either the starches or the proteins." In fact, an eight-ounce glass of milk already contains some nine grams of protein, some 20 percent of a typical woman's daily need.

Hay concludes that, for the worker, breakfast should consist of bread with butter or honey, coffee, and a dish of soaked dates, figs or raisins. Breakfast for the sedentary person can omit the bread. At any meal, if the wrong combinations are used, one will suffer not only from acidosis, but also from "insufficient drainage." Acidosis, he also warned, could come from keeping digesting food in the bowels for more than 24 hours.

Eventually, by the 1930's, Dr. Hay opened a sanitarium called *Hay-ven* in the Poconos of Pennsylvania. There the patient could try such recipes as *Pale Moon Cocktail* or *Hay's Happy Highball*, made without alcohol. He could assay *Easter Bunny Salad* or *Fountain of Youth Salad*. And following this he could have a succulent main dish—perhaps Dr. Hay's *Parcel Post Asparagus* with his *Startled Chicken*.

The object was to avoid mixing protein and carbohydrate at the same meal—rather difficult if one uses food-composition tables, which show us that virtually all of our foods have some protein, carbohydrate and fat in combination. Indeed, the modern medical idea about combining foods is simple: "Any two foods which may be eaten separately may be eaten together." The axiom includes alcoholic beverage.

So popular were the combining rules of Hay and others in the 1920's and 1930's, however, that they were seriously tested in a study of 200 people who were ill, together with a large group of normals. When the foods were separated as Hay prescribed, no improvement in health was seen. When hamburger and potato were dangerously combined, the well did not become sick. The investigator, Dr. Martin Rehfuss of Philadelphia, could find no significant differences among the test groups which could be attributed to diet.

McCann went on writing. He published *Thirty Cent Bread,* which among other things attacked canning and advocated killing all cattle to make grain cheaper. In 1918 he wrote *This Famishing World*. His publisher advertised that his writings were, "compelling, mortifying, vengeful blows that smash the easy plausibility . . . stripping the . . . display of scholarship to the bone."

Was he taken seriously? In 1922, Fordham University awarded him an honorary doctorate of law. Now "*Dr.* McCann," he was more believable than ever. In 1923, he moved to the *New*

York Evening Mail and opened his own Alfred W. McCann Laboratories. There, for a suitable fee, a manufacturer could have his product studied "impartially." Amazingly, no product analyzed was found to be harmful, and the Laboratory endorsed everything from cigars to chicken though McCann approved of neither tobacco nor meat of any kind. However, lots of food which the Lab was not paid to analyze proved dangerous indeed.

He also invented "kidneycide," which described what happened to you if you ate anything except what he recommended: you ended up in a state of "acidosis." He decided that if one consumed 80 grams of protein a day, one was in danger of acidosis. (Today, it appears that even deprived Americans eat as much and more.) McCann wrote, "When we eat the flesh of an animal we eat the end-products of the animal's life processes . . . the animal sweat, dead cells, toxic waste . . . Meat tends toward excessive intestinal putrefaction . . ."

He found unusual sources for documentation; for example, he wrote that, "Most of the kidneycides of America have never heard of Anthony Bassler or the *American Journal of Electrotherapeutics and Radiology.*" He was probably correct.

More and more, McCann was heard on the radio, which was fast becoming a feature of every American home. His highest drama on his broadcasts dealt with the heart. Heart attacks, he warned, were nothing more than the result of prolonged acidosis. That acidosis could be avoided.

Give up meat, he urged. Abandon the deadly trap of refined sugar, which produced the heart-killing acid blood. Do you not fear, he asked, the toll of leaking lime salts which must result? Will you wait until acidosis strikes you dead?

In 1931, McCann was making one of his usual hour-long broadcasts, reiterating the usual themes, warning that only his truth could stop the slaughter of the heart. He had no sooner gone off the air when suddenly he slumped forward in his chair.

He was dead at 52. Much of his fame died with him. Yet today the *American Dictionary of Biography* still remembers Alfred Watterson McCann as a "pure food crusader."

14

The Drinks Are
on the Hauser

As word got around, crowds began to form in the sacred corner of
Paris, crowds large enough so that *Figaro* felt obligated to report
the incident the next day. It was true. *Maxim's*—not the best
French restaurant perhaps, but probably the longest standing
symbol of Gallic *haute cuisine*—was festooned with vegetables, a
strange and astonishingly gaudy display for what had always been
a conservative establishment.

But even more shocking than the salad facade was what went
on inside. There was a lavish private party, and its main feature
was a vegetable-juice bar. A "Hauser Bar" it was called, for the
party was in honor of Gayelord Hauser, perhaps history's most
influential exponent of liquid nutrition.

"Ca c'est fou!" (That is crazy!) Hauser himself reports the
curious French as saying. "But," he adds, "it was no crazier than I
am."

Born in 1895—the year Daniel Palmer founded his school of chiropractic, a time when the first cereal flake ads were appearing, when Horace Fletcher was learning to chew, when Macfadden's *Physical Culture* was still just an idea—Hauser survives at this writing, as a link between that dim, pre-vitamin day and our own. A tall (six feet, four inches), lean (he goes on a laxative-and-liquid regimen whenever his weight rises to 205 pounds) and handsome man, Hauser is not only the creator of a number of food-and-health ideas, but also an extraordinary popularizer of them. For he enlisted to his support the celebrities of the Western world.

What John Harvey Kellogg accomplished by turning The San at Battle Creek into a fashionable spa, Hauser did with little more than his charm. For example, he recalls one of his lectures, arranged in Paris by Lady Elsie Mendl at her Avenue d'Iena salon, at which the audience consisted solely of the Duchess of Windsor, Lady Duff Cooper, Princess Aspasia of Greece, Princess Karputhala of India, Lady Cavendish (Fred Astaire's sister and original dancing partner), Lady Carnarvon, Madame de Saint Hardouin (once the French Ambassadress to Istanbul), Madame Dubonnet (whose family's *apéritifs* are so widely drunk) and one or two others. When the journals of fashion and society reported on these and similar ladies, they also dutifully reported their use of Hauser secrets of youth and beauty.

For lesser folk (and bigger newsstand circulation) any number of 1930's movie stars served the purpose—from comedienne Billie Burke to Greta Garbo, whose curious vegetable-laden diet habits were learned mainly under Hauser's tutelage. Perhaps more than anyone else, Hauser built the popular link between special foods and beauty. In New York, Dorothy Gray hired one of Hauser's assistants to open a "beauty bar." Helena Rubenstein initiated a "food for beauty" restaurant. Ann Delafield used Hauser methods to set up her Success School at Richard Hudnut's New York salon, and later directed the Main Chance Farms of Elizabeth Arden (among the most costly and famed of the so-called "fat farms"). While Hauser—at this writing 81 years old—is not today so well known, his ideas are fundamental still in both the health-food and fashion worlds.

His beginnings were not so auspicious. Born Eugen Ben-

jamin Gellert Hauser, he came to America in 1911, the year
Casimir Funk's pigeons got well. At once he entered a hospital in
Chicago; he had tuberculosis of the hip. "A boy lay dying . . ."
Hauser begins his *Treasury of Secrets.* "Send this boy home," he
quotes the doctors. "There is nothing more we can do for him."

"So," writes Hauser, "the unhappy boy was sent back home
to die in the Swiss mountains. There a miracle happened."

The miracle came in the form of an old missionary, who told
young Eugen Benjamin, "If you keep on eating dead foods, you
certainly will die. Only living foods can make a living body."

"Living foods" is a term still much used. Its meaning is
obscure, but it is usually in a context which suggests that foods
which have been cooked or processed have been "killed." Young
Hauser followed the old missionary's vague advice, lived and
renounced orthodox medicine for "natural" healing.

"Once I got on my feet I decided to make nutrition my life's
work," says Hauser. "It was an arduous task 60 years ago (he is
writing in 1973) because there were no nutrition schools then.
However, after World War I, I was. . . able to visit those clinics
devoted to diet therapy."

Hauser's exact training is not clear. He maintains, "I am a
doctor, not of medicine, but of natural science. I have taken my
inspiration from the teachings of Hippocrates . . . Father
Kneipp, Hindhede [a vegetarian author of the 19th century who
was often quoted by Dr. Kellogg], Bircher-Benner* and other
great teachers. . . ."

Other than getting up at 6 A.M. to hear Bircher-Benner's
lectures—the only time of day when the good doctor imparted his
findings—Hauser seems to have learned a European variety of
chiropractic manipulation which is sometimes known as *naprapathy.* For a time, Hauser also learned from Sir Arbuthnot Lane
(remember *Lane's Kink* and the wholesale surgery to remove
sections of the intestine in which putrefaction was causing disease?), ". . . under whose auspices I lectured in England." Hauser

---

*Dr. Max Bircher-Benner, proprietor of a Zurich sanitorium where
patients received the *Frisch Kost* ("fresh food") diet of vegetables, juices, milk
and *Muesli,* a mixture of grain and dried fruit which is probably the first version of
the modern granola.

especially endorses Lane's New Health Society, which taught Englishmen to avoid sweets and starches and get more protein—a confusing injunction when one thinks of Lane's vision of meat-putrefaction as the cause of so much disease. But then, consistency is not always the hallmark of foodism.

In 1922, at age 27, Hauser returned to Chicago and opened an office. At one point, this office appears to have been a place for *naprapathic* manipulation and massage. Later, in the 1950's, however, he refers to this as "my first food clinic," and in 1973, he says that he "began with a dietetic school in Chicago."

One of Hauser's mentors was Benedict Lust, who through a long career established treatment centers in Switzerland, then in Butler, New Jersey, and in Tangerine, Florida. Lust applied a number of theories, but perhaps most significant were *Nahrungswissenschaft* (which might be translated as "food science") and *Zone Therapy.* On the surface, Lust's ideas look traditional enough. "The *natural* system for curing disease," he writes, ". . . is based on a return to Nature in regulating the diet, breathing, exercising, bathing and the employment of various other *natural* forces to eliminate the poisonous substances in the system. . . ."

In practice, however, Lust was a big user of "health cocktails," mainly made of vegetable juices. The editor and publisher of *Nature's Path* magazine explains, "There is something more behind these health, raw juice cocktails than simply satisfying the palate . . . When people form the health cocktail habit, they put liquid life into their bodies."*

A confidant of Bernarr Macfadden, Lust was also an advertiser in *Physical Culture,* and wrote a book on *Zone Therapy.* This was a system invented by two Connecticut physicians, Drs. William H. Fitzgerald and Edwin F. Bowers. It was introduced (and heartily endorsed) by *Everybody's Magazine,* the editor of which was Bruce Barton, the second "B" in advertising's famous B.B.D. & O.

---

*John Lust, editor of *Nature's Path* magazine, reports this in *Drink Your Troubles Away,* a book much used in health-food stores to help sell juices and juicers.

According to Lust, the human body is divided into sections. And if one pushed on the appropriate part, one could clear up trouble in a related section. Fingers and toes were especially good places to push. To cure a goiter, for example, one had only to press on the first and second fingers. "One of the most effective means of treating partial deafness," we are told, "is to clamp a spring clothes pin on the tip of the third finger, on the side involved in the ear trouble."

In childbirth, Lust advises pushing metal combs against the backs of the mother's hands. Also, he says that, "Rubber bands around the great toe and the second toe afford a gratifying help." (Dr. LaMaze, of natural childbirth fame, has apparently not read this work.)

To stop falling hair, one rubs one's fingernails together. Mouth pressure is a very fine technique for dealing with headaches and menstrual difficulties, and Bowers and Fitzgerald report that in "several hundred cases of whooping cough, we have not yet seen a failure." Their treatment was pressing for five minutes at the back of the throat.

There is current interest in what is now called—especially by devotees of such Oriental eating systems as *macrobiotics*— "acupressure." It seems to be remarkably like Zone Therapy. Of "acupressure," we may say that there is one real reason for momentary effectiveness; it is hard for the mind to perceive two sensations at once with clarity. This is why the movie cowboy bites on the bullet when in pain. It is why meaningless "white noise" played through earphones has seemed to relieve pain for dental patients. Beyond this, there is no medical rationale.

We now have some idea of the broad reaches of Gayelord Hauser's education. "People," he writes, ". . . came to me as a last resort. Many were skeptical about 'food science,' as I then called it. I had to work fast to convince them. . . ."

In response to this burden, Hauser invented his "Seven-Day Elimination Diet." (Sometimes he refers to this as a "Seven-Day Housecleaning.") Since this diet is believed by Hauser to be his best-known, it may be worth considering in some detail—also because it helps us to understand what it was that so many of the rich, titled and cinematically-revered were getting from Hauser.

Breakfast is a glass of fruit juice and a cup or two of herb tea. At midmorning, "if you want something more substantial," you can have some yogurt and a few bits of carrot, green pepper, cauliflower and celery. For lunch there is *Hot Hauser Broth* (a brew of cabbage, celery, parsley and carrot in water, with a little tomato juice and honey), but just a cup. Then there is a little yogurt, a little salad, and hot tea with lemon. Mid-afternoon permits you some fruit or vegetable juice. Dinner provides more *Hauser Broth,* some vegetable and salad and another cup of herb tea. Finally you may go off to bed with some nice herbal laxative and even, if you are hungry for some reason, a little juice.

Hauser described this diet as "a feast." The procedure gives the body a chance to clean itself up inside and to heal itself. Won't you be hungry? Hauser doesn't think so. He and his students do this for seven days, twice a year, and they are not hungry, he assures us.

In fact, he cites an even stricter regimen which does not provoke hunger—the one he encountered on his own visit to a modern German "fasting" sanitarium, Dr. Buchinger's place at Überlingen. With 150 rooms, every one was occupied at the time (one of them by the circus' John Ringling North).

The head physician started Hauser off with a "fruit day," which meant that he could eat two pounds of fruit. Next day the nurse appeared in the morning with a pitcher of *Bitter-Wasser* (bitter water), "a terrible tasting laxative drink," of which he was compelled to drink "every drop." Knowing that this was "a terrific laxative. . . I stayed close to my room."

The rest of the day's food consisted of a morning cup of mint tea, a lunch cup of clear vegetable broth, an afternoon cup of herb tea with honey and an evening glass of fruit juice. Hauser insists that he never felt hungry. But he does say that author Ludwig Bemmelmans tried the sanitarium and quickly checked out.

Hauser's housecleaning diet brought him so much trade that he soon had to hire ten assistants. Soon he was on a regular lecture schedule, had a syndicated newspaper column (King Features Syndicate) and had begun the first of the books which eventually would be translated into 27 languages.

Many Chicago physicians were not much pleased by Gayelord's rapid success. The late Dr. Morris Fishbein, then editor of the *Journal of the American Medical Association*, looked into Hauser's writings and commented in his book, *Your Diet and Your Health*: "He has a system of diet which he sells to people who are interested in remarkable systems of eating, and he also sells what he calls the 'zigzag' system for weight reduction. In this system most of the reduction is brought about by driving the body to rapid elimination*, using various salts and cathartics. He also has some of the salts for sale and their names are such that they must be bought in the form in which he sells them, rather than in any of the common forms in which they are generally available in drugstores."

(At one time, Hauser did appear to have an interest in a firm which made health products. He sometimes sold these with and through his lectures and books. However, in the 1930's, as we shall see, new Federal laws extended the definition of "labels" to include written materials which traveled, interstate, with products. In recent years, Hauser has been careful not to recommend specific brands very much.** In fact, his *Treasury of Secrets* carries the disclaimer: "This book was not written or published as a labeling device for any product endorsed by Gayelord Hauser. Any attempt by a manufacturer, retailer, or salesman to use this book in conjunction with the sale of any product whatsoever shall be considered against the wishes of both author and publisher.")

Some Hauser observers have cynically accused the healer—whose formal schooling appears to have been, in this country, at the Chicago College of Naprapathy—of name-dropping. In fact, he is conservative about the use of his clients' names.

In 1927, he prepared a talk about beauty through diet and began to lecture in Hollywood. Soon he met Garbo, through conductor Leopold Stokowski. She was already following a strict

*In fairness, it should be said that Hauser's latest reducing plans do not now include laxatives, although he does mention them in connection with his own and others' weight-reducing efforts.

**In 1934, FDA acted against Modern Health Products (Carl Hauser, president). In 1937 FDA seized three of the Modern Health Products—sold under false claims.

diet, mainly of boiled vegetables. Her visage was notoriously sad at the time, her mien remote. Hauser diagnosed her as "suffering from overtiredness and insomnia." He lectured her on her folly and "coaxed her back to intelligent eating . . . I insisted on a balanced diet."

Soon, in her solitary dressing room, he exults, she was eating vegetables, but *raw*. And she had begun to include in her bowl of what the French call *crudités*, "bits of ham, chicken, cottage cheese and wheat germ."

The result? Soon Garbo made her classic *Ninotchka*. The publicity featured the line, "Garbo laughs!" And Hauser won congratulations.

Gayelord was soon circulating widely in Hollywood. He was given the task "to sustain the gorgeousness of twelve showgirls" in a film called *The All-American Coed*. At mid-afternoon they were drooping. He set up for them what was called "the first beauty bar in Hollywood." They drank such things as orange juice with raw egg yolk and Hauser's "Hi-Vi booster," tomato juice with celery-flavored yeast and lemon juice. Again his stock rose, enough so that he could order the cameras stopped while everyone took what might be called a "Hauser break."

He got national attention. And few people welcomed the bubble-bursting of such as Dr. Fishbein, who wrote, to little avail: "Mr. Hauser is convinced apparently that appendicitis can be cured by diets or starvation, and the most dangerous advice he gives is to take some of his laxatives . . . when suffering from appendicitis . . .

"Hauser also goes so far as to recommend eating onions as a cure for cancer, and he says that deafness can be cured by taking some of his system of elimination. His whole system of diet is based on misconceptions and fallacies. . . ."

As his reputation grew he gained access to a number of famed healers. For example, he exhibits special pride in the comments of Dr. William Howard Hay—whom we will remember as the proprietor of *Hay-ven*, the physician who taught Americans to fear certain combinations of food. As Gayelord reports Hay's opinions: "Hauser . . . I like your gospel of 'living foods.' If people were given natural foods, their appetites would be natural; they would not constantly overeat . . . Never weaken in your conviction that natural food is best for man's health and happiness."

Clearly, Hauser is proud to show us that he belongs to a great tradition of food and healing.

Some special quality made Gayelord Hauser stand out. Ceaselessly, he changed, improved. In 1951, at the age of 56, he was as polished and handsome as ever. In that year he wrote perhaps his most powerful book, *Look Younger, Live Longer.* It is this book which is usually credited with starting the passion for blackstrap molasses.

Of the sticky stuff, he writes: "On the basis of a 2,000 calorie per day diet, it provides seven times as much iron as it does calories." The statement is subtle indeed. A calorie is a measure of the energy which food will provide. (It is really a *kilocalorie,* one thousand calories in the language of physics or chemistry, but the name has been shortened.) Iron is a mineral which, most importantly, is essential to the body's forming of hemoglobin, the protein in blood which transports oxygen; its need is measured in milligrams. Hauser's statement is a bit like going into a bank and asking for a pound of money, chocolate and strawberry. It is virtually meaningless to a nutritionist.

In truth, blackstrap is a fairly good source of iron, though not as good as Hauser implies. But in terms of B vitamins, it has some notable weaknesses. For example, as a source of riboflavin (vitamin B-2), blackstrap has .04 mg. in a tablespoon. The U.S. RDA is 1.7 mg. per day. So it would take 42.5 tablespoons of blackstrap to provide a day's recommendation for riboflavin. As for niacin—of which we shall see that shortages are virtually unknown in the U.S.—there are 0.4 mg. in a tablespoon. The U.S. RDA is 20 mg. So the daily recommendation for niacin would require 50 table-spoons of molasses. The thiamin (vitamin B-1) content of black-strap is .02 mg. per tablespoon. The U.S. RDA for thiamin is 1.5 mg. Thus, to get our daily recommended thiamin would take 75 tablespoons, or over 3,200 calories of molasses a day. The reader is left to his own judgment. Is blackstrap molasses, as Hauser claims, a "wonder food?"

Look Younger, Live Longer sold at a lusty rate. The Hearst newspapers syndicated it. The *Saturday Evening Post* ran bits under the title, *You Can Live to be 100, He Says.* (Note the last two words; they embody a familiar magazine gambit of declining responsibility for the nutrition information which is presented.) *The Reader's Digest* condensed it.

Unhappily, the reading public takes little interest in such details as food-composition tables. They assume that publications which they trust do such things for them. Much more convincing, and much more widely known, than Dr. Fishbein's critiques were the endorsements of important people. Lady Mendl appeared on Hauser's lecture platforms. No less a figure than the Baron Phillipe de Rothschild became the European distributor for Hauser products. The Duchess of Windsor wrote the introduction to the French edition of his work.

Blackstrap molasses, at best a quaint sort of product, sold to a few country grandmothers at the rate of some 500 gallons a month until Gayelord became its champion. Once Hauser's book was out, sales increased a hundred fold. And they continue to this day. Requests for reprints of the *Reader's Digest* article set a record.

The Food and Drug Administration—which does read food-composition tables, and which became aware that the Hauser book was being displayed with molasses—seized a quantity of the books, construing them as labeling for *Plantation Blackstrap Molasses.* Such seizures are publicized by the Federal government, so that the populace will be aware of what has been done; they are published among the FDA's *Notices of Judgment.* Unfortunately, these are perhaps even less widely read than are the food-composition tables.

What the public seemed to prefer were energetic Hauser instructions such as those in a chapter called "The Time Is Now." In this chapter, Hauser refers to the nutritional deficiency diseases, such as beri-beri and pellagra. Then he asks, "Can we, in the face of these discoveries, say that we will wait? No, the time is NOW . . . All the vital factors of foods that we know about should be meticulously included in our diet. Yesterday it was said of some that 'their need in human nutrition was not established;' today they show promise of rescuing us from dreaded diseases . . ."

The diseases of which he speaks are the "degenerative diseases." He refers chiefly to cancer, arthritis and heart disease, for which, largely, we have no good answers.

As *his* answers, Hauser offers "wonder foods"—skim milk, brewer's yeast, wheat germ, and blackstrap molasses. There was, and is, no evidence that these foods supply anything which is not obtained from a diet of ordinary foods. There was, and is, no reason to believe that these foods will spare us from the diseases which medicine cannot consistently cure by more scientific means.

Why has the FDA been concerned about mis-statements of the nutrient content of such foods as blackstrap molasses? First, when claims are made for the nutrient values of a food, the consumer should be able to expect that he will get these values, since he is paying for them. There is really no difference between overstating the B-vitamin content of molasses and falsely claiming five times the real horsepower for a car.

Second, there is a major concept of consumer nutrition at stake—that there is no single food which is essential to life or health. The nutrients needed for man's health are widely available almost everywhere on the globe, despite the fact that local flora and fauna may differ radically. For example, the protein of alligator steak will support our needs as well as that of beef—or giraffe chops, armadillo burgers, roast seal, or fricassee of termite. The Samoan may use taro root for his starch much as the Vietnamese uses rice, the inland Chinese uses millet, or the American eats his French fries.

To sell a product by implying that one cannot get good nutrition without it—or that one will get some sort of supernutrition *with* it—is false science and unscrupulous business. It misleads and confuses, and so makes it more difficult to understand the facts of nutrition. Man could not have arisen, survived and flourished everywhere on the earth if the raw materials for his body chemistry were really so hard to find.

Finally, there is the widely misunderstood relationship between foods, their nutrients, and illness. The fact that the absence or short supply of a nutrient can cause a certain illness does not mean that illness implies a shortage of nutrients. Indeed, the extreme odds are that when illness occurs in our society it is *not* the result of malnutrition.

True nutritional deficiency disease is not easy to produce. The shortage of the nutrient in the diet must be profound, and it must persist for some time.

The simple rule is this: Nutrients can relieve illness only when that illness has been caused by a shortage of those nutrients. Once the body's needs for a nutrient have been met, excess amounts of the nutrient accomplish nothing useful, and—we shall see—can cause harm.

Supposed "health" foods persuade people to spend needlessly large sums of money. The same nutrients are always available, much more cheaply, from foods in any supermarket, provided one knows what to buy. As an example, recall our look at raw sugar. At this writing, two pounds of ordinary table sugar cost about 40 cents; two pounds of one of the best-known brands of "raw" sugar cost $2.70. In other words, one pays six times as much money and gets "no significant difference" for it.

Such considerations led government officials to raise questions about the fact that Gayelord Hauser was a partner in Modern Products, Inc., while his writings and lectures recommended the items sold by the firm. The FDA action on Plantation Blackstrap Molasses included in the complaint a finding that the product, from which FDA said Hauser received royalties, was accompanied by the pamphlet, *Crude Black Molasses, the Natural Wonder Food.*

Incidentally, many health-food authors stress the natural calcium in blackstrap. Hauser calls attention to the importance of this mineral.* The calcium is important, and it is present in molasses—but most of it comes from the lime water used in refining sugar. Similarly, a good deal of the blackstrap's iron and copper come from contact with metals in the refining process.

Hauser does his best to keep up with the latest in public wishes and attitudes. When William Horatio Bates' book, *Cure of Imperfect Eyesight by Treatment without Glasses,* became a big seller, Hauser claimed that eyes could be improved by a mix of his diets and a combination of exercising and relaxing the eyes, à la Bates.

*He also says that calcium is found in few foods other than dairy products. "Green leafy vegetables," he says, "have calcium; but it is in an insoluble form that cannot pass into the blood." Not so; one can easily use the calcium from greens.

The diets follow the pattern of Hauser's prescription for "a famous motion picture star," whose eyes burned and got red. He fed her vegetable broths, food yeast, liver, milk, "all the natural foods that restore health and beauty to the eyes."

When a nutritional deficiency really does exist, it is not a deficiency of one part of the body, but of the whole. If the "famous star's" eyes burned because she was extremely short of some nutrients—Hauser suggests that B vitamins and A were needed—those shortages would show up in other symptoms, too. For example, if the lady was deficient in thiamin (B-1), then her symptoms would have been part of beri-beri.

The rest of Hauser's treatment was to relax one's eyes and try to "see black." Physicians who specialize in diseases of the eye do not agree that such efforts will cure visual flaws, with the obvious exception of simple fatigue. Even sleep does not stop the movement of the eyes; the shallower levels of sleep are in fact designated as REM sleep, standing for rapid-eye-movement.

Hauser continued to leave no food unturned. He espoused careful chewing, and while he cautioned against extremes, he adds, "But believe me, basically, 'Fletcherizing' is sound."

Hauser explores other areas, too, as in his book *Types and Temperaments, with a Key to Foods,* which appeared early in his career and classified people according to chemical types. There are sulphur types, "fiery, spontaneous and talented," such as Norma Shearer. There are sodium types, such as Douglas Fairbanks and Billy Sunday. But, Hauser warns, there are complicating factors—different qualities in different parts of the same body—such as negative bodies and positive heads. These people had all better look out if they do not follow the special Hauser diet appropriate to their natural make-ups.

Hauser's appeal to beauty also is a command to diet, with the five natural wonder foods and a naturopathic plan of life. He offers his slant board, on which one lies, head down, feet up, for at least fifteen minutes a day.

He continues the grand tradition of baths, too—sun baths, air baths, sea baths, alternating baths, oil baths, and even "dry baths." One of his baths is for what he delicately refers to as the difficulty of the "tired husband." For this there are special "sitz" bathtubs, the "sitz" being pretty much what it sounds as if it is. If you don't have the special equipment—the tub, of course, not the "sitz"—then Hauser recommends that you partially fill an ordinary tub with cold water. You crouch down so that "only the feet and the 'sitz' are in the water." If one is short of time, he adds, one can "simply immerse the scrotum in . . . ice water."

Hauser's nutrition has become more and more "scientific," in keeping with the advances of science. As an example, he notes that *glutamic acid,* one of the amino acids which we get from proteins, has been found to be used in the chemistry of the brain. He tells us that when glutamic acid is "amply supplied in the diet," intelligence increases, learning is speeded up, and memory is keener. So when an elderly actress fears forgetting her lines, Hauser prescribes a mixture of milk, yeast and honey, with a tablet of glutamic acid, to be drunk every hour. He says that this, "produced a 'miracle' of memory . . ."

There are a couple of interesting scientific footnotes to this story. One is that glutamic acid is not one of the "essential" amino acids.* The body can make it in quantity, all by itself, from very common raw materials which are found in almost all diets. Secondly, glutamic acid is rather plentiful in an enormous number of food proteins and is consumed by most Americans to an extent far greater than the body can use. Finally, we observe that one of the "chemicals" added to foods, over the objections of most foodists, is MSG, the flavor enhancer. MSG is a salt of glutamic acid, often derived from grain protein. It is metabolized by the body to yield glutamic acid. It is also a seasoning standard, in very large quantities, in Chinese and Japanese cooking. If Hauser's claims are true, those of us who frequent Chinese restaurants ought to be mental giants.

In his concern about what is missing from food, and his enthusiasm for recipes and "wonder foods" to replace these nutrients, Hauser was among the first to single out and publicize one of the most powerful ideas in modern foodism—the "organic" concept.

The idea is that modern argicultural techniques produce crops which do not carry the nutrients we would expect. In a

*Essential amino acids are those which cannot be made by the body, so must be taken in from protein-source foods.

sense, it is envisioned that the plants themselves are fed on a deficient diet, and that hence the resulting crops are deficient as foods.

"Commercial fertilizers," he has written, "supplying phosphorus, nitrogen and potassium, force the growth of vegetables, but fail to furnish seventeen or more nutrients needed by healthy plants. As these plants are deficient in the missing nutrients, the animals and humans living on such plant foods likewise, suffer deficiencies . . . This chain reaction has resulted in a tremendous increase in disease among plants, animals and humans alike and *is exactly the reason why we must fortify our present diets.* . . ." (The italics are added.)

He is wrong. But he is not alone. In the earlier-mentioned government survey on food attitudes, a cross-section of Americans included not less than 85 percent who agreed with this idea except for college graduates, of whom 88 percent agreed.

It is the common practice of foodists, however, to suggest that there are really two kinds of nutrition—one of orthodox science and another which represents a sort of rebellion against science. Their favorite line seems to be, "Nutrition is a controversial matter, a matter of personal belief."

This position has grown in popularity from the moment when scientists began to penetrate the chemical veil which had obscured the truths of food and health. When virtually nothing was known of the chemical processes of life, intuition alone could guide the pen of the nutritionist. And no one could argue.

But beginning only about a century ago, experimenters began to understand the natural laws of human life and food—laws that were inviolable processes which could be analyzed, described and measured, as surely as those which applied to the apple falling on Newton's head. And just as surely as we know now how unlikely it is that an apple will fall *up*, so surely can we say what chemicals are and are not present, to a very tiny extent, in our soils.

This progress of knowledge has proven most inconvenient for the foodists. So we have the strangest paradox of nutrition.

In other studies of natural phenomena, we tend to place absolute faith in science. Boarding a jumbo jet, we believe it will fly safely. Buying an electronic calculator, we believe it will give us correct answers. We blandly stockpile, in our national backyard, enough nuclear explosives to blow the world apart. And few people doubt science's assurances of safety. In our homes, we separate explosive gases and oils from open flames with the flimsiest of shields, but we don't go to sleep fearful that our water heaters and furnaces might demolish us before dawn.

Yet when it comes to the chemical properties of a carrot, many of us seem to feel that they are beyond the understanding of science.

True, because of the infinite variety of life, we cannot say that we know all that there is to know about the carrot. Then neither do we know everything about the uranium atom or about gravity. But we know quite a lot about these things. Particularly, we often know enough about natural laws to say when an idea is false. Everyone knows that apples fall down, not up.

So it is against the background of this paradox that the vast majority of people believe Gayelord Hauser's statements about commercial fertilizers being the cause of a "tremendous increase in disease," even though science shakes its collective head in an emphatic *No*. Sadly, most of the public bases its nutrition behavior more on false concepts than on scientific facts. And so the public is largely deceived.

Let us see which ideas are known to be wrong, yet govern how most of us choose our food. For we now have entered upon the foodism of our own day.

15

Old Proteinaceous Joe
Or
Is There Sex after Dinner?

We all know someone like Joe Jenks—or so food writer Lelord Kordel says. Lelord—whose ten books, innumerable lectures and products have had a considerable effect on America's nutrition thinking since the 1930's—describes Old Joe as healthy, energetic and about 100 years old.

It is by now not surprising to learn that Joe has reached his lively superannuation by eating as Nature intended. But what makes Kordel different from the others who tell us what Nature had in mind is that he emphasizes a different nutrient. For Kordel was among the first to inspire the modern preoccupation with *protein.*

Kordel derives his basic nutrition concepts from the highest authority. When he was nine years old, he asked his mother: "Do people die because they don't eat the right stuff?"

The good Polish lady, who had brought Lelord to America when he was only five years old, replied: ". . . Thousands of them every day. Only it is called by some fancy name."

The source of Kordel's essential theory that, "Nature is the only healing force," is clear. But his idea of *how* Nature heals with protein is less evident.

One of his publishers, Belmont Books, tell us that Lelord was a student of von Liebig, one of the truly great men of chemistry. However, von Liebig was a German. Lelord's first five years of life, in Warsaw, would seem to have given him little time to commute to von Liebig's laboratories in Germany. Moreover, another publisher notes that Kordel was, in 1968, "in his sixties," suggesting that Kordel was born in the first decade of this century. Unfortunately, by 1900, von Liebig had been dead for 27 years.

Nevertheless, as an interviewer for Award Books tells us: "Out of the wilderness of pain and needless human suffering had come a voice of authority, holding out great promise . . . For many years before his first health lecture in San Francisco (in 1938) Lelord Kordel had tirelessly carried on years of research . . . worked day and night to prove the facts which he was so sure did exist . . ."

Indeed, so great was Kordel's passion for helping people, that he was not content with hitting the bestseller lists. Early in his career, he was also president of Detroit Vital Foods. In 1946, he was given a $4,000 fine for misbranding supplements. In 1957, as a principal of Nutrition Enterprises, he agreed to a Federal Trade Commission consent order, which specified that he cease making some claims for "Super-Nutri-Way," another health-food supplement. In 1961, the Food and Drug Administration seized a batch of *Michigan Brand Korleen Tablets* and a bunch of Lelord's books—maintaining that the books made false and misleading claims for the supplement. Later in 1961, some 3,000 pounds of honey were impounded by Federal authorities from Detroit Vital Foods. The Food and Drug Administration said that the honey was "misbranded," because it was claimed to help prevent or cure rheumatism, heart disease, arthritis and "premature death."

Aging and lost sexual ability—the honey was claimed to cure the latter, too—have been two great concerns of Kordel's. And protein has long been his main preventive for both.

He is not alone.

Probably the most prevalent single false idea about food and health is the concept that the more protein we eat, the healthier we will be. Because this misconception can be quite destructive, it is worth looking closely at some of Kordel's writing on the subject. For his work typifies a trend.

"If you want to live longer," Kordel informs us, ". . . you must eat *more* of the foods rich in protein, vitamins and minerals." He explains that, "Old Joe and other near-centenarians like him are actually throwbacks to those old days when men and women lived prolonged, healthy, active lives as a matter of course."*

Kordel tells us that his protein program can "lift the burden of age from your tired, well-fed-yet-starved body like the touch of a magic wand." Most of us, he says, do not understand this. Instead, we, "have been seduced down the path to early and inevitable murder . . . of your youth, good looks, pep, radiant vitality . . . And the 'murderer' is none other than yourself, aided and abetted by the high-pressure advertising of unscrupulous, profit-conscious processors of devitalized and artificial foods."

To show us what Nature wants, Kordel takes us with him on a trip to Argentina. His host gallops him out to the *pampas,* to meet a number of *gauchos,* some of whom turn out to be 70 years old. They gallop through the dust like young men, shouting and wheeling their horses, leaving the saddle only when darkness falls.

What explains the vigor of the septuagenerian cowboys? The answer is seen at dinner time—as each geriatric *gaucho* cuts off a great chunk of roasting steer meat, scarcely cooked, and wolfs it down as his only dinner.

We find a number of such examples in Kordel's work. For instance, there is "Grandma X." She comes to one of his lectures in her wheelchair, suffering from, "hardened arteries, high blood pressure and coronary thrombosis." Also her sinuses bothered her.

Taking Kordel's advice, she starts eating lots of meat. Next time Kordel sees her, she is ambling down a street in Hollywood as a chipper tourist. And even her sinuses have cleared up.

*The longevity statistics for the U.S. show the opposite—that health and longevity are greater today.

In his book, *Eat Your Troubles Away*, Kordel tells us about "Joe T." He is 45. He is fat. He starts working out at home. Not only does this fail to help, but Kordel writes that, "All this exercise made him too tired at night to notice his wife's changing attitude toward him." (Kordel's delicacy does not escape us sophisticated readers. We know what he is trying to say. And it is a shame. Because supposedly protein would have prevented it.)

There was no need, we read, for Joe T to be fat. But he didn't know one of Kordel's basic nutritional laws, which goes: "Fat can be removed only when it is exchanged for muscle by eating the muscle-building materials furnished by proteins."

We shall see that while this idea is self-evident to Kordel, it is foreign to the knowledge of less imaginative nutritionists. Their scientific principle is that any of the four principal sources of body energy—protein, carbohydrate, fat or alcohol—can be converted to body fat with equal ease. Indeed, whatever of these nutrients cannot be put to work at once—providing energy which is burned, or building materials to make body structures or chemicals—will be converted to fat and stored.

In the case of "Tom S," Kordel becomes more explicit about protein and sexual survival. He informs us about the "climacteric" in men, which he defines as a "period of glandular upset," sometimes called *change of life*. (Medicine has no evidence that men undergo such a change.)

Tom S, in his fifties, became depressed. He was nervous and grumpy. "Nothing his experienced secretary did pleased him any longer . . . she quit in disgust after having served him for more than twenty years." Kordel explains that Tom's, "starved gonads had retaliated by suddenly depleting their supply of testosterone" (the male sex hormone). As a result, "every nerve, muscle and organ . . . had pleaded . . . for testosterone." What could have prevented this sad situation? Kordel says, "a diet rich in proteins . . ." (and also vitamins and minerals). He reminds us that we regularly read of men even in their nineties, who are "passing out cigars."

One of the nice things about protein, according to Kordel, is that it does not require much chewing. He says that one may safely swallow chunks of protein, but that vegetables, fruits, sugars and starches need very thorough chewing.*

This idea is partly based on a medical idea of former times, sometimes used to justify Fletcherizing. For the saliva does contain enzymes which begin to break sugars and starches apart for the body's use. But science has since learned that these salivary enzymes do not play a very prominent role in digestion. Most carbohydrate digestion takes place in the stomach and small intestine. The teeth are the body's chief means of breaking up foods into tiny bits, to enable digestive chemicals to reach as much food surface as possible. A lump of meat swallowed whole is not digested nearly as well.

Ultimately Kordel becomes quite blunt about food and sex. "It has long been known," he reports, "that some foods stimulate the sex glands . . . Among the more commonly recognized of such foods are eggs, oysters and red meats." These he says, do much of their work through their protein. And he stresses that, "there is another that should be added to the list—milk." Kordel may have sparked the slogan—painted on any number of milk tank trucks over the years—"Milk Drinkers Make Better Lovers."

This idea is troubling. For all across the nation, nutritionists press high-schoolers to abandon soda pop in favor of milk. If Kordel is right, these well-meaning nutrition specialists may be planting a sociological time bomb. Perhaps after all, if Kordel is right, colas and uncolas may have redeeming social values.

On the other hand, despite the legends, science has evidence of no aphrodisiac food or drink. Sex experts who have studied the allegedly aphrodisiac foods, attribute their supposed sexual powers to three factors. One is simple suggestion. Most impotence, after all, is psychological. The second is the odor, appearance or other association of the food with sexual secretions or organs, as in the case of oysters. Cattle testicles, for example, are known in some parts of the Southwest as "prairie oysters." And finally foods which seem to have a *diuretic* effect (urinary stimulation) may provide some genital sensation.

*Remember that virtually all foods are combinations of some amount of protein, carbohydrate and fat. Eating meat is not "eating protein."

Kordel backs his assertions about milk and sex with an undocumented story of Mahatma Gandhi, the Indian ascetic. Kordel says that Gandhi had no problem pursuing a life of chastity while on a diet of mainly fruit and nuts, but that once he added a little milk, he was in trouble.

Any number of foodists agree with Kordel's thesis that the "diets of a great majority of American families create the real causes underlying so much unhappy married life." And they agree when he adds, ". . . Consider the logic of safeguarding your marital happiness by making certain that your nervous system and your sexual glands are well fortified by protective foods . . ."

To Kordel, these protective foods are largely protein-rich animal-source foods. Sylvester Graham and Dr. Kellogg and the vast majority of the old foodists would have been appalled.

But today, when it comes to sex, strength and beauty—the magic passwords of our day—many modern foodists share his protein enthusiasm to the last bite of steak. As Adelle Davis sums it up in her *Diet for Better Sex,* there are three major precepts of eating for sex, and two of them involve protein: "When you eat a nutritious meal, high in proteins," she says, ". . . you will feel cheerful . . . full of vitality . . . and ready for any activity, including sex." Elsewhere, Adelle informs us that we cannot possibly get enough protein unless we drink a quart of milk a day— thus closing circle fully with Kordel.

Sex is not the only exercise for which protein is given undue credit. Contrary to the beliefs of most American consumers, protein needs increase little with an increase of activity. The truth is that one's protein need is almost entirely a function of one's size—and largely unrelated to activity.

But the thinking of most athletes and sports-minded, body-building Americans runs firmly counter to science here. The U.S. training table is likely to be a groaning board of meat, eggs and milk. Weight-lifters eat such foods in quantity—and then pop protein pills with almost every grunt and groan. Interviews of Olympic athletes reflect a strong tendency to seek extra protein, in the belief that other foods "make me soft inside."

A *Los Angeles Times* article recalls a thrift crusade of then UCLA football coach Tommy Prothro, who once brought a scale to the pre-game meal, determined to keep his players to 16 ounces of steak each. So much meat, in the scientific view, furnishes 50 percent more than a whole day's useful protein for the biggest defensive tackle—with no regard for other meals eaten during the day or for the protein in the eggs, milk, bread and other foods eaten with the steak. Incidentally, we might consider the fact that such a meal would probably not even have left the stomach for several hours—and that for the most part, the nutrients from the food would not be available until the game was over.

The ancient tradition that meat equals strength persists, despite evidence to the contrary. UCLA footballers, for example, still eat meals built around steaks, a few hours before the game. "Over the years," UCLA trainer Ducky Drake is quoted, "our teams have been pretty successful. We are aware of the studies on protein . . . but don't feel there's any reason to change."

Dr. Nathan Smith, the University of Washington physician who is one of the nation's leading authorities on sports nutrition, sums up the situation: "Hoping to increase body size and strength, many athletes have been attracted to high-protein diets and concentrated protein supplements. This blind belief in protein . . . goes back well before the advent of modern nutritional science . . . The use of high-protein diets . . . : widespread among certain groups of athletes, even though their diets ordinarily contain *three or four times* what the body needs for *optimal performance.*" (Italics added.)

Moreover, as is the case with excess of any nutrient, unusually high intakes of protein are not without hazards. Smith gives this example:

"Typical of many of the popular protein supplements is . . . *Super 96 Protein,* which one . . . football player took while attempting to gain weight. Instead, it ruined his appetite and produced severe diarrhea, resulting in actual weight loss. The label . . . indicates that it contains animal protein from . . . 'undenatured liver, pancreas, heart, spleen, mammary, ovarian and testicular substance.' This long list of slaughterhouse refuse certainly has no place in the diet of any individual . . ."

Smith is not alone. A recent Federal Trade Commission staff proposal called for the following warning label on all protein

supplements: "PROTEIN SUPPLEMENTS ARE UNNEC-
ESSARY FOR MOST AMERICANS. THE U.S. PUBLIC
HEALTH SERVICE HAS DETERMINED THAT THE
DAILY DIET OF MOST AMERICANS PROVIDES ADE-
QUATE PROTEIN."

FTC is referring to national surveys, largely at poverty
levels. Even these people were getting 60 to 100 percent more
protein than the National Research Council finds more than
adequate.

As a technical note, let us keep in mind that our requirements
for protein are really requirements for the essential amino acids
which are the real building blocks of which proteins are composed.
We eat proteins to get the "essential" amino acids which our
bodies cannot make. Studies show clearly that the typical American receives *five to seven times* as much of the essential amino acids
as he needs.

Nevertheless, coaches, trainers and athletes continue to
worry about amino acids. Consider a basic paper on nutrition
prepared at a western university for Olympic ski racers. It says,
"No one food has all ten essential amino acids." This idea is false.
Large numbers of foods contain *some* of each amino acid. Further,
all of the essential amino acids, in ample amounts, are found in
almost any animal-source food—meats, fishes, milks, eggs, and so
forth.

Finally, the Olympic team advice warns that, "some high
protein foods are relatively low in amino acids." Since proteins are
made of amino acids, this idea is harder to swallow than a
tablespoon of liver extract.

It is not only athletes who worship protein. In an article
called "How Lucy (Ball) Bounces," beauty adviser Lydia Lane
describes an interview in which she asks Lucille Ball, "where all
her energy comes from."

The two were sitting in Lucy's dressing room, sipping a
mixture of carrot, apple and celery juice. Referring to a jar of raw
gelatin on Lucy's dressing table, Lydia Lane quotes the veteran
comic: " 'I put this in fruit juice for a lift. It's pure protein and
practically tasteless.' "

Such gelatin is close to being pure protein. But its amino acids
are so poorly distributed that almost any other food has better

quality protein. In addition, protein is no more useful as a source of energy—which in nutritional terms means *fuel value and nothing else*—than ordinary table sugar. In fact, in the process by which the body uses gelatin for energy, the protein is a less efficient source, for it must first be converted to carbohydrate.

Isn't there some reason why the typical American should go to special lengths to seek out proteins and their amino acids? A number of supplement manufacturers insist that the requirements for protein, and for various amino acids, are set too low. But desirable protein intake is some 56 grams a day for the model American man and perhaps 46 grams for the American woman, more if they are larger. Even in poverty groups, intake actually is on the order of about 100 grams a day. And the richer folk often eat far more.

Says the FTC's staff report: "Protein deficiency is evidently a rare nutritional problem in the U.S. . . . Every expert in the field of nutrition consulted by the staff expressed the opinion that 'the overwhelming majority of Americans get more protein than they require for good health from their usual diets.' The clear consensus of these experts is that protein supplements are a fraud on the American public. (This poll of experts included experts who have been associated with the industry position on other issues.)"

Such reports have not dampened the enthusiasm of those who enjoy selling protein as though it were hard to get. For example, at most health-food stores you can get your daily supply of protein in supplements which furnish it for a cost of a mere $20 per day. Of course, you need not spend so much. You can go to Sears and get *Nutra-Pro Wafers (Lemon)*—each tablet of which is advertised to contain 1.2 grams of protein. The price is 100 tablets for only $3.50. And 100 tablets will give you slightly more protein than the typical adult in a poverty-level family gets each day (some 100 grams).

For the same price as the bargain supplement, you could get (at this writing) an enormous steak—only some 10 ounces of which would supply your whole protein need for the day, *plus* some valuable vitamins and minerals. And other food sources are much cheaper.

Yet Hoffman Products is reported by FTC to advertise: "Do

you consume enough protein? Did you know that a study by the National Research Council has indicated that there is a good chance you do not?"

In addition, FTC finds that many companies offer protein supplements as especially "energizing." Says the FTC staff, "Shaklee [a supplement maker which does much better than $100 million a year, hires astronauts as celebrity directors, but nevertheless seems to maintain a kind of folksy, little-guy image suitable to its door-to-door sales techniques] went so far as to represent that 'nothing refreshes and satisfies like a protein break.' "

FTC staffers, looking at such examples, have proposed a rule which begins:

"NO REPRESENTATION SHALL BE MADE, DIRECTLY OR BY IMPLICATION, THAT ANY PROTEIN SUPPLEMENT:

(a) CAN COUNTERACT OR DELAY THE EFFECTS OR SIGNS OF AGING OR SENILITY, INCLUDING BUT NOT LIMITED TO BALDNESS, THINNING HAIR, AGING SKIN AND DECREASED MENTAL AND PHYSICAL CAPABILITIES . . ."

"This investigation," they observe, "has included a review of all of the advertising and labeling of the over 80 companies involved in the sale and distribution of protein supplements. As demonstrated . . . it appears that this industry markets these products mainly by exploiting the public's ignorance of nutrition, diet, and related health problems and the public's unfounded fear of protein deficiency . . . protein deficiency is probably the least common of all major nutrient deficiencies in the United States."

Yet routine popular nutritional counsel advises more protein. For example, a reader of the *Detroit Free Press* asks that newspaper's *Action Line* the question: "The thing that impresses me most about the Olympics is how all the divers have flat stomachs . . . What's their secret?" The answer is:

"No secret at all, really, just hard work and proper diet. MSU (Michigan State University) diving coach John Narcy told Action Line that divers on his team do 50 situps a day . . . Also helps to grip weights behind head and do exercise on slant board." And, "Divers," he says, "stick pretty much to high protein . . . diets."

They are not alone. With them are all those others who are concerned about "flat stomachs"—from movie queens and television talk-show hosts to U.S. presidents. To the long list, we might also add most of the American public. For in recent years, protein has acquired a reputation as the secret of being slim.

Let us look now at some of the truth, and some of the consequences, of our national preoccupation with the round belly.

Jack Spratt would eat no fat,
His wife would eat no lean . . .

16

Mrs. Spratt's Millions
Or
Diet Is a Four-Letter Word

It had been a long time since anyone had seen an arm like pitcher Denny McClain's, with a fast ball that blew the very lint off his opponents' numbers. When he was only 24 years old, in 1968, he became the first major league hurler in more than three decades to win an awesome 31 games in a single season.

But by the spring of 1972, Charlie Finley, the hardheaded owner of the Oakland Athletics, spelled out the tragedy. He announced that he was optioning McClain to Birmingham, in the minor leagues. What had brought about the downfall of this pitching superstar? It was none of the usual pitching hazards—not bone chips or spurs, not unsuccessful surgery, not torn muscle. Instead, according to the press reports, McClain had tried to lose some weight.

There is reason to believe that for Denny McClain, as for most Americans, "diet" was a particularly repugnant four-letter word. For a true reducing diet is just one thing—a plan for eating in which the body gets less fuel than it needs. Such a diet, no matter what the freeswinging promotions tell us, tends to cause some hunger. And the loss of much body fat takes time—a good deal more time than most people think it does. So losing any appreciable amount of excess weight means being a little hungry for quite a while.

It is hardly surprising that most of us, when confronted with this truth, become susceptible to the wiles of anyone who says he has a shortcut. Where Denny McClain's advice came from, we do not know; but the Oakland team physician tells us that Denny tried using pills.

"He had," says Dr. Charles Hudson, "been taking diuretic pills for some time."

"Diuretic pills" are medications which stimulate the loss of body water through urination. By far, most of the weight of our bodies is water. And by far, most of this water is needed. For our cells must live in a salty inner sea. As with all body systems, there is room for error and adaptation. We can dry out a little or get a little too juicy. But only so much. Water is basic to the body's chemistry. When the needed water runs short, we are endangered. True dehydration is accompanied by discomforts of many kinds, by weakness, and finally by collapse.

"Mr. McClain," Dr. Hudson reports, "has been complaining of some loss of strength and cramping in his extremities . . ." The symptoms are typical. For the sportswriter, what they meant was that the steam was out of Denny's fast ball, and they were hitting his pitching all down the lineup.

True, as McClain lost water, he also lost weight. But that weight, sadly, had nothing to do with body fatness. The weight loss was a kind of illusion. And that illusion cost Denny McClain a great career.

There is no reason to think less of people who try the water-loss method, while avoiding real fat-reduction. For most Americans who seek to be slimmer choose some method which depends on nonsense. The tired old water trick recurs again and again. For example, in general, New Yorkers tend to be a wary, if not suspicious, lot. But a little more than a decade ago, offered the chance to buy a snappy plastic suit, the wearing of which would "just sweat away" excess poundage, many jumped at the chance. The principle of the plastic reducing suit was really no different from that of the water pills; the water merely leaves the body by different routes.

Eventually, the seller of the suit, a Brooklyn firm, was tapped with a postal fraud order and denied the use of the mails. But the incident suggests the persuasiveness of almost any idea which promises to remove fat—without actually making the remover feel hungry.

Arthur Summerfield, then Postmaster General of the United States, called the weight-reducing business, "the most widely practiced medical fraud today." (He was speaking in terms of postal frauds only; the health-food business as a whole, then as now, represented a much greater overall fraud.) But despite the repeated governmental assaults on such products as the *Steam Bath Suit* (as the sweating device was known), people still seem to believe in the basic idea.*

At the end of the 1960's the *Sauna Belt* emerged in national advertising, with full-page ads. (Full-page ads in the major national magazines indicate the extent of a product's success, since each full-page ad in the major magazines, tends to cost from $15,000 to well over $50,000.) The idea of the *Belt* was to sweat out, not the whole body, but just the troublesomely adipose midsection.

The myth was exploded. But early in the 1970's, *Trim-Jeans, Slim Shorts* and *Air Shorts* took over. Sold at between $6 and $14, the plastic pants were donned, then inflated with an air pump. "The shorts work," said *Newsweek*, "by trapping body heat between vinyl and skin; the heat, it is claimed, 'breaks down fatty tissue.'"

Doctors scoffed, some publicly. But Abercrombie and Fitch, a trusted store of the affluent, whose patrons might be expected to include people of considerable sophistication, proudly sold over 1,000 pairs in the first two weeks.

*An HEW study suggests that equating water loss with fat loss is perhaps the most pervasively believed of false reducing ideas.

What convinces the users of such devices? They actually do see the pointer on the scales go down. What they do not realize is that they carry just as much body fat as ever. Most have heard, for example, that boxers "sweat off" extra pounds before a weigh-in, with steam baths and exercising while bundled up. The weight, however, returns as soon as the boxer gets thirsty and drinks the needed water again.

So it is that the Council on Foods and Nutrition of the AMA describes the use of "water pills" as "irrational" in treating obesity. For making the scales go down by increased sweating or urination is about as meaningful as surreptitiously turning down the pointer when no one is looking. Steam cabinets, plastic belly bands, inflatable pants, saunas and exercise in heavy clothing are of the same value.

Indeed, the very great majority of all that Americans buy for fat reduction—from foods, to products, to services—is of similar low worth. The total price tag cannot be known exactly, but estimates run to the billions. For example, *Newsweek* guessed a few years ago that the bill for "belts and wheels, inflatable suits, stretch straps, electronic and battery-operated" reducing devices was $100 million a year. And this is just small change when we look at the big reducing picture.

To this we might add the fees paid to "fat farms," such as California's *Golden Door,* Elizabeth Arden's *Main Chance* or Texas' *Greenhouse*—or to "health salon" chains such as those of Jack La Lanne or Vic Tanny,* which number in the thousands. The rates for many of the "fat farms," which offer such treatments as herbal wraps for the overweight, approach $1,000 a week. The *Golden Door* however, with tips, runs to better than $200 a day. Owner Deborah Mazzanti boasts of such celebrity patrons as Debbie Reynolds, Kim Novak and Barbra Streisand. Some weeks are for men, such as some of the Watergate principals, who are said to have gone to the costly spa to recover from their travail among the herbal wraps and facials.

In an article in *Family Circle,* Deborah Mazzanti gives away some of her dieting secrets. The first week, for breakfast, you start

*When ample amounts of calorie-burning exercise are used, the gyms are useful.

out with a hot drink—"I would prefer you to drink a cereal coffee or herb tea," says Deborah. And with this you can have a little fruit.

Lunch brings you a wheat-germ cracker, thin, but a sumptuous three inches in diameter. And with this you feast on a cup of vegetable broth with an egg stirred into it and "a bit of grated romano cheese." This is one of several similar choices.

For dinner you can have some "low-calorie appetite-spoilers," such as vegetable broth, a little fruit and some carrot, radish and celery. There is a libation, too, of two tablespoons of fruit juice over ice in a champagne glass. Later, there is a main dish—say, six mushrooms stuffed with a few green peas and some cheese, served with a broiled tomato. Clearly, food cost does not explain the tab at the *Golden Door.*

Of course, there is more. You are encouraged to sing and whistle when possible, and five times a day to do some "Ha" breathing. (Remember Bernarr Macfadden?) And there is exercise, five-minute periods of it in the beginning.

In a moment, we shall examine exercise and its real effects on obesity. For one thing, it is the stock in trade of the salon chains which serve as the poor person's "fat farms." But those who offer weight reduction rarely rely on just one idea, so let us look at some of the popular concepts of fat removal.

The Pillar of Salt. It is a favorite recommendation of beauty experts that the dieter should not consume salt. John Robert Powers is one of many who gives such advice.

The idea is that salt helps the body to retain fluid; thus, if you eat salt, you become wetter—and heavier, but not fatter. Giving up *extra* salt is relatively harmless. The typical American dietary provides more salt than we need without adding more from the shaker. On the other hand, for normal people, it is fruitless to hope that abandoning table salt will have any effect on fatness.

Appetite Killers. In 1972, the Food and Drug Administration concluded a study of drugs used to limit appetite, and the final verdict was that *anorectics,* the medical term for such drugs, had "limited use in the treatment of obesity."

The drugs which have any real value are not available without a prescription. These are *amphetamines* and their chemical relatives. And even these stimulants are useful only for some people, and only for the first few weeks of reducing.

But from the start of our national preoccupation with obesity, beginning in the early 1950's, a broad assortment of drugs has been offered by physicians and promoters alike, with the promise of reduced appetite. For example, in 1956, one firm bought full-page ads for a product which was said to stop you from eating half way through a meal. It was claimed that you might lose 33 pounds without a hungry moment, and that the wonder drug had just been released by the Federal government for general use.

The company began to coin money. The drug was *phenylpropanolamine hydrochloride*—which, though it was related to the medically used appetite suppressants, had actually been released for over-the-counter sale in small amounts for other purposes. In fact, one may still see it in some trade preparations for colds.

In 1942, a researcher tried this drug, in *large* amounts, and found that it failed to reduce appetite. He also found many unpleasant side effects. The American Medical Association opinion was: "We doubt that (the allowable dosage) taken three times daily would exercise an appetite effect of any practical significance for the majority of obese users."

A month later, another company got on the bandwagon with a direct-mail offering: "Federal Health Authorities Now Release Safe Drug for Reducing That Limits the Ability of Your Body to Produce Sensations of Hunger." And it offered the same product through drugstores under another name.

There came another: "First No-Diet Reducing Wonder Drug Used Successfully by Thousands of Physicians! Lose As Many Pounds As You Like Without Diets of Any Kind!" Soon there was a deluge of brand names.

Six months later, the National Better Business Bureau issued a warning about the products. Three months after that, the Post Office issued its first fraud order on the items—and during the next year it issued some 70 more.

Moreover, the drug could be dangerous for some people, especially if they exceeded the amounts in the instructions. While it had to carry the warning that it was not to be taken by people with high blood pressure, heart disease, diabetes or thyroid disease, unless on a doctor's advice, the fact is that most people who have such conditions are not aware that they are so afflicted.

Testifying before a Congressional investigating committee, obesity expert Dr. Leon Hirsch said: "Those containing phenylpropanolamine could cause coronary attacks or cerebral hemmorhages in some people."

Some of the companies went out of business. But certain promoters whip up new businesses the way some people try new recipes, with new corporation papers and new trade names.

Other firms began to blend more than one "appetite killer" into their products. Take a drug which we might call "Slimmo." It contained phenylpropanolamine—in an amount about half that which failed to show appetite suppression in the 1942 experiments. It also had *benzocaine,* a weak anesthetic, which was supposed to anesthetize the nerves in the mouth that transmit taste. The promoter said he based this ingredient on the work of a Dr. William L. Gould. In truth, in Dr. Gould's experiments benzocaine was administered to *enhance* flavors!

The third ingredient was, and is, ammonium chloride. It is a mild diuretic, a weak version of the drugs that pitcher Denny McClain took, which made him urinate away some of his body fluid.

The maker of one of these triple-threat preparations became a big television advertiser in the early 1960's; it sold under the trade name *Regimen.* In commercials, models were shown week by week, supposedly losing weight without feeling hunger. In Federal court proceedings, the government presented evidence that the models had been on diets "verging on starvation" to achieve the televised results. The makers were convicted and fined.

The reader may assume that this conviction would end the problem. But advertisements for similar products are commonplace today. They are hustled in some of the nation's largest-circulation magazines and Sunday newspaper supplements and sold by some of the largest retail drugstore chains. They do not kill appetite in the 1970's any better than they did in the 1960's.

One added thought on phenylpropanolamines for appetite

suppression—the drug has been used for years by asthmatics, in much greater amounts. If the drug worked, FDA asked, why were not all these asthmatics living skeletons?

A short-lived product of the 1950's and early 1960's was the "bulker." This is a preparation—usually methyl cellulose—which is supposed to swell up and produce a "satisfied feeling."

The late Dr. Norman Jolliffe, of the New York City Health Department, ran a test on three groups of 40 people each. Only one of the groups got the methyl cellulose, in black coffee. A second group got black coffee, and a third got nothing at all. The result? The people who got nothing at all lost the most weight, more in fact than the other two groups combined.

"The real moral of the story," said Dr. Jolliffe, "may well be that people who thought they had a reducing crutch did not stay on their diets . . . They trusted to the crutch . . . Those who knew they were on their own stayed on their diets . . ."

One of the most successful diet products launched in the 1950's was based on common sense. Usually in the form of a candy, cookie or cracker, it derives from Mother's nutrition principle: "Don't eat that now! Do you want to spoil your dinner?"

It occurred to the producers that spoiling dinner was exactly what they wanted to do. The candy—one brand of which is the well-known *Ayds*—usually contains mostly sugar of one sort or another and gives you some 50 calories. Typically, you are instructed to eat it about half an hour before dinner with a hot drink. Of course, candy doesn't seem very scientific—it might even be compared to ordinary candy of 50 calories, which costs a great deal less—so vitamins and minerals are added. The justification for these micronutrients is that supposedly you eat less, so you won't get enough vitamins and minerals.

But when, in 1957, Representative Blatnik's House of Representatives committee investigated reducing products, Dr. S. William Kalb, an obesity expert, said of such candies and cookies: "Regardless of what formula is on here, the vitamins and minerals are just added as a come-on. It doesn't mean anything. It has no therapeutic value."

Nevertheless, the candies seem to help some people. For a

generation, *Ayds* has been a big buyer of magazine advertising. Touching stories of melting fat are told. Consider the lady who "gave up 87 pounds to get a good job," as it says in the headline. She tells how her obesity so put people off that she had to work in a boarding kennel, because, ". . . At least the animals didn't care." Then her aunt told her about *Ayds*. "I bought a box of the vanilla caramel kind . . . and I started on the *Ayds* plan." She says she felt less hungry and got so interested in her scale that she, "finally wore out the springs." The candy eaters always live happily ever after. This lady says, "Now I have a boy friend, a lot of store-bought clothes . . . Me, who grew up fat and never thought I could be thin."

Was Mother right about spoiling our appetites by eating before dinner? To an extent, yes. On the other hand, 50 calories is not a lot of food—perhaps equal to half an ounce, one bite, of prime steak. And the candies are merely food. Half of a modest potato, a cup of greens or half an apple would have the same effect. Except for one thing, which explains many a reducing testimonial. As Dr. Herbert Pollack, a noted clinical nutritionist puts it: "There are some suggestible people who can be given an empty capsule to swallow. If told this will destroy their appetites, they will lose all hunger. When any [over-the-counter] reducing pill works, it is for psychological reasons."

There is a little more to most of the reducing remedies than this. Note, as you read their ads, that they usually refer to "plans," not just products. This is because the pill or device usually comes with instructions that read something like, "Eat all you want, but be sure to avoid . . ." There follows a list of high-calorie foods.

Along with these remedies come some curious ideas about nutrition. Foodist thinking about fatness is characterized by one of Adelle Davis' statements to a magazine interviewer: "Obese people are obese because they're getting so few nutrients to build energy to keep fat worked off."

The obvious implication, that the way to get thinner is to eat *more* food, so that we will feel more energetic, burn more energy, and so use up our stored fat, is curious. So is another possible implication—that supplements can make us burn fat.

Let us look at some examples of this thinking—keeping in

mind the tradition that there is one healthful, "natural" way of eating.

The idea is well expressed by C.E. Burtis. In his book, *The Fountain of Youth, Longer Life through Natural Foods,* Burtis has a chapter called "Normal Weight? It's Easy!" Discussing patterns of eating which lead to obesity, the author says that, "they all share one factor in common. Chemical imbalance . . . The mere existence of a condition of overweight is in itself *prima facie* evidence of disturbed body chemistry . . ."

How do we normalize this chemistry and get thin? We follow Burtis' plan. Meats should be "under- rather than over-cooked." We should drink "milk that has been allowed to clabber (from certified raw milk *only;* soured pasteurized milk is unfit for human consumption)." We can have "fresh raw vegetable juices (but *no* fruit *juices*)." Potatoes are eliminated, "Except for *raw* russet—not red—potatoes, which after thorough scrubbing may be grated . . . into fresh raw vegetable salads, first removing any 'eyes,' " which are "poisonous."

Later, we can include a few of the forbidden items, but for now we must be very careful, eliminating almost all condiments except *oregano,* which is apparently not fattening.

In general, such authorities as Paavo O. Airola, N.D. agree with Burtis. Airola is a "naturopathic doctor," according to his publisher, *Arco,* which heralds his work as a report from "Europe's most progressive medical clinics." Airola's expertise is documented by none other than Dr. Frank S. Caprio, the venerable American sex expert, with at least ten volumes to his credit. In his introduction to Airola's book, *Sex and Nutrition,* Caprio hails the naturopath as a "famed European nutritionist," who, "writes with authority," and whose work, "merits wide distribution."

In his book, *Health Secrets from Europe,* in the chapter on "The European System of Preventing Heart Attacks," Airola writes a terse summary of the problem and the answer:

"Everyone agrees that the cause of obesity is overeating. But what causes overeating?

"Dr. T.L. Cleave, famous British scientist . . . explains what makes us 'civilized' people such compulsive eaters. He says that man . . . has an inborn instinct which guides him in his choice of the kind and amount of foods he should eat. He can trust this instinct with absolute confidence, *but only as long as he uses natural substances;* that is, the foods which occur naturally in his environment and are in their natural state."

This suggests that the Maine man should not eat California peaches, nor the Californian eat Norwegian sardines. Probably no fish should be consumed by the desert dweller, and the New Yorker should limit his diet to whatever he can grow on his windowsill.

The need for food in its "natural" state should present some problems for owners of health-food stores, who could not offer such processed stock items as blackstrap molasses, wheat germ, cold-pressed oils, and stone-ground wheat. Meat would have to be taken raw and bread not at all, since it must be manufactured. The person who follows this precept will have to spend much of his day browsing in the fields, perhaps pursuing one of Dr. Kellogg's goats.

Turning to other popular advice, we come on authoress Linda Clark. "In this era of devitalized foods," she writes, following what we begin to discern is a modern pattern, "you may have to eat many extra pounds of food in order to satisfy your body's needs and cravings for necessary vitamins and minerals." She tells of a man who "ate slice after slice of white bread." As soon as his wife started baking whole-wheat bread, however, he ate only one slice.

Clark says that one reason why people overeat is, "Dieting without vitamin-mineral supplementation." Some food authors are more explicit about vitamins as reducers. In *Let's Eat Right to Keep Fit,* Adelle Davis suggests taking vitamin C as a diuretic, to make the body lose water. With this idea, we have gone full circle.

If you don't want to buy supplements, pills, or plans to lose weight, you can buy gadgets. The March, 1961, issue of *Mademoiselle,* in an article called "Reach for an Expert" said: "Spot-reducing on a salon level can be an at-home achievement of your own with the new Verve Relaxicizor unit. One of their representatives will check you out with Beauty Belt placements and show you the many ways to use this electronic wonder."

The news was only 12 years old. The Relaxicizor, sold at

from $100 to $400, appeared in 1949. You used it by strapping contact pads onto fat spots of your body. It transmitted an electric current to the muscles, which was supposed to cause them to contract, making them firmer and you thinner. The charm was that you didn't actually have to do anything; you could lie back, watch TV, and twitch your bulges away.

Who would buy such a device? An estimated 400,000 Americans—yielding a gross of some $40 million to the producers.

In general, "spot reducing" doesn't work. Excess fat tends to be deposited largely just under the skin—where is largely a matter of heredity. The fact that you wiggle a muscle under the stored fat has no real effect on that storage depot. The muscle burns the fuel it gets from the bloodstream, or from storage in its own cells, rather than from fat which is close by.

Author Robert Sherrill quotes Food and Drug Administration Dr. Joe Davis on Relaxicizor: "They had started out saying the device would reduce weight, and we eventually got them to stop that advertising. Then they claimed it would reduce girth, and we got them to stop making that claim."

Later, we shall see why government moves slowly in such matters. Not until 1970, after some dangers of the gadget became apparent, was FDA successful in stopping its sale—after 21 years of marketing. In his decision, a Federal judge declared that the device could contribute to, "heart failure . . . gastrointestinal, orthopedic, muscular, neurological, vascular, dermatological, kidney, gynecological and pelvic disorders," along with possibly aggravating, "epilepsy, hernia, multiple sclerosis, spinal fusion, tubo-ovarian abscess, ulcers and varicose veins."

Massage—whether with hands, rollers, vibrators or any other device—does not make fat go away. In one study, a machine was applied to one leg of the subject and not the other, over a period of ten weeks. In the end, both legs still measured the same.

One illusion of exercise lies with a confusion between pounds and inches. When we increase muscle tone by exercise, our muscles stay slightly tensed, pulling fat in with them. You can see this effect by watching yourself pull in your tummy when you try on new trousers. You are just as fat as ever, but you appear to be narrower.

As the late Dr. Norman Jolliffe said, "As far as I know, there is no machine which can cause a patient to lose weight." He attributed any weight loss in reducing salons to prescribed diets, and a "psychological setting" which is "helpful to the dieter . . ."

Some commercials continue to show smiling patrons lying back on machines which bend and fold them. But it is the machine which is burning the energy (from a wall socket), not the patron.

Every "painless" reducing idea has a market. Consider the book *Cellulite: Those Lumps and Bulges You Couldn't Lose Before.* Author Nicole Ronsard, a salon owner, describes cellulite as "a gel-like substance made up of fat, water and wastes; trapped in lumpy, immovable pockets just below the skin. It cannot be lost by the usual regimen of diet and exercise." She says the lumps are caused by a mixture of tension, fatigue, eating habits, insufficient water, poor breathing, lack of exercise, and polluted air.

It would be tempting to see if the people of smoggy Los Angeles are lumpier than the inhabitants of airier cities. But the fact is that scientists know of no such substance as cellulite. Asked to evaluate the book, one professor of endocrinology, Dr. Charles Lucas, opined that the best thing was "the picture of the pretty lady on the cover."

Ms. Ronsard advocates, among other things, rubbing the lumps in a special way. A number of authors on natural healing feel this helps the figure. Linda Clark recommends a technique for massaging improvement into facial muscles, with a subsequent increase in firmness, saying, "sagging lines and double chins may improve."

This method, called *Profile Symmetry,* "developed as the result of observing a cat cure a muscle wound by licking it gently and methodically. An expert staff of trained muscle technicians have applied this technique to humans. They time the gentle massage to the heartbeat, and at the same time exercise the muscles beneath the surface to increase their tone, circulation and normal tension." One gets the impression, since Ms. Clark refers here to the possibility of "home exercises," that this particular exercise would require a very close friend, if the natural method is used.

If the reducer does not want to be exercised, he might try being "wrapped." There are endless trade names for this. They usually guarantee the loss of inches, not pounds. As *Newsweek* reports on this booming business: "The naked customer is marked and measured by a white-smocked technician, who then takes rolls of wet linen and firmly wraps her . . . from the ankles up, pressing the fat upward."

The customer reclines, is soaked with a secret liquid—one example costs $12 a quart at 112 *Trim-A-Way* salons, but others are said to be merely solutions of cheap Epsom or other salts—and then gets into a plastic suit for 90 minutes. On being unwrapped, the customer is quickly measured, to see how many inches the expensive (often $25) treatment has taken away. Some operators claim the treatment forces water out of the fat. Is this possible? Authority Dr. Morton Glenn, when asked by *Newsweek,* said the idea is "wishful thinking."

Why does the method seem to work? In many cases, diets are given. On a temporary basis, you have only to squeeze one arm, or even a finger, tightly for a minute or two, and you will see that it is temporarily smaller.

The technique concerns some physicians, who fear possible dangers to patients with varicose veins or other forms of vascular disease.

The wrapping concept was part of the idea behind the *Sauna Belt.* But here the squeeze was combined with voluntary exercise. The idea is credited to a California spa owner named Jack Feather, who sprained his knee, wrapped an Ace bandage on it and noticed that when the elasticized cloth came off, his knee seemed narrower. Soon Feather began to wrap the arms of women customers, and then their waists, while they exercised at his establishment. By 1962, the bandage had become a rubber belt. And by 1968 it was getting heavy advertising. In the next six years, Feather is said to have sold 600,000 belts at $10 each with the offer, "If you do not lose one to three inches from your waistline in just three days . . . you may . . . receive an immediate refund."

In a Post Office hearing, Dr. Sedgwick Mead, of the Kaiser Foundation Rehabilitation Center Hospital, appearing as an expert witness for the government, summed up the general medical view of many such devices, when he testified: "There is no really successful way of reducing the waistline without reducing body weight as a whole . . . inert fatty substance cannot be in any way . . . decreased in volume by massage, compression or exercise."

Yet the women's magazines keep discovering such treatments. Current beauty stories often differ little from one in *Mademoiselle* a decade ago, which read: "For months now we've been hearing miracle stories from models about the Ben Benne Salon in New York, whose specialty is REDUCING LEGS . . . first the legs are massaged for an hour . . . then they are wrapped from heel to hip in tight, cocoon-like tapes . . . saturated with a special dehydrating solution. The tapes are left on two hours while you rest . . . and definitely produce a change in measurements."

Newer ads and ideas for "dietless" reducing—which usually turn out to be accompanied by rather strict diets—are more difficult to deal with. (We shall see that even the seemingly easier enforcement cases, such as that of the *Sauna Belt,* backed with 14,000 complaints of failure, usually fail.)

Most of the newer exercises and related systems do not include much exercise, however. After all, the typical buyer does not really want a lot of effort, or he would simply cut down on food and move around more. But mild exercise of short duration really uses little energy. Says Dr. Herbert Pollack, "Half an hour of special arm and leg exercises, for example, might be very tiring, but they would burn very few calories, perhaps those in a teaspoon or two of sugar. You could lose far more weight by spending that half hour in a leisurely walk."

There is a fairly simple rationale which applies to exercise and weight control. First, it must apply to the whole body, not just one spot. For example, at the University of California, Drs. Grant Gwinup and Terry Steinberg measured the forearms of professional tennis players, who are, in a sense, one-armed athletes. If spot reduction through exercise were possible, one could be certain that the playing arms of the tennis pros, put to daily hard use, should have much less fat than the non-playing arms, which are used mainly for balance, for tossing up the ball and for shading the eyes from the sun.

The researchers found that the playing arm was bigger, for it was more muscular. But by measuring with skinfold calipers, they found that the amount of fat under the skin was essentially the same in both arms.

The mathematics of energy hinge on the formula that a pound of body fat represents some 3,500 calories—either in extra food eaten or in extra energy burned. These mathematics are unchanging.

The ability of mankind to fatten is a basic mechanism of survival, because our requirement for fuel is constant. A steady flow of energy is required to fuel life processes—the functions of the heart, the lungs, the brain, and so on. Should we run out of fuel, these organs would stop at once, and we would die.

So the body must have fuel reserves. Otherwise, skipping breakfast could mean death. The body developed the trick of tucking away a reserve of fuel to deal with this danger. The storage process begins in the womb, mainly during the last two months of gestation.

So losing fat is a matter of tipping the fuel scales, so that we burn more than we take in. Because this simple equation is immutable, we can test the truth of any weight-reduction claim.

Consider a direct-mail ad for *Fat Fighters.* "Fat Fighters," the ad says, "is almost a miracle." And this, we see, is true. It would have to be to deliver on the promise that this "simple, sensible way to lose weight without crash or fad diets" makes it possible for us to, "lose up to 5 lbs. in one day, 10 lbs. in a weekend, 20 lbs. in a week!"

To lose five pounds in a day, we must burn 17,500 calories of fuel more than we ingest. Let us assume that we eat nothing all day. Typical American adult fuel need is between 2,400 and 3,000 calories daily. To lose *one* pound, therefore, we must eat nothing all day, and have a larger than normal calorie need.

The ad promises a five-pound loss in a day. Assuming that nothing at all is eaten, and that there is normal physical activity, we can figure how heavy we must be before a day's starvation will make us five pounds (17,500 calories) less fat. The promise is possible, if only we weigh about 1,029 pounds.*

*Based on the fact that the more we weigh, the more calories we burn.

But perhaps this method depends upon burning up more fuel, increasing our activity. Let us see what vigorous activity, such as bicycling or swimming at competition speed, will do. For the average man, either of these activities burns between eight and nine extra calories per minute, or between 480 and 540 calories per hour. To lose five pounds in a day by racing with a bicycle, to the extent that one burns up 17,500 extra calories, takes some 35 nonstop hours. By swimming hard, we could accomplish the same thing in only 32 hours—still hard to do in a day.

Or, we can use our knowledge of calorie requirements to calculate a situation in which the ad would work—a 352-pound young male who does not eat anything while racing a bicycle for 24 hours. However, it does not seem likely that this program would be followed very long.

These mathematics apply no matter what method is used for weight control. Even "the miraculous Slim-Through-Sleep Plan," designed by Frank Rocco, R.H., must conform to the laws of energy. Usually, when slimming is promised while you sleep, either a record is at work with hypnotic suggestion, or a diuretic pill is at work, with kidneys and bladder the targets.

If it is a device, it doesn't matter whether it is the *Skinny Dipper* ($50), the *Trim Twist Exercise Jogger* ($9.95), or a rubber mat on rollers called the *Treadmill* ($235); the energy *you* must deliver to lose a pound is the same.

For example, in his recent nutrition text, the author calculated the energy values inherent in claims for the Joe Weider ("Builder of Beautiful Bodies since 1936") "5" Minute Body Shaper ($7.98 plus $1.00 for shipping and handling). The ads, which have been many, include such headlines as, "They had to pay me to show a photo of myself 14 days ago . . . Not now!" The pictures in the ads are mainly of attractive ladies with exposed navels. In the ad referred to above, a lady is shown twice. The first time, her shoulders are slumped, causing her naval to fall forward (along with other anterior structures which are loosely encased in a bikini top). In the second picture not only are the lady's shoulders pulled back tightly, drawing up her navel and causing her anterior structures to rise up quite a lot, but she also has a big smile. The captions say that she now has a waist, after 14 days, which is seven inches smaller.

The exerciser itself is a system of pulleys which you attach to a door, and then—lying down—pull at with your hands and feet. The author's calculations, with generous allowances for energy burn, showed that if a typical lady used the Shaper 10 minutes a day, with 352 arm and leg raisings per minute, she could burn 70 to 80 calories. Thus, she could by such frenetic movement lose a pound of fat in 44 days.

To lose ten pounds in 14 days, as the lady says she did, she would have to speed up a bit. She would have to move her arms and legs 11,062 times a minute.*

Such numbers become tedious. But they show that weight reduction has no magic.

Grapefruit diets keep reappearing, with the implication that grapefruit dissolves body fat. Grapefruit is often combined with eggs in such diets. We can see why grapefruit in large quantities might produce an illusion of weight loss, especially when, as is the case in some plans, additional vitamin C is added to the grapefruit. Excess vitamin C stimulates the kidneys. Eggs, however, do not. The grapefruit-and-egg diet enables the reducer to stop being just a fat person and become a fat person who uses restrooms a lot—and nothing more.

But the grapefruit-and-eggs diets (one Congressional committee counted more than 50) continue. Typical of such menus is one proposed by salon-keeper Jack La Lanne.

"Let's throw the fat away," Jack suggests. For seven days, he recommends a breakfast of two eggs, grapefruit and coffee. (Coffee, it should be noted, also has diuretic properties.) Then there is a lunch of two or three eggs, tomatoes and coffee, followed by a dinner of two eggs, salad, toast (one slice), grapefruit and coffee.

Along with his material suggestions, La Lanne urges, "Use plenty of Vitamin F-in-G—Faith in God." This injunction takes us to quite another plane, one with which the author is not willing to take issue.

*Such quickness is not within the potential of many—except perhaps for hummingbirds, which are rarely obese.

Indeed, so desperate can be the wish to grow slim, and so difficult the trial imposed by energy's laws, that some have literally fallen upon divine support. In Laguna Hills, California, Joan Cavanaugh found help in faith and lost 90 pounds. From her experience came an organization called PACE*WEIGH. This non-denominational, non-profit organization has had its effect, as have others like it. Says member Lupe Rocha, "I had tried every diet ever invented. With PACE*WEIGH I came to see that my overeating was a spiritual problem." And she lost 50 pounds.

"I consider myself very fortunate," says Ms. Rocha. "In the Old Testament gluttons were stoned to death."

Indeed, in our own time, people who are fat are still put to a kind of social death, if only by themselves. Unfairly, they are treated as gluttons. They shouldn't be. The mathematics of energy contradict popular belief—this time, the idea that fatness means gluttony.

Suppose that we eat only ten extra calories a day beyond our energy needs—an amount provided by little more than half a teaspoon of sugar. In a year, this will add a pound. In 20 years, it will add more than 20 pounds. 20 pounds can drive us from the bikini and lead us to wear our shirts outside our belts at every opportunity. But it is scarcely gluttony.

Heredity, we have learned, is certainly involved. So is the pattern of early parental feeding. For either or both can contribute to the development of more of the cells in which humans store fat, apparently making it much more likely that we will fatten.

Apart from the medical price of obesity, the drive to avoid the stigma of gluttony is powerful. And any number of healers are ready to offer a quick road to slimness.

Not the least appealing of these is Abraham Friedman, M.D. He has an especially attractive way to help. A physician who says that for 25 years he has limited his practice to weight control, Friedman's thinking may be summed up in two of his maxims, much repeated on television. One is: "Reach for your mate instead of your plate." The other is: "Make love, not fat."

The *Ladies' Home Journal,* always quick to bring to its readers the latest wonders of science, presented its condensation of the book with the injunction: "Don't snicker!"

Dr. Friedman's insights begin with the premise that, at bedtime, many of us may be used to eating a snack of "about 700 calories for food and beverage. Now, by substituting sex for this snack," says Friedman, "you are actually saving those 700 calories—besides burning up the additional 200 calories worked off during sexual intercourse."

Friedman, too, applies some mathematics of energy. "Every three times you substitute sex for a 700-calorie snack," he writes, "you'll lose more than one pound."*

(Here it may be meaningful to observe that, in the *Journal* article, there is a picture of Mrs. Friedman and the spare doctor. In the caption, it says that he has "lost 16 pounds since their marriage and attributes the weight loss to practicing what he preaches in this article." According to Dr. Friedman's own data, this would suggest that 48 times they have substituted love for eating. For the sake of their marriage, one may well hope that either (a) they have not been married long or that (b) neither is inclined to snack.)

We might also consider that 700 calories make rather a large snack. For many women, this much fuel might be about a third of daily total calories.

Once more, we might reflect on two possibilities which derive from our energy mathematics. First, checking on the doctor's estimation that 200 calories are burned during sexual intercourse, we note that this is the amount of energy consumed by an hour and ten minutes of moderate canoeing, more than half an hour of waltzing, roughly half an hour of tennis (keeping in mind a study which shows that a professional set of tennis involves no more than six minutes of true action) or some 22 minutes of actual football play.

Returning to our energy mathematics, and to Friedman's estimation of 900 calories saved per marital engagement (700 in food, 200 in love), let us explore two sets of conditions. In one, we might assume that the 700-calorie snack is an extra for his reader, beyond normal bodily need.

---

*Actually, Friedman has miscalculated. Three of these combinations, at 900 calories per instance, would lead to only 2,700 calories lost, not the 3,500 which equal a pound. Unless, of course, Friedman is assuming some very energetic foreplay—say, on racing bikes.

In this case, we find that, without sex, there is a steady gain of one pound every five days, or some 73 pounds gained every year.

Alternatively, the 700-calorie snack might be a regular part of food intake, with which there has been no regular weight gain. In such a case, it is disturbing to speculate on the fate of an affectionate young woman of average size. Before marriage, she would have been consuming about a third of her needed calories before bedtime. After marriage, this part of her fuel would be omitted.

Within two years of the honeymoon, this amorous young thing would *disappear entirely*.

With such hazards and such difficulties of weight control as we have seen here, it is no surprise that the majority of Americans turn to faddish meal plans which promise to make us slim.

17

Protomania
Or
Richard Nixon's Diet Revolution

At the height of his power, Richard M. Nixon could command virtually anything he wanted—at the very least, for lunch. But when noon came at the White House, he held both his appetite and his power in check. His routine order was a dish of cottage cheese, with ketchup on it.

The reason for this odd lunch was not that Mr. Nixon liked cottage cheese so much. In fact, as Patricia Nixon told a *Ladies' Home Journal* reporter, "The only food that Dick really doesn't like is cottage cheese . . . He forces himself to eat it. He puts ketchup on it to make it more palatable."

Mr. Nixon's motive was nutritional. He had a tendency to grow plump. And someone had told him that if he ate cottage cheese and other "protein" foods, he would stay slim. The longer his administration lasted, the more of the White House staff began

217

to eat the same lunch. And while there were sweeping changes when Gerald Ford took over, one of the few Nixonian institutions which remained was the cottage cheese and ketchup. For Mr. Ford, too, had to watch his weight.

Perhaps no single idea about weight control has taken hold in so many minds as the belief that foods high in protein make us thin. The idea is quite false. And while there is no good reason why ordinary folk should have doubted so widespread an idea, it is striking that a man with a personal staff physician and with the best of the nation's scientific advice at hand for the first sign of sniffle or acid indigestion, should follow this pointless and unsafe nutrition advice.

The nation's faith in protein has ancient roots. It probably began with the belief in Greek and Roman times, that meat makes muscle. Linda Clark helps keep the myth alive: "High calorie foods are usually the sweets and carbohydrates and not only upset the digestion but put on flabby fat. Protein, on the other hand . . . puts on solid, hard, healthy muscles."

In the minds of many there are two magical pathways for food in the body. Carbohydrates go straight into the fat, and proteins go to the muscles. This is fallacy. We have seen that there are four major sources of energy to fuel the body—carbohydrate, fat, protein and alcohol. And we have seen that there is an energy balance, with excess calories of fuel being converted to fat and stored. It does not matter where the fuel comes from.

Isn't protein somehow more reluctant to be turned into fat? Not at all. Only so much protein can be put to use in body chemicals and structures. Any excess—and we have observed that virtually all Americans consume far more than they need—is simply burned up for fuel or stored as fat. But there are phenomena which conceal this truth and seem to confirm the magic of protein.

In the fall of 1972, a New York physician named Dr. Robert Atkins published a book about how to be slim, *Dr. Atkins' Diet Revolution,* written with the help of Ruth West, author of such works as *Stop Dieting, Start Losing.* In five months the Atkins book had sold 660,000 copies at $6.95. At one point, the publisher, David McKay Co., was ordering 100,000 copies a week. By late the following summer, after only 11 months, the book had sold "well over a million copies" in the expensive hardcover version and spent 40 weeks on the bestseller lists.

Curiously, the *Revolution* was not so very revolutionary. Its theme was old—to lose weight, eat a lot of foods high in protein and scarcely any which are high in carbohydrate. In 1864, William Banting published a bestselling pamphlet called *A Letter on Corpulence, Addressed to the Public,* with the same advice.

Banting was 66 when he wrote *Letter,* "about 5 feet 5 inches in stature, and in August last . . . weighed 202 pounds." And he couldn't seem to do anything about it. "I have tried sea air and bathing in various localities, with much walking exercise; taken gallons of physic and liquor potassae . . .; riding on horseback; the waters and climate of Leamington many times, as well as those of Cheltenham and Harrogate frequently; . . . and have spared no trouble nor expense in consultations with the best authorities in the land . . . without any permanent remedy . . ."

Banting suffered a lot with his fat, at one time having to go downstairs backwards to avoid pain in his leg joints. Then once when his doctor was out of town, he went to a surgeon named William Harvey. Harvey gave him diet advice, taking away "bread, butter, milk, sugar, beer and potatoes. These, said my excellent adviser, contain starch and saccharine (sweet) matter,* tending to create fat, and should be avoided altogether." Banting was told to eat a lot of beef, mutton, kidneys, fish, poultry and game, with here and there an ounce of dry toast, a daily low-starch, low-sugar vegetable, a little fruit and some wine. He got thinner, and, . . . "Most thankful to Almighty Providence for mercies received and determined to press the case into public notice as a token of gratitude."

The flurry of interest in the *Letter* soon faded away. But it came to popular notice again at the end of the century, when the Earl of Salisbury's weight problem led his doctors to rediscover it and prescribe a diet mainly of meat. The core of the diet was a big patty of chopped beef; thus do we get our name for Salisbury Steak.

The diet has been brought back into vogue repeatedly ever

*The inclusion of butter as a source of much sugar and/or starch suggests the nutritional ignorance of the time.

since. And in the last 20 years, the frequency has been astonishing. Every new version has seemed to sell furiously, reaching a climax with Atkins' and West's book, which was called by the trade press, "the fastest selling book of all time." But perhaps the main question is, why does the plan seem to work?

There are three principal reasons. In its "Study of Health Practices and Opinions," FDA found that about half of Americans were concerned about their weight, and that half of these had been on a reducing diet recently. Authorities say that few people stay on their diets very long; they tend to crash-diet for a short time, expect heroic results and then watch their weight creep up again—in what Dr. Jean Mayer has labeled, "The Rhythm Method of Girth Control." The high-protein diet is admirably suited to such quick dips into abstemiousness; for it seems to give instant results.

Quick weight loss has very limited possibilities. As we have seen, even if we stop eating entirely, we can lose each day only an amount of fat equal to the energy we burn—for typical Americans, between 2,000 and 3,000 calories, less than the 3,500 calories of one lost pound.

So even with exercise, it is hard to lose a pound a day. Half a pound is a good loss. Yet most diet ads seem to promise at least a pound a day. And "Weight Loss By The Hour" advertises: "8 A.M. . . . 126 Pounds! 8 P.M. . . . 124 Pounds! 8 A.M. . . . Tomorrow 122 Pounds!"

How can this be? The answer lies with the old water game. You don't have to take pills to lose water. You have only to change your metabolism. Normally, carbohydrates provide the basic energy source for the body—especially the energy essential to such organs as brain, heart and lungs. This is why glucose, a simple sugar, is dripped into the blood vessels of surgical patients who cannot eat. When proteins and fats are the main energy sources, the body must convert protein to carbohydrate and use fats for energy by a special chemistry.

In a sense, carbohydrate is a very "clean" fuel. Its waste products are carbon dioxide gas and water. But when protein and fat replace the carbohydrate as the fuel supply, there are other waste products. The kidneys flush them out in the urine, using much water to do the job. And the scales go down rapidly.

For many people, this avoids some of the discouragement of reducing. For there is a tendency to retain extra fluid when we start to lose fat. So when we are really getting thinner, we may not see the scales go down for from one to three weeks. We think we have failed. The retained fluid also makes us look as plump as ever. A week of such seeming failure is enough to make a lot of people give up. "I starved and didn't lose a pound," they say.

The water loss of the high protein diet has no more to do with stored fat than has the sweat in a Steambath Suit. We have not thinned; we have been desiccated, like a dehydrated mashed potato. Add water, and we are plump and juicy again.

Along with the deceptiveness of this water loss, there is also danger. It stems from the condition that provokes the water loss, the bodily state known as ketosis.

This is a chemical condition which results from the change of fuel. Dr. Atkins has his readers check their urine with "keto sticks" to make sure that they are in this state, which can be a key problem for the undiagnosed, untreated diabetic, who cannot use carbohydrates efficiently. It is one of the things that makes the diabetic sick. It is also one of the problems of the starving mariner on a raft, helping to account for his confusion and nausea.

Keeping the body in a ketotic state may make long-term protein dieters less interested in eating. But ketosis is also a reason why warning statements about "high protein" diets were issued by the Council on Foods and Nutrition. They cautioned against the real hazards of such diets for those with high blood pressure and other cardiovascular disease, for people with kidney disease and for pregnant women, to name a few.

Yet ketosis was not the only source of medical concern. For the "high protein" diet incorporates another illusion.

This second illusion is perhaps the most serious hazard involved. And it begins with the simple chemical fact that "high protein" diets are mainly composed, not of protein, but of fat. Indeed, using ordinary foods, it is not really possible to choose a diet in which protein is the main nutrient.

For even such "high protein" foods as beef are rarely more than 20 to 30 percent protein. Nearly all the remaining calories are in *fat*. "High protein" dieters are generally on very high fat diets.

A fatty diet has three key health effects. First, it is a primary cause of the *ketosis* and water loss. Second, it makes the foods consumed a compact source of many calories—shutting most foods from plants out of the diet and leading to shortages of the nutrients we need to get from plants. And, thirdly, it may be involved in heart and blood-vessel disease.

On the other hand, the fatness of "high protein" eating is one thing which makes it attractive to so many. For the fatty substances in foods are the main carriers of flavor. And it is fat we speak of when we say that foods are "rich." So fatty meats and sauces and the like are considered by most to be the luxury foods.

Isn't it nice to believe Atkins and West when they write: "On this diet you are allowed to eat truly luxurious foods without limit—for example, lobster with butter sauce, and not merely hamburgers, but rich tasting cheeseburgers . . . as long as you don't take in carbohydrates, you can eat any amount of this 'fattening food' and it won't put a single pound of fat on you."

For all these reasons, *protomania* in weight control seems to come back stronger in each of its endless reincarnations.

For example, Atkins' co-author, Ruth West, had written much the same thing in her 1956 dieting book. The publisher's blurb reads in part: ". . . This method is based on the de-calorized, high-protein system. Excess protein not only gives you energy, helps keep complexions clear, hair sparkling, health at top form, but also speeds slimming . . . the presence of excess protein makes it possible for your body's metabolism to burn up unwanted fat."

The book hardly went unsold. E.P. Dutton and Co. gave it six hardcover printings, and Bantam Books started its paperback version in 1957 and reached the eighth paperback printing in 1962. But it could scarcely match the Atkins book.

The first modern impetus for the diet began with an article in *Industrial Medicine* in June of 1949. Drs. Gehrmann and Pennington reported on its use with Du Pont Company personnel. Magazines such as *Holiday* picked up the idea.

Then came the so-called Air Force Diet, in 1960, essentially the same thing, published by a Canadian firm. While this was very popular, protomania really got rolling with the publication of Dr.

Herman Taller's *Calories Don't Count.* Taller's book had an added emphasis, which was to be its eventual downfall; he recommended adding oils to the diet, especially *safflower oil.*

In the late 1950's safflower oil had begun to enjoy a vogue for the prevention of heart disease. Known as *Carthamus tinctorius,* safflower has long been used and cultivated in China, India, Egypt and the south of Europe, partly for medicinal purposes, but mainly as a yellow dye, which is why it is also known as "bastard saffron."

Some African doctors, experimenting with oils high in polyunsaturated fatty acids, found that they seemed to produce a drop in blood cholesterol. Safflower oil is high in polyunsaturates, and the safflower was being grown and pressed locally. There are other oils which are not significantly different in their content of polyunsaturated fatty acids, and which are cheaper.* But safflower had a nice, unfamiliar ring and quickly took the foodists' fancy. Unhappily, it was soon found that the reduction in blood cholesterol level was temporary.

But safflower's name for health was established. Production of the plant boomed, particularly in California. For one thing, safflower seeds mature in midsummer, when cotton and other oilseed crops are not keeping the oil mills busy. Furthermore, the yield is very high; in California, safflower yields over 2,000 pounds of seed per acre. And the residue after pressing makes a good 20 percent protein cattle feed.

When Herman Taller put out his high protein, low-carbohydrate diet, he included the taking of two safflower oil capsules before each meal. Thus were combined safflower's association with weight reduction and its name for lowering cholesterol. The market boomed. By 1962, over half a million acres were under cultivation in California, with a seed potential of over a billion pounds.

When *Calories Don't Count* first appeared, the oil was not easy to get—especially in capsules. And the book said to use capsules. On September 27, 1961, the day *Calories Don't Count* was published, CDC Pharmaceuticals (the reader may guess what CDC stands for) started business operations. The business was making capsules of safflower oil.

*Corn oil, for example.

The book was a smash. And the first 11 printings contained a commercial announcement for the CDC capsules, manufactured by Cove Vitamin and Pharmaceutical, Inc., of Glen Cove, New York. As then FDA Commissioner George Larrick explains: "This was the basis of an attempted crash promotion of safflower oil as an aid in reducing and to lower blood cholesterol, treat arteriosclerosis and heartburn, increase resistance to colds and sinus trouble, improve sexual drive, and for other purposes."

FDA began to investigate and found what Larrick calls ". . . a surprising story. This best selling book had been edited in such a way as to promote and sell these worthless . . . capsules. Dr. Taller had prepared a draft and the publisher had it revised 'in more of a mail order inspirational technique' . . . This manuscript was then sent to the office of Kenneth Beirn, an employee of the General Development Corporation. When returned it contained the commercial announcement mentioning Cove as a source of the capsules. Cove and others then established a closed corporation, the CDC . . . to market the capsules for which the book would create a demand. Financial interests in the new company were acquired by a limited group including Cove, Dr. Taller, Beirn and others. Two vice presidents of the publishing company (Simon and Schuster) acquired options to purchase stock."

The capsules and the book were seized where they were sold together, the book being construed as mislabeling for the oil. The drug company filed, but then withdrew, an answer to the Federal charges. Says Larrick, ". . . because the publishers and the author refused to support the health and diet claims made in the book."

The reader might suspect that this made publishers gun-shy about such books. On the contrary; what they had seen was a lesson in success, a lesson of 2 million books sold.

McKay, the publisher of Atkins' book, sold some 1,100,000 copies in hardcover alone during the first year. The authors' royalties are unknown. But the publishing convention is 15 percent of the retail price of a hardcover book. If this was true for Atkins and West, then the hardcover royalty on *Revolution,* in the first year, should have been $1.04 per book, or some $1,144,000. This, of course, is only an estimate.

The publisher would have discounted the books to stores at

about 40 percent. So its *gross* take should have been $4.17 per copy, or about $4.5 million before costs. Again, if conventions were followed, the hardcover publisher got half the proceeds from the paperback version which has sold several times as many. The usual paperback royalty is 10 percent of retail price.

Even on a much more modest scale, a diet or health-food book remains a good investment. Small wonder that some of our best publishers are unperturbed by medical criticism. Indeed, the more attacked a book is today, the better it is likely to sell. It is hard to find a distinguished publisher which has not given us an undistinguished book on nutrition.*

The theme of *Calories Don't Count* was printed indelibly in the public mind. Never mind that a bean, a potato, a slice of bread really had only a few calories. It wasn't the calories that counted; it was the fact that carbohydrates were "fattening." The idea was quickly reinforced.

For example, there was soon *The Drinking Man's Diet.* It was addressed to the businessman: "Your personal and social responsibilities, not to speak of your tastes, call for a good deal of eating and drinking . . . Your health—or so you have heard the authorities claim—demands that you cut down to a semi-starvation diet which is bound to leave you short-tempered and anti-social. Our diet wipes out the dilemma . . . It can be summed up in one sentence: EAT LESS THAN SIXTY GRAMS OF CARBOHYDRATE A DAY. That's all there is to it."

In 1965, the year after the *Drinking Man's Diet* took hold, Carlton Fredericks entered the lists with *Dr. Carlton Fredericks' Low-Carbohydrate Diet.* The cover featured the slogan, "The book that started the diet the whole country is talking about!" The reader may draw his own conclusions about this statement.

Fredericks gives much space to Banting's *Letter on Corpulence.* And then he acknowledges Taller's contributions. "Dr. Herman Taller," he writes, "reapplied the principle, which became famous in his book *Calories Don't Count.*" Fredericks now speaks of the "abuse" given the book by medicine, and says that it

---

*For example, despite all the medical outcry about Atkins' book, another publisher was quick to take his *Superenergy Diet,* and *Family Circle* published a condensation of it.

actually had "scientific validity." He adds that, "To understand
the motivations for the slander," we should read "the last chapter
in this book."

The last chapter turns out to be written by Herman
Goodman, M.D. It portrays Fredericks as a victim of Federal
persecution. "What was the sin?" asks Goodman. "Dr. Fredericks
sat at his microphone. He told the truth about science, nutrition
and big business . . . Toes stepped on? You bet!" Goodman says
that "the word" went out, "from a coalition of government
agencies, trade associations, business bureaus, university nutrition
departments." He adds that the media and "scientific societies,
medical and dental organizations, dietetic associations joined." He
also says that there were "no legal charges."

The FDA has another view. According to its statements,
Fredericks (who was Harold Fredericks Caplan in college)
graduated from the University of Alabama in 1931 as an English
major. FDA says that Fredericks was hired by U.S. Vitamin
Corporation in 1937, ". . . to write advertising copy . . . Later,
Fredericks was sent out to give talks to promote the sale of
vitamins . . ."

In the 1940's, Fredericks began to make radio broadcasts and
write books. According to an article in *The Reporter,* he answered
listeners' inquiries on stationery headed, "Institute of Nutrition
Research, Carlton Fredericks, Executive Director." The magazine quotes a typical form letter for such replies, which asks for
$3.00 for a supplement called FOOD-EX, which the company
would mail.

In 1945, the State of New York brought Fredericks into
court. *The Reporter* story says that three investigators had appoint-
ments with Fredericks, and that one described an array of
symptoms. "Defendant said that I was lacking certain vitamins
. . . that mine was not an odd case, that he had many patients with
similar complaints . . ." According to *The Reporter,* Fredericks
charged a $10 fee and prescribed a diet. He was fined $500, for the
illegal practice of medicine.

He got his Ph.D. from New York University's School of
Education in 1955, writing his thesis about listeners' responses "to
a Series of Educational Radio Programs."

In 1960, Fredericks had been listed as "chief consultant" to a firm called Foods Plus, Inc., when FDA seized some 200,000 bottles of its products, charging "false and misleading" labeling. Indeed, Fredericks has had a series of problems with Federal agencies, including the Food and Drug Administration, the Federal Communications Commission and the Federal Trade Commission. To understand the tenor of these "persecutions," we might note a March 4, 1962 ruling, in which a Federal court in New Jersey upheld a seizure and injunction case filed by FDA against 42 Foods Plus, Inc. products. This decision was a landmark, because it was the first time that a broadcast was construed to be labeling of a product.

In his decision, Judge Reynier J. Wortendyke, Jr. found that Fredericks had recommended, "various vitamins and dietary supplements as remedies and/or preventives for human ailments which included the following: Respiratory diseases, circulatory diseases, cystic mastitis, club feet, paradentosis, neuritis, lowered thyroid activity, disturbed elimination, high blood pressure, strokes, rheumatic fever, tooth decay, allergies, damaged brain and nerve cells in children, multiple sclerosis, hardening of the arteries, lack of mental resistance to house-to-house salesmen, varicose veins, vertigo, mental disorders, lack of resistance to cancer, epilepsy, shingles, Bell's palsy, amyotrophic lateral sclerosis, lack of resistance to radiation, arthritis, gray hair, rheumatoid arthritis, mongolian idiotism, lupus erythematosus, sexual frigidity, heart disease, muscular dystrophy, coronary thrombosis, cerebral palsy, nervous system diseases, Peyronie's disease, angina, diminished vigor, nervousness, glossitis, tartar on teeth, infertility in women, lack of mental alertness, for longer life, for tightening loose teeth, for pain and discomfort in glandular cycles, scleraderma, bursitis, and premenstrual tension, backache and cramps."

The resulting Federal injunction did not apply to Fredericks personally. For he had terminated his contract with the company. But such were his claims.

Such is the quality of support given to the high-protein diet. In 1967, it was given a big lift by a book called *The Doctor's Quick Weight Loss Diet,* by Dr. Irwin Stillman, of Coney Island, and writer Samm Sinclair Baker * The book refired the national

---

*Their success inspired them to author a series of books of similar value, such as diet advice to teenagers.

imagination. And why would it not? The idea had always worked.

The opening case histories are inspiring. "In one case, a woman who had 'tried everything' without being able to reduce, dropped 25 pounds the first week on the Quick Weight Loss Diet, 67 pounds in 4 months . . . She . . . has improved her health and has achieved a lovely slim figure, to the amazement and delight of her family and friends . . . Neither she nor any other of my patients, not a single one, suffered ill effects from quick and dramatic weight losses. Every one of them enjoyed a new glow of healthy vigor and vitality . . . and each undoubtedly added years of life . . ."

Who could resist such a promise? Yet if we apply our energy mathematics, we see that a weight loss of 25 pounds in a week requires eating some 12,500 calories per day less than one's body burns. This, we see, is entirely possible—as long as the patient fasts entirely and weighs 735 pounds to start.* Of course, we are told that the lady has lost 67 pounds in all, and that she now has a "lovely slim figure." If the lady did weigh 735 pounds to begin, this means she now weighs 668 pounds. With every concession to poetic license, it is hard to envision a lady weighing 668 pounds as having a lovely slim figure, unless of course, she is rather tall.

But Dr. Stillman adds to our problems of credulity by saying, "You can eat as much of fine foods on the list as you need to satisfy your hunger."

The list of approved foods is very explicit. And Stillman says, in capital letters, "NOTHING ELSE IS PERMITTED ON THIS DIET—NOTHING! IF IT'S NOT MENTIONED IN THE PRECEDING LIST, DON'T EAT OR DRINK IT." We see that we may eat all we wish of ". . . beef, lamb and veal, with the fat trimmed off, chicken and turkey with the skin removed, all lean fish, such as flounder, haddock, cod and perch, eggs which are not fried, cottage cheese, farmer cheese and pot cheese made with skim milk," and all the water we can hold, but at least eight glasses a day.

The diet and the book made a howling success. It hammered home the idea, once more, that carbohydrates made you fat and protein let you get slim again. Total copies sold to date are said to exceed five million.

*The heavier the person, the more calories he burns merely by being alive.

Meanwhile, Dr. Atkins was waiting his turn. He was working for a physician who was medical consultant to A.T. & T., the telephone company. According to *New York* magazine, in 1963, Atkins had to have his picture taken for identification. (After all, the telephone people can't be too careful about who will ask their executives to remove their trousers and cough.) Atkins saw in the photo that he had three chins, where one should have been. He decided he had to do something, and he picked up on the old Pennington diet from Du Pont. He later told *New York* that, "after just six weeks on his diet he lost 28 pounds." He went on to say, "I don't get much exercise and I have a weakness for French fries."

Atkins claims that in 1964 his diet worked for 65 telephone executives. In 1966, the plan was written up in *Harper's Bazaar.* It caught on. Never mind that the comments of genuine authorities were typified by those of Dr. Jules Hirsch, of the Rockefeller Institute, one of the world's leading researchers in obesity, who called the diet, "the most unutterable nonsense I ever saw in my life."

The *New York* article records some of Atkins' regrets. "I admit," he is quoted, "kidney stones are a conceivable complication . . . They are very rare among my patients . . . Increased cholesterol? . . . of the thousands of people on my diet, only 30 percent of them show any increase.* Of these, only 8 percent have a significant increase that could be a problem." (So if all Americans took his advice, there woud be significant cholesterol increases for only 18,400,000 people.) ". . . There's one other point that I'm very sorry about. I recommended the diet during pregnancy. I now understand that ketosis during pregnancy could result in fetal damage."

From the mid-1960's on, a veritable flood of books on the same theme appeared, each with its own small wrinkle. For example, there was Sidney Petrie's *Martinis & Whipped Cream, The New Carbo-Cal Way to Lose Weight and Stay Slim.* Written in association with Robert B. Stone, the book flatly states that, "The carbohydrate calorie is more fattening than any other kind of calorie," an idea for which science has no support. But from this

---

*Atkins said in 1972 that he had given the diet to 10,000 people. So he would have raised the cholesterols of only 3,000 patients.

concept comes the "carbo-cal" list. It turns out to be nothing more than a listing of the number of calories derived from carbohydrate in the listed foods.

The public's appetite for such books seems insatiable. *Martinis & Whipped Cream* is said by the publishers to have sold 150,000 copies at $5.95 in hardcover. While small compared to Atkins' sales, the reader should appreciate that this number represents a very great publishing success. Sales of Barbara Kraus' list of *Calories and Carbohydrates* in 7,500 foods have also been high. *The Boston Police Diet,* essentially similar, had a nice flurry.

And from all these books, the magazines took a huge supply of diet articles. One author kept track of seven large-circulation magazines for two years. *(Harper's Bazaar, Mademoiselle, Good Housekeeping, Ladies' Home Journal, Vogue, Seventeen and Redbook.)* In the first 12 months, from March of 1969 to February of 1970, these journals carried 26 diet articles. In the following year, they carried 38.

While some of these articles were sound—*Redbook* and *Good Housekeeping* have had responsible nutrition reporting for some years—most were gimmick-oriented reports, such as "Chewing Your Way to Health," "Sexual Vitality," "Peace" and "Hot Dog Diet The Three Star Way."

Such magazine launchings can reverberate for years. *Harper's Bazaar,* which gave Atkins a national audience, started another movement in 1962. This came from an Italian physician named Dr. A.T.W. Simeons, who told of the wondrous results of injecting dieters with a hormone called HCG *(human chorionic gonadotropin),* produced by the outer covering of the fertilized ovum.

The American Medical Association's Department of Drugs cited a double-blind study in which HCG had no more effect on weight reduction than did injections of salt water. The drug experts concluded that they found, "no scientific evidence from controlled experiments to justify the use of HCG in the treatment of obesity."

Physician-nutritionist Dr. William McGanity, of the University of Texas, also pointed out, in answer to a question addressed to the *Journal of the AMA,* that the HCG injections were being accompanied by a 500-calorie a day diet. Such a diet is of course extremely limited. It is quite hard to get adequate nutrition even from a 1200 calorie diet.

There is certainly little question that any adult who weighed more than 30 pounds would lose weight on a 500-calorie daily diet. (On the other hand, few people of this weight would be on a diet.) Even a rather small woman requires some 2,000 calories a day and cannot be adequately nourished with 500 calories of food, in terms of all needed nutrients.

Nevertheless, many people have patronized chains of weight-reducing clinics which use HCG. Most of these, sadly, are owned or directed by medical doctors.

Both ridicule and serious professional criticism have been directed at the method, and at such clinics, for more than 13 years. Yet they continued to boom—despite such statements as one from the AMA, that, "because of the unproven usefulness of HCG it would appear that there is an ethical question raised when any physician engages in such a weight loss scheme. There may even be legal questions involved."

The Federal government felt there were legal questions. In 1975 the Federal Trade Commission finally ordered two such clinics in Los Angeles to stop advertising the therapy. At about the same time, FDA ordered the following addition to the "Indications" in all HCG labeling:

"HCG has not been demonstrated to be effective adjunctive therapy in the treatment of obesity. There is no substantial evidence that it increases weight loss beyond that resulting from caloric restriction, that it causes more attractive or 'normal' distribution of fat, or that it decreases the hunger and discomfort associated with calorie restricted diets."

Book and magazine publishers continue to offer new "discoveries" in weight control and in general nutrition—often the same ones over and over again. Magazines and newspapers continue to accept spurious ads for eating and exercising systems.

Part of the publishing problem may be simple innocence. It is hard to believe, but the very people who disseminate so much nutrition information have little or no valid knowledge on the subject, and often do not think that they need to get any.

It is interesting, in this light, to read *Cosmo* editor Helen Gurley Brown's introduction to *Cosmopolitan's Super Diets & Exercise Guide.* "The reason I don't balloon up is because . . . I *diet.* And diet simply means eating sensibly . . . Once in a while I will *have* . . . along with other 'baddies' like fettucini Alfredo and buttered corn muffins . . . some Swiss chocolate—but most of the time I'll be good. . . . I virtually exist on high-protein, low-calorie foods—I do like health foods . . ." And she tells us that she has learned from the *Guide,* "how to cook for my husband David and myself when he's on a more rigorous no-carbohydrate regimen than I am . . ." Thus, the nutritional sophistication of much of the press.

The *Guide* follows the popular pattern of turning to celebrities as nutrition experts. Here is some typical celebrity nutrition advice. Rod Steiger is quoted on losing thirty pounds: ". . . This is the diet that did it. Breakfast was my biggest meal: two eggs, poached; sausages; black coffee . . . Six or seven cold shrimps for lunch. Dinner was cold chicken with crisp lettuce (no dressing)."

It is not hard to see the roots of Steiger's belief—or that his eating makes for very poor nutrition, as all the "protein" reducing schemes must be. But let us check through *Cosmo's* lists of good diet examples to notice how consistent is the pattern.

Says David Niven, "I won't eat nonsense foods . . . I'll eat a man-sized steak." Says Joan Crawford, ". . . fruit for breakfast . . . or a boiled egg. Midmorning . . . cheese. For lunch, a slice of boiled chicken . . . one or two whole tomatoes . . . No bread ever." Says Patti Page, "No starches, bread or sweets." Says Katharine Ross, "High protein . . . cakes, pies, chocolates are *verboten.*" Says Eva Gabor, "I crash-diet with grapefruit, pots of coffee, a teeny steak or bite of chicken, and a lettuce leaf or two . . . I usually go to a health spa for a weekend and let them take over." Says Nancy Reagan, "The Governor and I . . . when we dine out at political banquets, we push the mashed potatoes into a far corner of our plates." *Et cetera.*

To be sold, both books and magazines must be promoted. Enter newspapers, TV and radio. In one ten-day period soon after his book came out, Atkins appeared in Los Angeles, San Francisco, Denver and New York. He did 34 newspaper interviews, one for a magazine, 12 radio and nine television shows locally and *The Merv Griffin Show.*

"It has to be damn worthwhile for me to leave my office, and I expect every minute to be filled when I do," he told an interviewer. This is quite understandable. In a *Women's Wear Daily* interview, Atkins said that he and his partner, Dr. Ira Mason, had an office which required the services of ten nurses and 23 rooms. If 23 rooms are needed to hold the patients two physicians are examining, one can estimate quite a high volume of patients. Atkins said that they treated perhaps 500 patients a week.

New York magazine reported that each patient comes in first for a $125 work-up and then pays a substantial sum for each regular visit. Simple mathematics tell us that Atkins and partner must see far more than 1,000 patients a year on a regular basis. If we guess that each of these may come in from 10 to 40 times a year, we can posit a tidy income. When we put diet books by physicians in perspective, it may be worth considering one inevitable advertising effect of such authorship. And this is why medical ethics set some rather tight standards on self-promotion for physicians. Television, book and magazine promotion of special diet methods by physicians is easily interpreted by the public as an ad saying, "Have I got a diet for you!"

Some 20 years ago, Representative Blatnik's Congressional investigations concluded that, "The advertising of so-called obesity remedies or weight-reducing products is an area fraught with deception and outright fraud . . .

"These alleged . . . remedies . . . usually promise an unsuspecting public virtual automatic weight reduction by way of statements such as 'no diet reducing' or 'eat plenty and reduce' or similar claims . . ."

Eager for the sensational, most book publishers and magazine editors suspend not only good sense but all investigative responsibility as well. With a plethora of scientific information available to them from the nation's regulatory agencies and research institutions, these media arbiters prefer not to ask any questions when they find a hot new diet idea.

Since 1949, as we have seen, "high-protein" reducing has been a national fad. In 1976, *Forbes* magazine gave its verdict.

Malcolm Forbes himself made the appraisal. He needed to lose "a dozen pounds." So he, "checked all the stuff and guff on the subject." His conclusion? "Low carbohydrate is where it's at, fellow obesities."

He expounds: "You can almost literally stuff yourself with steaks and every meat, fowl, fish—fried, sautéed or richly sauced . . . Out are sugars, starches . . . Anyone who remains as brainwashed as we all were . . . on the low-calorie approach is either unaware, masochistic or taking the advice of those who are . . ."

How important is it that Malcolm Forbes and so many others who have the public ear believe in this nutritional myth? The fact is that high-protein eating is not only ineffective for weight control. It also represents a harmful nutritive pattern—one with health implications far beyond the national plague of fatness.

18

Swing Low, Sweet Glucose Tolerance

In 1970, the American Osteopathic College of Preventive Medicine conferred its first honorary membership upon Carlton Fredericks, "a leading nutritionist for over 30 years."

In celebration of this honor, Fredericks presented a talk based on his then recent book, *Low Blood Sugar and You.* According to the organization's publication, *The D.O.* (Doctor of Osteopathy), Fredericks urged that patients who showed signs of "emotional disturbances, depression, excessive perspiration, mental cloudiness, fatigue, suicidal tendencies, incoordination, exhaustion, drowsiness and headaches" should be considered to suffer from hypoglycemia, or "low blood sugar."

Such a patient, *The D.O.* reports, "should be put on a high-fat, high-protein diet . . . This type of diet . . . helps to correct low blood sugar . . . Dr. Fredericks also spoke of a number of uninvestigated areas in which hypoglycemia may be a factor, including asthma and alcoholism. He noted that it was an osteopathic physician who first devised a high-fat high-protein diet for epileptic control." And he went on to advise the osteopaths about therapy—telling them about a liver supplement he had made up.

Fredericks was scarcely alone in raising an alarm about low blood sugar. Within a generation the management of hypoglycemia has become a major medical enterprise—surprising when one realizes that the problem has little reality.

In 1973, a joint statement of physicians and scientists appeared in the *Journal of the AMA*. It was prepared by the Council on Foods and Nutrition in concert with the American Diabetes Association and the Endocrine Society. It began:

"Recent publicity in the popular press has led the public to believe that the occurrence of hypoglycemia is widespread in this country and that many of the symptoms that affect the American population are not recognized as being caused by this condition. These claims are not supported by medical evidence . . ."

What sort of publicity? As an example, in November of 1971, a lady named Mary Scott Welch told the millions of readers of the *Ladies' Home Journal:* "If you're not really sick but you don't feel really great either, maybe you have *HYPO-GLYCEMIA.*" The reader who has followed foodism through the centuries can see what a bonanza this might be—a "disease" in which you aren't actually ill.

The *Journal* lists a dozen cases as a starter, cases which, we might as well say at once, correlate very nicely with some classic symptoms of neurosis. We are told about Helen, who "feels tired all the time"; Paula, who is "constantly on edge"; George, who "wakes up at 4 A.M."; Lydia, who "can't concentrate well"; Yvette, who used to "make beautiful love," but hasn't had it so good of late; Ed, who is apathetic and is "turning into a blob"; Meg, whose doctor "says her light-headed spells are imaginary." And more.

The trouble? As we pointed out before, glucose is the primary fuel of the body. The glucose which circulates in the blood to feed vital organs is known as the *blood sugar.* The *Journal* and an armload of other popular magazines tell us that many people use up their blood sugar too fast. Such people are supposedly injured by a diet which contains a lot of carbohydrate (sugars and starches).

Fredericks posited several causes of the vulnerability to his osteopathic audience, the primary one being "hyperinsulinism." In other words, low blood sugar is supposed to be a kind of mirror image of diabetes.* So if diabetics tend to produce too little insulin to use up the sugar in their blood, "hypoglycemics" have too much insulin; they burn up blood sugar fast and run out of fuel. Fredericks and his fellow believers say that "hypoglycemics" should put more fat and protein into their blood, so that the "excess insulin" can't cause their fuel to be used up so quickly.

Mary Scott Welch takes us with her into the private precincts of the doctor's office, and the bloodstream of a lady known as Lucy, a department store buyer and mother of three. Ms. Welch meets Lucy through a Dr. Alan Cott—a medical paperback author on food and health. Lucy was having temper tantrums and making bad buys. Dr. Cott ordered a Glucose Tolerance Test (GCT).

GCTs are cited by healers and patients alike as absolute evidence of low blood sugar. Ordinarily used to identify diabetics, the GCT requires an overnight fast, followed by a jolt of sugar water in the morning at the lab. For possible diabetics, the test is most meaningful. The diabetic usually cannot handle a sudden onslaught of sugar; his blood sugar level bounces upward and comes down very slowly.

After the big swig of sugar, hourly blood samples are checked. Ms. Welch tells us that Lucy's test showed that she had a "clearcut physiological reason for the tears and temper, the self-doubt and indecisiveness, the agitation and sleeplessness."

How did the doctor identify this reason?

"We watched the impersonal numbers take on immediate . . . meaning: 75, 180, 125, 100, 50, 75, 78. Here was the profile of hypoglycemia."**

---

*One health-food journal calls it "diabetes upside down."

**The numbers of a GCT refer to the milligrams of sugar found in each 100 grams of blood, or milligrams/percent.

But was it? Ms. Welch, presumably informed by Dr. Cott, describes as "normal" a GCT in which 100 milligrams/percent is the fasting level, in which the high is 160 and within three hours there is a return to 100.

Actually, 60 may be a normal fasting level. And "normal" blood sugars may well dip below this. Indeed, one of the nation's foremost authorities on the subject, Dr. Thaddeus Danowski, of the University of Pittsburgh's School of Medicine, has found that perhaps 20 to 25 percent of "normals" show levels between 45 and 60.

Setting the "normal" levels for such a test at 100 is akin to deciding that 98.6 degrees is abnormally low body temperature. It is putting that minimum at least 67 percent higher than it should be. If this error were applied to body temperature, anything lower than about 165 degrees would be abnormally low.

Mary Welch tells us that treatment for Lucy is to cut back on sugars and starches and eat more protein. This therapy is credited to Dr. E. M. Abrahamson, "noted blood sugar specialist."

Apparently, Mary Welch closed her article before a review of the subject by *Consumer Reports* appeared in mid-1971. It noted big sales of Dr. Abrahamson's book (written with A. W. Pezet).

According to *Consumer Reports* the book, written 20 years before, had gone through 23 printings and sold over 200,000 copies in hardcover. Pyramid Books had described Abrahamson/Pezet's work, titled *Body, Mind, and Sugar,* as, "A Brilliant Medical Advance!" and called low blood sugar, "an illness that affects 10 to 30 million Americans!" It had been reviewed by the late *New York Herald Tribune* as "A valuable contribution to the vast subject of human nutrition."

The book blames most suicide, murder, and alcoholism on low blood sugar. Abrahamson and Pezet (described as a writer "of both fiction and nonfiction") decry low blood sugar as responsible "for the moral breakdown that underlies all delinquency and crime."

According to *Consumer Reports,* "The authors conceded that their views were not accepted . . . but this they said was 'largely because most doctors have not yet had time to read the literature.' "

While Abrahamson recommended only dietary change, Dr. John Tintera (of Yonkers, New York) treated "the problem" differently. He began to inject ACE (adrenal cortical extract, a hormone mix taken from the adrenal glands of animals). Tintera said low blood sugar also caused mental disorders and allergies. And in 1958, he said so in *Woman's Day*.

The Westchester County Medical Society censured Dr. Tintera for the article, but the censure seems to have had little effect. Tintera became, according to *Consumer Reports,* "the fountainhead for much of the erroneous information disseminated by the Hypoglycemia Foundation."

Tintera began a trend of giving ACE as treatment for low blood sugar. For example, his local medical society received a complaint from a young professor, *Consumer Reports* tells us. Tintera had given him injections of ACE for low blood sugar, once a week for seven months, and "allegedly told the young man that he would need the injections the rest of his life. After having spent hundreds of dollars on ACE, the young man entered a hospital for a series of tests, which revealed no abnormalities." Since that time, Dr. Rachmiel Levine, a leading authority on the body's use of carbohydrates, has described ACE treatments for low blood sugar as "acute remunerative therapy."

Low blood sugar has become a darling of foodism. *Newsweek* notes that health columnist Dr. Peter Steincrohn called it "the most commonly misdiagnosed disease." It observes that "Mrs. Marilyn Light, a former hypoglycemic who runs the Hypoglycemia Foundation from her home in Mount Vernon, N.Y., estimates that one in five Americans suffers from the disorder . . ." It adds that there are supposedly "500-odd physician members" of the Foundation.

For well over a generation, the threats and promises concerning hypoglycemia have steadily mounted. There is Dr. Samuel Homola's book, *Naturally Youthful Health and Vitality,* in which he says: "If you suffer from fatigue, weakness, headache, irregular heartbeat, dizziness, trembling, cold sweats, inability to think, excessive hunger, depression, mental illness or any number of 'nervous' ailments for which there appears no apparent cause, you may be suffering from hypoglycemia." And Dr. Atkins assures us that, "The commonest reason for a patient to walk into a doctor's office is that he has hypoglycemia which hasn't been diagnosed."

In itself, hypoglycemia is not merely a figment of an acquisitive medical imagination; but neither is it a disease, nor even a disorder. When a patient's sugar levels are low, the doctor merely has a sign of possible trouble. If he finds the sign, he should look for the cause.

All of us have low blood sugar whenever we go too long without food. How much discomfort is experienced seems to vary from individual to individual, and for the same person from day to day. Some of the discomfort is physical and some is emotional. The person who is very anxious about his food responds to the physical symptoms of hunger with more fear and anger. Consequently, he is more likely to experience cold sweats, trembling, headache, even panic.

Why? First, let us observe the psychiatric axiom that food has the deepest sort of symbolic meaning for all of us. Second, the anxious person not only takes a delay of feeding badly, but his anxiety can actually have the effect of depressing blood sugar. And finally, anxiety can produce nearly all the symptoms attributed to low blood sugar by popular writers.

If we review the supposed signs, we see that they have a large emotional component. For example, a mail-order ad for Dr. J. Frank Hurdle's book, *Low Blood Sugar, a Doctor's Guide to Its Effective Control,* says that its program for "Blood Sugar Balance will lift you to *new heights of superior health and vitality."* The ad says the program will make us "A NEW PERSON . . . when your resistance to disease is multiplied a hundred times . . . when you are virtually free of headaches, tensions, sleeplessness, and all kinds of mental upsets . . ."

In another book, *Goodby Allergies,* elderly Oklahoma Judge Tom R. Blaine (who says he is a cured hypoglycemic) tells us that he now requires people in divorce cases to take glucose tolerance tests. He claims that marriages can be saved by diet. A publication of the Hypoglycemia Foundation, *Delinquent Glands, Not Juvenile Delinquents,* claims that, "controlling hypoglycemia . . . could do much to . . . reduce alcoholism and drug addiction; to combat juvenile delinquency, mental retardation, chronic fatigue . . ."

Looking again at the ad for Dr. Hurdle's book, two cases are cited. One is of "a middle-aged man who trembled so violently that he was convinced he had Parkinson's disease." Another is of a "woman suffering from a supposed 'severe reaction to menopause' characterized by depression and unwarranted fears . . . sleeplessness, nausea and overall misery."

Could too much carbohydrate and too little protein really be at the root of all these emotional and physical changes? Says the joint statement of the three scientific societies: "There is no good evidence that hypoglycemia causes depression, chronic fatigue, allergies, nervous breakdowns, alcoholism, juvenile delinquency, childhood behavior problems, drug addiction or inadequate sexual performance."

The statement adds that, "a great many patients . . . anxiety reactions present . . . similar symptoms." Indeed, if we consult a good text in psychiatry, and if we compare the signs of *anxiety neurosis*—considered by many to be the most common form of neurosis in our society—to the symptoms held out in popular books on hypoglycemia, the two patterns match beautifully.

In *Clinical Manifestations of Disorders,* Dr. Louis Linn lists some of the typical physical signs of anxiety neurosis and of its acute manifestation, *anxiety reaction:* "There is hypersensitivity to ordinary sights and sounds, as a result of which startle reactions occur frequently . . . Cardiac palpitation, breathlessness, giddiness, nausea, dryness of mouth, diarrhea, compulsive eating, urinary frequency, seminal emissions, blurring of vision, general physical weakness . . . may occur chronically."

Foodists have a simple response. "How do you know that anxiety symptoms don't come from eating carbohydrates?" Indeed, they seem to have convinced much of the American public that this is exactly what happens. The link between carbohydrate and wayward emotion seems to be well accepted.

Consider the intimate tale of actress Suzanne Pleshette's personal life, as revealed in *Family Circle.* "During the filming of *A Rage to Live,* she was uncharacteristically quiet and very tired. Her doctor diagnosed her condition as hypoglycemia." Suzanne says, "I was frightened . . . I'd never before been sick in my life." She now is on a "high protein" diet and says she feels better.

Suzanne shares some of the secrets learned from her low blood sugar, such as ". . . a wonderful trick with potatoes. I bake them, scoop out the inside, which is only carbohydrate and makes you fat, and throw it away. Then I charbroil the skins, which are nearly all protein . . . I even phone the restaurants . . . and ask them to save the potato jackets for us when we go out to dinner."

Unfortunately, there is not much protein in potato jackets; they are mainly carbohydrate, too.

Johnny Carson's television viewers are often treated to the advice of an Oregon pediatrician named Dr. Lendon Smith. Recently, Smith took his homely counsel to another network—to ABC's *A.M.* show in Los Angeles (where Jack La Lanne is the fitness expert, and Carlton Fredericks is billed as "*A.M.*'s nutritionist"). When a viewer phoned in a question about hard-to-manage teenage emotions, Dr. Smith promptly recommended that the parent check to see if the youngster had eaten sugar or starch in the preceding three hours. Host Regis Philbin sagely nodded his agreement.

It is hard to have any understanding of life chemistry and still view carbohydrates as poisons. Let us see why.

All the energy of life comes from just one source, the sun. Humans have no way to take in this energy directly. But plants can trap solar energy by using it to combine carbon dioxide and water.

The product of this combination is a "hydrated carbon"—or *carbohydrate.* Sugars are the basic forms of carbohydrates.

Glucose (dextrose) is the most common basic sugar in food. Then comes *fructose* (fruit sugar). These are found in virtually all plants, separately and in combinations.

One of the most common combinations is a molecule of each of these two. That makes *sucrose,* the sugar you see in your sugar bowl (whether the bowl holds raw sugar, white or brown). Sucrose is also present naturally in most plants.

Plants can string glucose molecules together in chains of hundreds. This makes a more compact storage form for energy—as in the berries of wheat or the kernels of corn. Such chains of sugars are the starches.

Plants employ "hydrated carbons" as the main raw materials of their chemistry. For carbon, hydrogen and oxygen (the elements one finds in carbohydrates) are the main elements of all life. 94 percent of your body is composed of them.*

It is in this light that scientists have trouble believing that carbohydrates make us sick or crazy.

But popular books seem to ignore the evidence. George Watson, Ph.D., author of *Nutrition and Your Mind*, writes, "What you eat determines your state of mind and, in a sense, the sort of person you are."

His publisher says the book tells how Watson has taught "hundreds of 'difficult' patients . . . which basic American 'super-market' foods . . . may actually be responsible for . . . headaches, nervousness . . . insomnia, claustrophobia, 'Christmas Blues,' sexual inhibitions, compulsive overeating and 'emotional' distur-bances."

The ads say Watson is "a leading chemical psychologist," though the jacket of the book says his field is "Philosophy of Science." In any event, *McCall's* describes the book as "a formida-ble feast for thought," and *Esquire* calls it "detailed and carefully documented."

Watson's hypothesis on food and emotion is actually fairly complex. To keep on a steady keel, he says, we must know what our "psychochemical type" is. Some people, for example, seem to get a little strange eating carbohydrates, while some others seem to get a bit odd by *not* eating them.

The basic concept is made clear in *Cosmopolitan*'s summary of the book. There is a big picture of two cartoon ladies. One has frizzy hair, staring eyes, a frown, large hips, a low bust and is eating a hamburger and French fries with soda pop and pie à la mode. She says, "I eat the food that's *wrong* for me, and I'm bad-tempered, anxious, fearful, suspicious and upset!"

The other lady has long, wavy hair, mascara on her eyes, a nice smile, cute hips and a high bust. She is eating what looks to be an apple, salad, chicken and vegetables. She says, "I eat the food that's *right* for me, and I'm open, friendly, relaxed, cheerful, efficient, and serene!"

The choice looks pretty clear. What sensible *Cosmo* reader is

*The same three elements also compose fats and the vast bulk of protein molecules as well.

going to look at this picture and then eat pie à la mode, at the risk of becoming frizzy-haired and unlovable?

Attempts to justify the longstanding foodist indictment of "starch and sugar" have been made for generations. And most have been on rather weak grounds.

For example, Lelord Kordel explains that starches do their dirty work by clogging the bowel. They tend to get stuck. Then when the bowel is clogged, the poisons of digesting food stay inside us, making us feel awful.

Kordel tells of a man who suffered from both constipation and eye trouble. Kordel advised him to disdain starches and eat proteins. The man did and is quoted, in a state of both ocular and intestinal relief: "Life, it's wonderful—when your bowels and your eyes let you enjoy it!"

The latest popular nutrition seeks more complex explanations, not so easily challenged by common sense. Most of these newer ideas center about two kinds of carbohydrates—"refined" and "unrefined."

Perhaps the chief spokesmen for this approach are Drs. Emanuel Cheraskin and W.M. Ringsdorf, Jr., who both teach dentists at the University of Alabama. Cheraskin is a frequent lecturer at dental societies across the nation. There is a good chance that your dentist got his ideas about nutrition from one or both of them.

The pair are well known for their bestseller, *New Hope for Incurable Diseases.* This was presented by the publisher with such claims as, ". . . Multiple sclerosis, glaucoma, schizophrenia, alcoholism . . . aging . . . can be controlled or prevented with proper diet," and Bantam Books offered their bigger seller, *Psycho-Dietetics,* with the cover blurb that the book told how, "Changing your eating can relieve nervousness and irritability, reverse memory loss . . . help you achieve a happier . . . emotional life."

Publishing in the journal *Natural Food News* (a publication of Natural Food Associates of Atlanta, Texas), the Alabamans say that refined carbohydrates "contribute to a plethora of malnutrition."

They back up this statement with a bibliography of five references: studies by (1) Cheraskin, Ringsdorf and Clark (presented by Rodale Books), (2) Clark, Cheraskin and Ringsdorf, (3) Cheraskin and Ringsdorf, (4) Cheraskin and Ringsdorf again, and (5) Cheraskin, Ringsdorf and Brecher.

From such sources, and a few others (including Linus Pauling, who recommends taking a lot of vitamin C for colds; Roger Williams, whose latest book featured an endorsement by Adelle Davis; and John Yudkin, who says that sugar should be banned as a dangerous substance), the authors conclude that, "refined carbohydrates play a role in diabetes, hypoglycemia, gout, kidney stones, urinary infection, peptic ulcer, cardiovascular disease, dental caries, periodontal disease, overweight, intestinal cancer, diverticulosis, indigestion, hormonal disorders, oral and vaginal infections, osteoporosis, alcoholism and mental illness. In contrast, unrefined carbohydrates . . . do not contribute to these disorders."

Some of these connections with carbohydrate are very surprising. The reference to carbohydrates in vaginal infections is especially puzzling, whether refined or unrefined.

We must remember that ultimately human digestion puts our food through a very severe refining process. In terms of carbohydrates, for example, they cannot pass through the wall of the intestine and get into our bloodstream except as simple sugars. The long chains of starch, for example, must be broken apart into the individual glucose molecules. The sucrose of table sugar must be broken into one molecule of glucose and one of fructose.

The sugars go to the liver. There any sugar which is to be released into the blood is first changed by the liver into glucose—if, of course, it was not already glucose. The cells care no more about the original source and form of this fuel than your car cares whether the gasoline it gets was refined from Arabian or Texas oil.

J. Daniel Palm, the author of *Diet Away Your Stress, Tension and Anxiety*, says that glucose is bad stuff. His writings have helped to create a recent run on supplies of pure fructose. While there is some evidence that fructose may be converted to fat at a greater rate than other sugars, much of it is changed to glucose. The only improvement seems to be in the profits of the health-food store.

None of this should be taken to mean that we could live on nothing but sugar, or that there is no limit on how much sugar we can healthfully eat. We do need to get carbohydrates from other foods for the other nutrients which they contain. And one of the medical reasons why low-carbohydrate diets of any kind are unsafe is that they tend to eliminate important nutrients we should be getting from grains, vegetables, and fruits.

When nutritionists caution against eating too much pure sugar—we actually consume little pure starch—it is not because sugar is a poison. It is because unlike most other foods, pure sugar comes with no other nutrients. This is equally true even of somewhat impure sugar foods, such as honey, raw sugar and maple syrup.

Why are people so quick to believe that a basic nutrient such as carbohydrate is at the root of their emotional difficulties? Says Dr. Thaddeus Danowski: "It is easier to say, 'I have hypoglycemia' than to say, 'I can't cope.'"

The wish to believe can be very strong, however. Not long ago, the author had just completed a lecture at the University of Florida, when a nice lady in her fifties stopped him.

NICE LADY: I hope you won't think I'm rude, but you're wrong about low blood sugar being emotional. I had it, you see, and I felt just awful until I knew what it was.

AUTHOR: I'm glad you're feeling better.

NICE LADY: I am, and when it started, I thought I was going to die, really die. I was away from home and all, and I didn't know where to turn. But emotion had nothing to do with it, because it was all over.

AUTHOR: What was over?

NICE LADY: All the crying and everything. I was up in Georgia and having to go through all Mother's things and sell the house, after she passed away. In fact, I had just signed the papers that day, and I had been there for two months, so I wasn't emotional. It was over.

AUTHOR: It's a hard thing to do.

NICE LADY: Yes. But when I signed the papers, and I knew I was going home again, then it was all done. And that was the night it started.

AUTHOR: Started?

NICE LADY: All the symptoms. I was all packed up, you know, with all of Mother's things, and then I woke up in the middle of the night, and I couldn't breathe. My heart was pounding, and I felt so scared, and there was no reason, and I sat up in bed, and I was sure I was going to die. Well, I managed to phone the neighbor, and she came over and she got me to the hospital. And the doctor in the emergency room, he gave me a shot to relax me, and finally I could breathe again. But I didn't get over it until I found the *real* cause. Until then, even my husband thought I was going to die, because I kept on waking up and feeling cold and clammy, and not being able to breathe, after I got home.

AUTHOR: How did you find out what it was?

NICE LADY: One of my best friends, I told her, and she said the same thing happened after her father died, and she knew this doctor who could take care of it. I went to see him, and at first he couldn't find anything, and then he asked me what did I eat before I went to bed that night, and I remembered about the chocolate-covered peanuts. And you know what he said?

AUTHOR: No.

NICE LADY: He said it was the chocolate-covered peanuts. They're full of carbohydrates, you know, *refined* carbohydrates. It wasn't anything to do with emotions. It was the sugar and all. And that's what I want you to know—about the *real* low blood sugar, about people like me.

There is endless scientific evidence to refute the fad that carbohydrate consumption is somehow linked to the welter of unrecognized emotional disturbance which is one of the hallmarks of our culture. It may, however, be worthwhile to note a letter written a few years ago, when the fad began.

The letter is from Dr. Walter C. Alvarez, whose good sense made his newspaper column so well received, and whose long years at the Mayo Clinic had endowed him with the respect of his colleagues. Asked about hypoglycemia, Dr. Alvarez said that he thought he might have seen, "the first patient known to science with a *real* low blood sugar. He had a cancer of the beta cells in his pancreas."*

Among the, "hundreds of persons I have seen who had been told they had low blood sugar . . . my laboratory could not confirm it . . . not a single one had any sign of it. My feeling is that it is one of those diagnoses that a doctor makes if he wants to make a raft of money; also if he wants to get women with neuroses out of his office quickly, and very happy about what they have. They don't want a diagnosis of 'just nerves.' That makes them very angry."

*Indeed, when blood sugar is genuinely low, the cause may be early diabetes. Extremely low sugar may mean serious disease of the pancreas or liver.

19

How to Sell a Vitamin

Today, many a misguided customer spends $100 or even $200 a month on special foods, pills, tablets, capsules, and elixirs to bring vitamins into his life.

Recently, Dr. Thomas Jukes of the University of California's Space Science Laboratory made some calculations on the bulk, wholesale cost of those vitamins. A very ample month's supply of the ten vitamins most commonly found in supplements is worth less than six cents.

This helps to explain why so many people like to sell vitamins. But why people like to buy them, when they could easily come free with sensibly chosen meals, is harder to understand. The secret seems to rest with a literature of spurious fear and hope that has surrounded vitamins ever since they were given to the first pigeons—the avian, not the human ones.

Cathryn Elwood is a leader among vitamin stylists, as we can see in her book, *Feel Like a Million*. You can find the book in any of thousands of health-food stores. For it is one of those works which furnish both a party line for the hard-core foodist—and a sales pitch for the health-food store.

We have only to ask what it is to "feel like a million" to get a sample. It is, Cathryn Elwood tells us, "an exuberant state of dynamic health that brushes disease germs aside as easily as the hot sun melts away the frost; that knows no weariness or fatigue and that actually strikes off the day's duties with the greatest of ease. Every precious moment of life becomes a treasure . . ."

The promise gets more specific. If we try her program, Cathryn says, "Soon you will find your hair more luxuriant, your eyesight sharper, your skin more velvety, your arteries and heart more youthful, your blood redder, old life-filching fatigue beating a retreat; your senses will be keener, you will stand taller, with your head higher, just from sheer natural energy and the normal tone of stronger muscles . . . With all this . . . bills for doctor, dentist, psychiatrist, hospital, medicine, stimulant and sedative will go flying out the window, along with your sufferings, miseries, hurts, peeves, failures and problems."

The secrets are nutrients, of course, and the special foods—ordinary ones rarely do—which contain them. The function of each nutrient is shown in its relationship to illness. For instance, since a lack of certain B vitamins, such as niacin, can produce nervous symptoms, if we have such symptoms, we need only take *extra* niacin and be well.

Cathryn, like so many of her colleagues, is big on special mixes of wonder foods, with very specific product endorsement. For example, "The Lindberg Nutrition Service (a California chain of health-food stores) . . . has blended a super product which I'd like to see served daily in every home in America. It is desiccated liver, powdered molasses, brewer's yeast and skim-milk powder."

The promises continue. "How would you like to increase your . . . intelligence?" she asks. All we have to do, she says, is eat food with glutamic acid in it. And unless we happen to remember the names of the amino acids, we are not likely to recognize that glutamic acid is one of them, and one of the most plentiful in everyday foods.

Then she lays out a basic diet—beginning with three servings of leafy vegetables each day, cooked, plus a couple more eaten raw. To this we add a pint of vegetable juice and two large servings of fruit juice.

We should get our yogurt every day—Miss Elwood explains how Metchnikoff discovered that yogurt was the secret of long life for the Bulgarians—together with a half cup of bean sprouts, a half cup of wheat germ embryos, a tablespoon of peanut oil, kelp or fish, plus some protein sources. To make this all complete, we should spend an hour naked in the sun, for this is our most natural source of vitamin D, being careful not to take a bath for several hours thereafter, lest we wash the vitamin D away.

This is really all we need for daily nutrition—except for a few commonsense additions, such as three tablespoons of blackstrap molasses, a like amount of brewer's yeast, a few tablespoons of skim-milk powder with ground bone added for more calcium and a little lecithin.

If we must snack, we should try, "a hearty nibble on sprouts." And of course we should exercise, ending always, "with a favorite headstand or an upside-down rest on your beauty board."

In addition to this everyday wholesome eating, Miss Elwood tells us about extras for special problems. For arthritis, as an example, "Cherries in goodly amounts have helped some, as have melons." Bad arthritis may require a fundamental dietary alteration—such as the raw food diet, the all fresh green diet and the like.

(As a technical note, the Arthritis Foundation has for some 20 years warned that diet is generally unavailing as a cure for arthritis—with the exception of special dietary restriction of *purines,* in cases of gout.)

In true traditional style, when Miss Elwood gives dietary instruction, she avoids the use of cold, simple facts. Let us join her as she has just returned from a funeral. A young father has died prematurely of a heart attack. Miss Elwood goes to the home of the widow, who is now bereft of all but small children.

It is lunch time. Miss Elwood sits idly at table while the new widow prepares the noon meal. A little tyke waits for the food, pounding his spoon for attention, unaware that Daddy will not be coming home again.

At last Mother appears with a dish in her hand. And on the dish is a fried hamburger.

"Like a dirge," Miss Elwood writes, "my thoughts ran round and round: 'A living melodrama this . . . she killed him but she loved him. There on the table is mute evidence of her weapon. And now she is crippling her beautiful children.

" 'Silently, slowly . . . the children of the man she loved and killed. Oh God, please show us how to put this vitally important message over to these kind, loving, but nutritionally ignorant people. My eyes scanned the table again, hoping to find one little milligram of vitamin E. Not one.'

". . . If only I could tell them how vitamin E prevents muscles from becoming riddled with holes and torn with lesions that fill with water. This was the cause of their Daddy's enlarged heart . . . Her own ignorance of food, about vitamin E and whole grains, about food and health is the cause of her sorrow."

Vitamin E has in recent years become the focus of many such harrowing tales of the foodist bookshelf. And indeed, some of the threats and promises are valid—for laboratory animals, but not for people.

As a *British Medical Journal* editorial concludes: "For as long as we can remember, vitamin E has danced before us like a will-o'-the-wisp, promising cure of everything from Depuytren's contracture to infertility. Yet when it comes to writing a prescription, vitamin E must be one of the most rarely used therapeutic agents . . . Many . . . even doubt whether it is a vitamin at all."

The excitement began in 1922, at the University of California. Drs. H.M. Evans and K.S. Bishop were feeding rats special diets free of a certain fat fraction. The rats could not reproduce. When green leafy foods were added to the diets, normal fertility resumed. The rats proved to have been missing vitamin E.

In the early 1930's, when these experiments were little known, the Shute family, in Windsor, Ontario, became curious about vitamin E. Dr. James Shute was interested in a study of menstrual problems, and seems to have connected them with the infertility of female rats which lacked vitamin E. Shute's eldest son, Dr. Evan, got involved and also Evan's younger brother, Dr. Wilfred. The story is fuzzy, but apparently, some of the people in the menstrual experiment showed some signs of relief from blood-vessel disease, after taking E.

The Shute family began to make surprising claims for the vitamin. And then *Time* ran a story about the claims. Soon some inferred, without any basis, that the vitamin not only restored fertility, but also did wonders for heart disease and sexual potency. And the floodgate opened. Today, Wilfred Shute's book, *Vitamin E for Ailing & Healthy Hearts,* claiming success with 30,000 patients, is still a big seller. Said Dr. Wilfred: "I hope this book will be the means of making available to all sufferers from heart disease the help they deserve—a proved, successful treatment."

Sadly there is not much chance that it has, or will. As noted clinical nutritionist Dr. Robert Hodges sums up the medical evidence: "Recent studies completed by Anderson . . . in Toronto and others at the National Institutes of Health in Bethesda fail to provide convincing evidence of the effectiveness of vitamin E . . . This echoes the results of similar studies throughout the world, all showing almost uniformly disappointing results . . ."

Dr. John Bieri of the National Institutes of Health, former president of the American Institute of Nutrition, confirms these conclusions: "Claims for beneficial effects of supplemental vitamin E are largely based on unwarranted extrapolation of animal studies to the human situation, or to misunderstanding . . . *There is no clinical condition in which vitamin E has been clearly proved to be beneficial.*" (Emphasis added.)

None of this seems to be heard, or believed, by foodists. In 1974, the Food and Nutrition Board cut the RDA (Recommended Dietary Allowance) for vitamin E in half—from 30 units a day to 15 units. And no one seemed to notice. Adelle Davis was still taking *1,500* units a day and urging everyone to follow suit.

The enthusiasts keep pointing out that vitamin E has brought babies to happy rat mothers, that its lack caused blood problems and symptoms like those of muscular dystrophy in monkeys, produced brain damage in chickens and heart attacks in calves. The scientists keep saying that none of this happens with people. But no one seems to hear them.

Between 1953 and 1961, the National Research Council sponsored studies of volunteers whose vitamin E was severely restricted. For six years, they were given "tests designed to reveal any changes in mental or physical health . . . No apparent change was caused by the low dietary levels [of E]." In fact, so available is vitamin E in the American diet, and so little seems to be needed, that true vitamin E deficiency has not been observed (in humans) by physicians in the U.S.

As the U.S. Food and Drug Administration sums it up: "There is no scientific evidence that vitamin E will do any of the dramatic things that are being claimed for it."

Yet the claims go on. By 1972, Mennen was advertising, "Vitamin E, incredibly, is a deodorant."

Authorities agreed that it was indeed incredible. And these ads stopped. Not so all the rest.

The vitamin was supposed to combat the effects of smog. Why? Experiments by Dr. Aloys Tappel showed that animals which got *no vitamin E at all* were more susceptible to smog hazards than those which got ample amounts.*

But *Prevention* enthused: "When factory smokestacks belch their black contaminants into the air, when automobiles send exhausts streaming out over highways and cities, jet engines trail engine debris over landscapes coast to coast . . . Run, do not walk, to the nearest vitamin shelf and stoke up on . . . vitamin E!"

Health-food books pound away at the need for vitamin E, and producers of wheat germ and wheat germ oil (good vitamin E sources) do not discourage them. What is the logic of those who push the vitamin?

A good example comes from *Everything You Want to Know about Wheat Germ,* by P.E. Norris. As nutrition writer Carlson Wade puts matters in the book's preface, "All those concerned with using Nature's foods for healing and for prolongation of life, should know what wheat germ can do to help create cellular-tissue rejuvenation in the body and mind." Wade refers to E as "precious youth and stamina-building." He says that "the fertility-virility power of vitamin E as found in wheat germ, makes this a 'must food' for everyone, male and female."**

---

*Given with chemical anti-oxidants of the type commonly used to retard rancidity in foods, additives which are severely attacked by foodists.

**It is unclear why women would want the "virility power" of vitamin E.

Norris takes it from there. He says that wheat germ is the richest known source of vitamin E. Quite untrue. Gram for gram, some seed oils have three times as much. And he adds that lack of E "is the cause of sterility, abortion, impotence, loss of virility, sundry sexual disorders, some forms of paralysis and other ills."

Norris implies that a lot of supposedly E-related health problems arose after white bread got going. And he says, "In India, where . . . little white bread is eaten, the people seem as fertile as ever . . . the population increases at the rate of 5–6 millions each year." He adds that the Russians eat nice dark bread, too, and that it is, "responsible for the tremendous fertility of the Russians. Between 1930 and 1940 the Russian population increased by 24 million, whereas the population of *all the other countries in Europe* increased by only 32 million." He is particularly sad about Britain, where he says that the introduction of white flour came in "1870 when the birth rate was about 36 per thousand. The more popular white flour became, the faster the birth rate fell, till in 1940 it reached . . . about 14 per thousand."

This is very convincing to foodists, but not to scientists, who observe that there is more to reproduction than bread. One can also note that India has fewer television sets than we do, and that Western birth rates have tended to decline with the increasing ownership of dishwashers and steam irons. Does this mean that sending steam irons to India would solve its population explosion?

Similar arguments are advanced about cancer and heart disease. True, these diseases have increased since the turn of the century. But so has the longevity of Americans and Europeans. And these are largely diseases of older people. Moreover, our diagnostic abilities have improved dramatically.

Nevertheless, Shute (who also is part of the Alsleben Shute Foundation for Nutritional Research, the object of which is in large part to teach the public "self-protection through personal preventive medicine") joins in the arguments about E and heart disease. He actually writes that, "Coronary thrombosis . . . is the greatest single killer in the world today . . . coronary thrombosis was unknown as a disease entity in 1900 and apparently hardly existed at that time."

Shute's conclusion? "It is irrefutable that when new and

more efficient milling methods were introduced . . . the diet of Western man lost its only significant source of vitamin E. With the loss of this natural anti-thrombin, coronary thrombosis appeared on the scene."

There are rare instances in which vitamin E really is used medically, as with some premature infants and in diseases in which fat cannot be absorbed. But even when E is used medically, the amounts given are small. And the reader who decides to try generous doses on himself, thinking they can't hurt, is wrong. All vitamins can be toxic at excess levels, and fat-soluble vitamins are especially harmful. For the surpluses are stored, not excreted as water-soluble vitamins.

UCLA's Dr. Roslyn Alfin-Slater, who has chaired the Food and Nutrition Board committee on the vitamin, reports that excessive intake in animal studies has resulted in, "depressed growth, interference with thyroid function, increased requirements for vitamins D and K and higher lipid (fat) and cholesterol levels in the liver. In humans, supplements of vitamin E above 400 units per day revealed . . . complaints of nausea, intestinal distress, fatigue, flu-like symptoms and a variety of non-specific complaints."

Dr. Victor Herbert, who is Clinical Professor of Pathology and Medicine at Columbia's College of Physicians and Surgeons, reports "possible undesirable effects" to include, "headaches, nausea, fatigue, giddiness, blurred vision, inflammation of the mouth, chapping of the lips, intestinal disturbances, muscle weakness . . . increased bleeding tendency, degenerative changes, and reduced human gonadal (sex gland) function (i.e. just the opposite of the increased function claimed by those making money pushing megadoses of vitamin E)."

Such medical reports are rejected by foodists—with some strange reasoning.

Consider, for example, Dr. Miles Robinson's introduction to one of the books which has done most to promote vitamin E— Herbert Bailey's *Vitamin E: Your Key to a Healthy Heart.* Robinson notes that, "The author of this book has some severe criticisms of those presently in control of official medical groups, such as the American Medical Association, and governmental agencies, such as the Food and Drug Administration, for their indifference to vitamin E." Explaining this "indifference" on the part of the AMA, for example, he says: "Probably the chief and insidious reason for this is that the AMA has been much corrupted." The corruption is said to come through, "income from drug companies which advertise in its many journals."*

Author Bailey's statements are stronger. He discovered the magic of vitamin E by treating his own heart disease with it. He advises that doctors will probably tell patients not to count on the vitamin for heart problems, and urges them to, "follow exactly the same course I did back in 1957—take vitamin E anyway. It's nontoxic."

Bailey's book is subtitled, "The Suppressed Record of the Curative Values of this Remarkable Vitamin." And he devotes a chapter to this suppression. "Alas," he says, anticipating objections to the idea that physicians, who devote themselves to healing could deliberately deny known cures to patients, "the orthodox thinkers have become so . . . rigid, so fanatic that some members . . . would rather die than consciously admit a wrong . . ." He says that Canadian and American Federal agencies tried to "destroy . . . crush anything and anyone daring to present views opposing . . ."

One finds the same protests about "suppression" throughout the foodist literature. They are legion in discussions of vitamin C.

Probably the only vitamin more popular than vitamin E is L-ascorbic acid, or vitamin C. The story of scurvy, and of the British seamen who suffered from it until the ships began to carry limes and other fresh fruits and vegetables, is perhaps the best known vitamin tale.

Nutritionists have pointed up the need for vitamin C-rich foods since long before the discovery of the vitamin itself, in 1928, and its later isolation. It is a very simple chemical, which can be made from ordinary glucose by the body of almost any animal— except the ringtail and some other monkeys, the guinea pig, an Indian fruit-eating bat and man.

---

*It should be noted, as Dr. Thomas Jukes has pointed out, that a number of these drug companies sell vitamin E, so they are not likely to conspire to keep people from buying the vitamin.

The human need for vitamin C attracted the early interest of the nation's citrus-fruit producers, who began to advertise citrus as the morning's source of vitamin C—until vitamin C and orange juice became almost synonymous in the public mind. Their success led them to pursue other nutritional ideas about oranges, too. For a time, they thought they had hold of two more winners, bioflavonoids and vitamin P.

In the early 1950's, one citrus marketer began to supply writers with releases saying that not only vitamin C, but also vitamin P and Bioflavonoids might cure or prevent infections such as the common cold. The idea was mainly that certain membranes appeared to be weakened in vitamin C deficiency—as evidenced by some of the hemorrhaging in scurvy—and that this weakening might let germs take hold.

Very quickly, the American Chemical Society concluded that there really was no vitamin P. Medicine and biochemistry concluded that the bioflavonoids in oranges supplied no nutritional need. The anti-cold properties of vitamin C were rejected by the researchers themselves. But the public went on remembering some of the early promotion.

Then in 1966, Mr. Irwin Stone wrote a letter to Dr. Linus Pauling. He had heard Pauling say that he would like to live another 15 or 20 years. "He said," writes Pauling, "that he would like to see me remain in good health for the next *fifty* years, and that he was . . . sending me . . . his high-level ascorbic acid regimen."

Pauling is an unusual man, at this writing 75 years old, a biochemist who in 1954 received the Nobel Prize for his work on the nature of chemical bonds. Soon after, he became very politically active in anti-war movements, writing the book, *No More War*. It was probably an important time for such thinking, but it was politically, an albatross. He was treated unfairly not only by politicians, but by scientific colleagues. This probably did not help his disappointment when, after years of work, he was beaten by a team of young scientists to the discovery of the structure of DNA, the secret of heredity. Pauling was certainly gracious about this scientific defeat, but he must surely have felt a little disheartened. The DNA discovery won a 1962 Nobel for the young researchers. In that year, Linus also won the prize a second time—but for peace, not for chemistry.

In any event, in 1966, while Pauling acknowledges his realization that Mr. Stone was exaggerating about vitamin C, he and his wife tried it; so some aspect of Stone's promise must have interested him. "We noticed," he reports, "an increased feeling of well-being, and especially a striking decrease in the number of colds that we caught, and in their severity."

The ultimate result was a book, *Vitamin C and the Common Cold*, and a very popular fad. But we may infer that Pauling was really interested in more than colds: "I estimate that complete control of the common cold and associated disorders would increase the average life expectancy by two or three years. The improvement in the general state of health resulting from ingesting the optimum amount of ascorbic acid might lead to an equal additional increase . . ."

In his 1970 book, and in more recent speaking and writing, Dr. Pauling enlarges on the promise of vitamin C. Dr. Thomas Jukes has compiled a list of vitamin C uses proposed by Pauling, which includes, "treating the New Year's Day hangover, virus diseases, bacterial infections, for the prevention and treatment of cancer, the common cold, vertebral disc lesions, for the healing of wounds, fractures and burns, protection against heart disease, for increasing mental alertness . . . for decreasing age-specific morbidity and mortality as much as 75 percent . . ."

How is all this to be done? Pauling recommends that all adults should be taking extra vitamin C every day, from 4 to 10 *grams* (4,000 to 10,000 milligrams), for many health purposes. The combined thinking of the Food and Nutrition Board sets a desirable intake of this vitamin for most adults at 45 milligrams a day. In other words Pauling thinks we should be getting from 100 to more than 200 times as much as nutrition science finds to be ample. Remember, too, that only about 10 milligrams a day, about a fourth of the FNB recommendation, prevents scurvy.

In other words, Pauling urges us to try eating more than three to six months' supply of vitamin C daily.

And if we feel a cold coming on? He urges that we carry some 500 mg. tablets with us and take a couple at once, and then take 1,000 mg. every hour. (This is a little less, at least, than the recommendation of North Carolina's Dr. Fred R. Klenner, who in his popular book, *The Key to Good Health: Vitamin C,* prescribes 1,500 mg. every hour for the first 10 hours, then 1,000 mg. an hour for the second day.)

How did Pauling arrive at such enormous intakes as normal and desirable for humans? He explains that he, "checked the amounts of various vitamins present in 110 raw, natural plant foods . . ." Then he calculates how much vitamin C would be present in 2,500 calories of such foods, "corresponding to one day's food for an adult."

Pauling has somehow estimated that man once had the ability to make his own vitamin C, but lost it 25 million years ago. He appears to have deduced that this loss of ability took place because man was getting plenty of C-rich plant foods. He then describes a "natural" intake of vitamin C which would have required the eating of some rather large volumes of food.

The average for the 110 raw, natural plant foods Pauling examines is some 2,300 mg. in 2,500 calories of them. (The 2,500 calories represent a typical energy need for a day, as supplied by the total day's food.) However, he notes that some of the richest sources—he gives the example of peppers, "hot or sweet, green or red"—would provide some 9,400 mg. of vitamin C in 2,500 calories.

This sounds reasonable, until we apply nutritional mathematics. These tell us that Pauling's early man would have gotten only 49 calories from a cup of green chili peppers. To get 2,500 calories, he would have needed 51 cups a day.

If we take a more modest C source, such as snap beans, they have 31 calories per cup. So 2,500 calories would be provided by 22.5 pounds a day.

But Pauling has overlooked the decline in man's energy expenditure in recent years. As recently as 1900, a man needed 4,000 daily calories. So even a 1900 man would have needed over 129 cups of string beans a day, 45 pounds of hot green peppers or 71 quart jars of spinach. We can see how hard life must have been in the old days, if Pauling is right.

What good does so much ascorbic acid do? The American

Academy of Pediatrics has expressed one of the milder reactions: "There is no acceptable scientific evidence that ascorbic acid will prevent the common cold." The Academy's Committee on Drugs advises doctors, "Any chemical compound, including water, may produce toxicity if taken in sufficient quantity. This is especially true for the fetus, infant and child . . . Physicians who care for children need only recall the experiences with vitamins A and D to recognize the danger in reasoning 'that if one unit is good, two must be better' . . . There is not sufficient evidence that ascorbic acid in doses recommended by Dr. Pauling is either safe or efficacious in the prevention or treatment of the common cold. Until such data are available, ascorbic acid should not be used for this purpose."

What do pediatricians fear in massive doses of vitamin C? Columbia's Dr. Herbert recently reviewed the known hazards. For despite such repeated statements as that of Adelle Davis ("There is no such thing as a toxic C."), there have been untoward incidents. For example, babies of mothers who took massive amounts of C during pregnancy have developed actual signs of scurvy when they no longer received so much C after birth.

Says Herbert: "The pushers of large doses of C do not bother to inform the public that large doses . . . can produce 'rebound scurvy' . . . The machinery of the body for destroying C is sharply speeded up when one is taking megadoses. This speeded-up machinery will then continue to function at high speed when one goes back to normal doses, and one may suffer . . . a transient case of scurvy, with swelling and bleeding of the gums, loosening of the teeth, muscular pain and skin roughening . . .

"There is also evidence . . . of . . . adverse effects on growing bone, inaccurate tests for sugar in diabetics causing them to take dangerously wrong doses of insulin, and false negative tests for blood in the stool . . . kidney problems . . . menstrual bleeding in pregnant women . . ." Herbert also notes that such doses can produce blood-cell damage in people with a certain enzyme lack—a lack found in 13 percent of American black males, some Orientals and some males of Mediterranean origin."

Hodges, of the University of California, also lists many hazards, including interference with bodily use of copper.

Exponents of vitamin regimes do not take such criticism lightly. Dr. E.V. Shute, the vitamin E man, summarily rejects negative research in a long appendix in Herbert Bailey's adoring book (*Vitamin E: Your Key to a Healthy Heart*): "In this series, only 20 percent were helped [by vitamin E]. There must therefore be something wrong with the arrangement of the experiment, or with the observations."

Pauling is even more argumentative about the refutations of his vitamin C ideas. In some late editions of his book, he adds whole chapters of argument with the medical community, focusing on three sets of experiments which were his main evidence on cold prevention and cure. One study was the work of Cowan, Diehl and Baker, who in 1942 had published results of a study with Minnesota students.

Pauling says that in the summary part of their paper, "they suppressed . . . facts." The researchers' summary said in part, "This controlled study yields no indication that . . . large doses of vitamin C . . . have any important effect on the number or severity of infections . . ."

When Pauling published his book, Diehl wrote to the *New York Times,* saying that his 30-year-old experiment showed no positive result. At the time of the study, Diehl and the others had nothing to gain by declaring failure. Indeed, they might have made quite a name by claiming success. Yet Pauling accuses them of bad judgment and omission, and implies that they are guilty of negligence in not experimenting further.

"A similar misrepresentation of their observations . . . was made by Glazebrook and Thomson (1942) . . ." writes Pauling. These two Scottish researchers used some 1,500 students in their test. Pauling gives much weight to their work as proof of his ideas. The Scots concluded, however, that, "the incidences of common cold and tonsillitis were the same in the two groups." Pauling says this is "contrary to the facts."

A third foundation stone of Pauling's claims for C is the work of Dahlberg, Engel and Rydin (1944), with 2525 soldiers. Again, the researchers summarize that, "no difference could be found as regards frequency or duration of colds, degrees of fever, etc."

"This statement," protests Pauling, "is not true." He attacks all the experimenters for "misrepresentation and incorrect description of . . . observations." Then he attacks *Consumer Reports* for reporting what such scientists have found, rather than doing their own research, as they had with the quality of disposable diapers.

Dr. Reginald Passmore reviewed the old studies and wrote, "I have reread the original accounts . . . carefully. Pauling's comments, while factual and accurate, *seem in no way to invalidate the original interpretation . . . by their authors, which was that the ascorbic acid had no practical effect.*"

Pauling still argues. He says that he has heard of some new trials to be conducted in the 1971–2 winter. They were. They did not confirm his thinking. Even one which seemed to show that Navajo children had slightly less severe colds has recently been declared by the experimenters themselves to have been in error.

It is hard not to sympathize with Pauling as a good and well-meaning man, who hates war and pain and disease. He seems himself now to be in some pain, as must Nobelist Metchnikoff have been when his yogurt for long life was derided.

Not long ago, a biochemist friend of both the author's and Pauling was having lunch with the latter. "Linus," the biochemist asked the grand man of Cal Tech, "is it really true that you and your wife don't have colds any more?"

He turned to answer with his benign smile and his open, honest eyes. "It is true," he said. "We don't get colds at all." Then, with the thoroughness of the disciplined scientist he added a footnote. "Just," said Dr. Pauling, "sniffles."

20

My Mother Squeaked
Or
How to Write
about Health Foods

Early in the 1960's, the author was waiting to tape a radio interview when he was introduced to Dr. Dan Dale Alexander, author of *Arthritis and Common Sense*. At that time, over half a million copies of his book had sold—not surprising, since well over 10 million Americans suffer from some form of arthritis at any given time, and medicine has had only limited success in treating it.

The author asked Dr. Alexander—a big, ample, pleasant man with an almost cherubic smile—how he had come upon the nutritional discoveries of his book, which supposedly explained both cause and cure of arthritis.

"My mother squeaked," smiled Dr. Alexander. "She had arthritis so bad she squeaked. I wanted to help her."

What did he do? He studied the problem and concluded that, "You can eat your way into arthritis and you can eat your way out

265

again." He explained some basic, commonsense decisions he had reached. What would you do, after all, if a door squeaked—or a wheel on your car?

Oil it, of course. Without going into great detail about Alexander's methods, he recommends eating a lot of oil, which goes to the joints and lubricates them. He urges avoiding the drinking of water with meals containing oil, because the water and oil won't mix and the water will wash the oil from the joints. Water, he says, should be taken only when the stomach is empty, and then it shouldn't be too cold, as ice water also has a bad effect on the joints.

The present tense is used here, because the book still sells, and Alexander still writes and lectures—even though the book, first published in 1950, met stiff criticism from science, and its advertising met some stiff opposition from the law.

Dan Dale began, more than 25 years ago, by publishing the book himself, 500 copies. Then he went out to sell it. Even when it began to sell, he needed some help. So publication was assumed by Witkower Press of Hartford, Connecticut, a firm formed especially for this project. Alexander owned 50 percent of the press with his wife, Edith, and was president. Bernard Witkower owned the other half and was secretary-treasurer.

Additionally, Alexander drew the usual 15 percent royalty against the retail price of the book, then $3.95. By early 1957, the 500,000 copy total had been reached, representing some $295,000 in royalties. Perhaps he got as much again as half owner of the publishing house.

This is a good living, though not perhaps as sumptuous as it may sound. For Alexander, like many of his colleagues, worked full time at the book, selling it with lecture tours, television shows, interviews in the press, autograph parties, and all the rest. Ads appeared in profusion as Alexander and Witkower discovered that the book was highly promotable—it was claimed that after just one major TV show, 65,000 copies sold.

Here are excerpts from some of the ads:

"Here's how victims of arthritis across America have won their fight against this dread disease."

"After 15 years of scientific research, Dan Dale Alexander, Ph.D., will discuss his new method of combating arthritis."

"This expert has spent his entire lifetime specializing on just one disease—arthritis!"

". . . A complete analysis of the causes . . . guide toward . . . recovery."

"Laboratory tests by the author developed a plan and a dietary regimen which have brought health to arthritics . . . caused their pains to disappear."

"Unlike present 'cures' supposedly caused by costly miracle drugs this book gives . . . an inexpensive corrective diet which lubricates the patient's joints . . ."

The ads were important to the law because they formed the only basis for legal action. True, scientific complaints about the book itself were many. Yet nothing can legally be done about the publication of ideas. The book was not a label for any particular branded product, so FDA could not act. There would have had to be some item such as "Alexander's Arthritis Oil." And the book would have had to travel in interstate commerce with the oil, acting as a label.

For example, shortly after Pauling's vitamin C book came out, the then powerful *Life* magazine ran a piece on "The Vitamin C Mania." The article was led by a large photo of a man named Louis A. Tuvin, ". . . who owns the oldest vitamin shop in New York City." Tuvin was hunched, in dark glasses, behind his counter, with a great stack of Pauling books on one side and big bottles of vitamin C on the other. *Life* said that in four months Tuvin had sold 40 million C tablets.

No action could be taken on this or many hundreds of similar sales techniques. The book was just a book. The pills were just vitamin C, sold by all sorts of people, though actually—like most vitamins—manufactured by only a few. But the packagers were safe.

Life found only three U.S. sources of C, making some 9 million pounds of it a year—Charles Pfizer & Co., Merck & Co., and Hoffman-La Roche. Immediately following publication of Pauling's book, the nation ran out of the vitamin. Some 3 million pounds more had to be imported from Japan and Germany, with some drug brokers getting doubled prices.

Since Witkower Press was selling a product, under Federal Trade Commission law, ads for the book had to meet a canon of truth. On September 7, 1956, FTC issued a complaint, charging that ads for the Alexander book were "false, misleading, deceptive."

The FTC Hearing Examiner, James A. Purcell, raised questions about Dr. Alexander's credentials. Reported Purcell:

"Alexander was graduated from the Norwich Free Academy, of Norwich, Conn. in June of 1937, as a member of a total class of 353 students in which he ranked #313. He thereafter entered Trinity College of Hartford, Conn., in March of 1945 and took one course during that semester which was a pre-college course in mathematics offering no scholastic credits; in September of 1945, he started his pre-medical courses of which he did not complete even his first semester, was placed on academic probation because of failure in two of the required courses and in fact did not earn any semester hour credits or any college credits whatsoever at Trinity College.

Alexander has no earned degree on any subject from any college or institution of learning . . ."

Advertising and interviews gave another impression. A typical claim was that, "as guest of the Army and Navy General Hospital of Hot Springs, Arkansas, [he] had further opportunity to observe results of therapeutic treatment by the services."

FTC found Alexander had been there by self-invitation, spending less than a day and having no scientific discussion with officials.

Ads also said, "Attendance at the International Congress of Rheumatic Diseases at the Mayo Clinic, in Rochester, Minn., finally convinced Mr. Alexander that his theory of cure by diet was superior to . . . potentially harmful drug treatments now in use . . ."

Again, he visited by self-invitation and was not known to have attended any scientific meetings or discussions.

FTC said his Ph.D. was unearned. He did have one from St. Andrews Ecumenical University College in London. But FTC said Alexander had never been there and didn't know if the College was authorized to confer degrees. Said the National Better Business Bureau: "His only knowledge of the existence of such a university college was based upon his having seen it 'in print emblazoned on his diploma.' He denied that he had paid a consideration for the degree but he 'sent a check of $100 in appreciation thereof' *prior* to receiving it . . .

"As for the degree of 'Doctor of Arts and Oratory' from Staley College of the Spoken Word, Brookline, Mass., it was found that this degree . . . was an outright purchase . . . inasmuch as he made a 'contribution' of $1,000 to the college prior to its conferment."

For years the Arthritis Foundation medical director and staff found the book galling and said Alexander's ideas were wrong, that the diet had no effect (with one possible, technical exception of very minor importance to arthritics as a whole). A series of experts told FTC that Alexander's ideas had no value. The hearing examiner decided that, "the book . . . is but a thesis by Alexander, predicated of unsupportable and unprovable postulates and amounts to nothing more than a collection and summation of the author's theories concerning arthritis, rheumatism and related diseases, all of which yet remain pure theory."

With the legal see-saw which follows such hearings, it was not until October, 1960, four years later, that FTC issued an order to cease representing that the book offered, "an adequate, effective or reliable treatment for the symptoms and manifestations of any kind of arthritis, rheumatism, or related condition, or rheumatic fever, or will afford any relief from aches, pains, stiffness, swelling or other discomforts thereof."

You might think that this would have stopped the book. What did the press do, for example? With all the hearing materials and investigations on public record, but before the final order, the *Los Angeles Times,* the West's biggest newspaper, proudly presented the book in more than 15 truncated installments.

Did the *Times* publish in ignorance? Perhaps at first. But immediately formal protests were made by the local Arthritis and Rheumatism Foundation and by physicians. For delay in treatment of arthritics can mean irreversible damage. Ineffective self-treatment can mean permanent crippling. The *Times* said it could not stop running the book.

With the facts known, publishers did not stop publishing, booksellers did not stop selling, newspapers were happy to take its advertising, radio and TV stations welcomed the lively interviews. Just the other day, a San Diego radio station was telling its listeners about a lecture by Dan Dale Alexander, presumably as a public-service announcement. A few weeks later, 26 years after he had first published his book, Dan Alexander was the honored guest on *Mayor Sam*, a television interview show in Los Angeles, conducted by former city mayor Sam Yorty.

Dan had discovered that his diets and his oil could also stop the common cold and had published accordingly. Moreover, he had decided that there were irritating and non-irritating car-bohydrates, which affected health. (Honey, for example, is not irritating. But you can always tell a sugar-eater; he gets coarse pores on his cheeks.)

Dan said that everyone should have a tablespoon of oil an hour before breakfast. He asked Mayor Sam if he had tried this. The political veteran shook his head somewhat sourly. No, he hadn't tried it. He would stick to his usual morning drink—honey, almonds and water beaten in a blender. Dan smiled and urged the oil again, cod liver oil. It was wonderful. It was why he had begun to call himself, "The Codfather."

It is important to observe that Alexander's big book was a rarity—because of its 42 weeks on the bestseller lists, and because he published it himself. But there are similar, though often less successful, books by the barrel.

Commented then FDA Commissioner Charles Crawford, some time ago, "To put it bluntly, false and misleading information about nutrition may be disseminated freely to the public without fear of any legal measures such as apply to false labeling or advertising." Only its use in advertising had made Alexander's book vulnerable to the law.

Only ethics can impel a publisher to check the ideas presented to him—for more than sales potential—against scientific knowledge and possible public harm. For weeks, the author and six lawyer fellow panelists at the White House Conference on

Nutrition labored to find some legally feasible solution. The best they could come up with was a plaintive, "Please—don't."

Arthritis was a big field for foodism, beginning in the 1950's and continuing into the 1960's. Since then, improvements in medical treatment have somewhat attenuated the flow of diet schemes to cure it.

In 1958, a major publisher, Holt, came into the field with *Folk Medicine: A Vermont Doctor's Guide to Good Health*, by D. C. Jarvis, M.D.

The jacket said: "Dr. Jarvis provides a new theory on the treatment and prevention of diseases ranging from the common cold to arthritis; from kidney troubles to digestive disorders . . . and many others which often defy conventional medical diagnosis and treatment . . . Folk medicine . . . boasts two simple remedies which can be obtained and applied anywhere. Each of these, honey and apple cider vinegar, has an outstanding record in the fight against human ills."

The record consists mainly of Dr. Jarvis' use of honey and vinegar on un-named Vermonters, chickens and cows—except, of course, for the example of Elisha Perkins' use of vinegar with his tractors.

As an example of Jarvis' science, he says that one reason apple cider vinegar is so good a curative is that it has so much potassium. A whole cup of cider vinegar—which is a lot of vinegar if you are thinking of imbibing the stuff—has 240 milligrams of potassium. This is not much potassium in the fruit and vegetable world. An ordinary potato of the same weight as the cup of vinegar has three times as much. And Jarvis calls for only two teaspoons of vinegar in, for example, weight reduction. He says, "The apple cider vinegar will have made it possible to burn the fat in the body instead of storing it . . ."

Hundreds of thousands bought the book. Magazines ran articles, hyping the sales. *Life* said, "It has made a powerful impression on the U.S. public."

What so impressed? Jarvis, an ear, nose and throat man, says there are three European types—Nordic, Alpine and Mediterranean—each having a "natural" diet. The Nordic should eat fish and kelp, avoid wheat bread and eat only rye. If he doesn't, he will feel just awful. He also describes *plus* and *minus* people. Whatever you are, you must eat accordingly.

(He does not face the dilemma of a child with, say, a Nordic father and Mediterranean mother. Presumably, his life will be a hopeless vacillation between kelp and wheat bread.)

If you have violated your type, honey and vinegar may help. He explains that we are always shifting from alkaline to acid and back. Life is great when you are acid and very grim when you are alkaline.

How do you know your state? You keep an eye on your urine, testing it for acid and alkaline once or twice a day. For example, "The pain of paranasal sinusitis is associated with an alkaline urine reaction. As a rule, one can shift the reaction to acid, relieving the pain, by taking one teaspoonful of apple cider vinegar . . . each hour for seven doses."

Alkaline on awakening shows you lack energy. If you have turned alkaline overnight, "it would be wise to take a hand bath of apple cider vinegar and water."

Later: "It will surprise some people . . . that, in getting rid of your chronic fatigue, you must seriously consider ceasing to use soap . . . Being alkaline, soap helps to create in your body the very chronic fatigue you wish to get rid of."

Migraine? "Two teaspoonfuls of honey taken at each meal may well prevent an attack." He says that honey causes an acid reaction, unlike cane or maple sugar. This, he adds, is why a real Vermonter always eats pickles with his maple syrup. Honey is also supposed to help high blood pressure, because it is, "a magnet for water."

Acid, he finds, is especially important for arthritis. Like Alexander, he has done research on the subject. "I . . . studied methods used by plumbers in freeing the inside of the furnace water compartment from deposited calcium." (Sure enough, vinegar will dissolve away calcium deposits, if you are a pipe.)

Honey is shown as the cure for bedwetting, sleeplessness, muscle cramps and the runny nose. And there is also helpful information about bladder stones in minks, cow eyes that water, producing milk with a prize herd, and the art of chewing leaves. No wonder the publisher said, "The astonishing facts FOLK

MEDICINE discloses offer tried and proved relief for a multitude of nagging complaints, and promise for zestful life."

Interviewed, Jarvis said, "I don't know why it (folk medicine) helps. Only scientific medicine can tell us that."

Scientific medicine gnashed its teeth. Dr. Philip White of the Council on Foods and Nutrition said Jarvis had, "combined honey and vinegar and given the mixture some pretty fanciful properties. Certainly there is nothing in honey or vinegar which support the claims made."

A typical comment came from Harvard's distinguished nutritionist, Dr. Fredrick Stare, who said, "This claptrap is strictly for those gullible birds stung by the honeybee."

Scientific criticism flooded the press. Even the *Reader's Digest* revealed the nonsense, in some 20 million copies. Holt could hardly have been unaware. Yet it ordered up some new printings and published a sequel, *Arthritis and Folk Medicine.*

Neighbors of Jarvis in Vermont began to batch up honey and vinegar and bottle it for sale. FDA seized some, but the fad went on.

Late in 1960, after two years of advertising, FTC finally ordered that Holt, in marketing *Folk Medicine,* "or any other book or books of the same . . . content, material or methods," cease and desist from representing that the method promulgated in the books:

"1. Constitutes an adequate, effective or reliable treatment for the common cold, arthritis, kidney trouble, digestive disorders, high blood pressure . . . obesity, chronic fatigue, headaches . . . , hay fever, asthma, dizziness, run down feelings, lack of energy, lack of fertility, sinus infections . . . or diseases which defy conventional medical diagnosis and treatment;

"2. Arrests the progress of, corrects the underlying causes of, prevents or cures . . ." (a similar long list);

"3. Prevents or cures sickness, maintains good health or prolongs the lifespan;

"4. Gives vigor . . .

"5. Has been scientifically tested."

A generation later, the two Jarvis books still sell, and help to explain why apple cider vinegar is sold in every health-food store in the land. And vinegar's reputation for healthfulness continues, as it remains part of many fad diets—such as the supposed obesity remedy of Lecithin, cider vinegar, B-6 and kelp.

Rarely would these books become so popular without the enthusiastic publication of condensations by the press. Some magazines seem to depend heavily on such excerpts for sales, just as, in a kind of literary symbiosis, the book publishers depend upon the magazines to spread the ideas and generate interest in the books.

Moreover, not one major national magazine has failed to use a kind of nutrition sensationalism, whether taken from books or not, to boost its sales. And the more a magazine depends on newstand sales—rather than subscriptions—the more eager its editors seem to be to seek out new eating schemes.

Family Circle, has no subscriptions and some 8 million copies per issue sold in the supermarkets—with a reputation for concern about public interest, and an image of responsibility attaching to the fact that the stolid *New York Times* owns it. After all, the recipes work, the home hints make the ink come out of the carpet, and if you try to make the Mickey Mouse Bicentennial toaster cover out of your husband's old argyle socks, it will probably come out all right.

But the nutrition stories have tended to be startling ever since the late 1960's, when *Family Circle* helped to launch Dr. Stillman's several low-carbohydrate reducing plans and his books. At one point you could even send in for a personalized diet plan created by a computer which had been taught to think like Stillman.

The low-blood-sugar fad got a big push from a *Family Circle* story. For advice on energy, the magazine turned to Beatrice Trum Hunter, of natural cookery renown. "Adequate protein is what most people lack," Ms. Hunter explains. "A protein breakfast of eggs and meat will carry you through the day, and your blood sugar is more apt to stay at a high level. If you want a between-meals snack, I'd rather see you eat a handful of pumpkin or sunflower seeds—anything with the one food with everything you need. You know how many people are tired all the time, or have little ailments. The change in their energy levels with natural foods is wonderful." These statements run counter to the scientific truth.

In 1971, *Family Circle* took up vitamin E in a big way. "Does vitamin E retard aging?" ran the headlines. "Protect fertility? Subdue cancer cells? Speed the healing of burns? Prevent ulcers? Clinical tests have shown that it promises all of these—and more."

The author of the article was the "scientific writer", Ruth Winter, who wrote *Beware of the Food You Eat,* actually a "revised, updated" edition of *Poisons in Your Food.* ("Have you had your poisons today?" the publisher, Signet, asks . . . "It is now impossible to eat an ordinary meal . . . that is not adulterated with . . . poisons.")

Ruth Winter asks how come great-grandfather always had "the energy to cope," while his descendants do not? She says maybe it was the vitamin E in his food. She adds that, "Obviously, we're not getting enough."

She outlines all the "proven" wonders of the vitamin, such as improving the speed and staying power of racehorses, along with their fertility. She concludes: "Enthusiasts . . . claim that it holds promise of helping practically every ailment under the sun. *No matter how extravagant these claims, they can all be held to have some basis in fact . . .*" (Emphasis added.)

So the real secret of energy, we can see, is protein—or perhaps natural eating—or it may be a low carbohydrate diet—or taking more vitamin E. Or is the answer as proposed in a 1973 *Family Circle* article about the "High Energy Diet," Dr. Watson's tests for whether you are a slow or fast food burner?

The magazine even offers to make you beautiful with nutrition. An article by Mary Ann Crenshaw, author of *The Natural Way to Beauty,* tells how to "Feed Your Skin, Hair and Nails—from Within." How? The section, "Protein-hungry hair," suggests one approach, and a second section, "Vitamin E for Hair," follows with another. We also learn how to be calm. Calcium is described as, "one of nature's own tranquilizers." This is why we should drink warm milk before sleep. "Remember all those tales about warm milk before bedtime for a sound sleep? Surprise! They were all true." Again, science can find no support for these ideas.

In 1975, one of this magazine's contributions to nutrition education was an article called "The Miracle Vitamin That Can Lower Cholesterol." The author, Lawrence Galton, has long written a responsible column of medical news. *Family Circle* sent Galton to England and announced that "a significant new development" had occurred at Pinderfields Hospital, in Wakefield, through the work of Dr. Constance Spittle.

The story is complex, but Spittle says she made the find after she had been living for a while on nothing but fruits, and later, some added vegetables. While on this diet, Dr. Spittle gave some blood to a patient and collapsed. She decided that this was because she had eaten "no protein for a month. I had had no fat either." Technically, this is not true. Vegetables and fruits are sparse sources of protein in many cases, and pretty good sources in others. The fat content would have been quite low, but there would have been some.

Spittle's blood was checked, and she saw that her cholesterol was down, as was to be expected on such a diet. Experimenting, she now turned to a "high-cholesterol diet along with a lot of fruits and vegetables." We can only speculate about what she ate. But it is a good guess that the cholesterol might have come from eggs, meats and other animal products. Spittle says that her cholesterol count stayed down. She concluded that something in the fruits and vegetables—she decided it was vitamin C—did the trick.

(Contrary to what many people believe, however, cholesterol does not always rise, or rise much, when more cholesterol is eaten. For example, in studies of selected volunteers, the Drs. Slater showed that adding two eggs a day to the diets of carefully chosen people did not cause cholesterol to go up significantly.)

Vitamin C authority Dr. Robert Hodges has commented on the matter: "Much of Dr. Spittle's evidence is inferential, and she appears to misinterpret the biochemical facts regarding vitamin C . . . There is certainly no evidence that if you take ample vitamin C 'the cholesterol will come off the artery walls into the bloodstream.' "

Hodges sums up: ". . . The 'Spittles affair' is a good lesson in the harm of patients obtaining medical advice from lay publications . . . A couple of medical editors took the untested clinical findings and unpublished suppositions of a rural English doctor . . . in an effort to boost circulation."

There is a further lesson in a 1976 venture of the magazine, *Dr. Frank's No-Aging Diet.* It was adapted from a book of the same name, by Dr. Benjamin Frank and Philip Miele. *Family Circle* heralds it as, "The first diet based on the scientific breakthrough of our time."

Why so? Because the diet supposedly leads you to eat more RNA and DNA, the molecules which carry the blueprints of heredity. "The quality of these nucleic acids deteriorates as we age," says Frank. "This leads to the creation of faulty cells." What to do? There are, "high-quality RNA and DNA that can be supplied from outside the body to nourish our cells and return them to a healthy state."

Frank put 16 patients on such a diet, and in a week or so they returned with glowing reports. They started getting younger looking. "Wrinkles of the forehead smooth out . . . Then the deep lines from the nostrils to the corner of the mouth become shallower and the 'crow's feet' at the corners of the eye begin to lighten . . . the back of the hands and elbows become smoother. Calluses on the feet . . . may . . . begin to disappear."

Frank says that at 70 or 80, "age may appear to regress by 10 to 15 years; at age 60, about 10 years; and at age 30 to 50, five years or more."

What do we have to eat? Four days a week, a can of small sardines, one day salmon, one day lobster or other shellfish, liver once a week, along with beets or borscht, and so on. Small sardines, the Norwegian type, began to disappear from the nation's grocery shelves.

The idea of eating RNA and DNA to grow younger sounds appealing. But it quarrels with two scientific facts from the start. First, RNA and DNA are proteins. Digestion tends to break them apart—into the amino acids of which they are made. So they are unlikely even to get to the cells intact.

Secondly, heredity is specific. That is, the cells get their instructions for making chemicals and reproducing themselves from DNA and RNA. So even if by a miracle, the nucleic acids could get to our cells, the effects would be strange indeed. For the instructions given by DNA and RNA from sardines, for example, are for the cells of sardines. If Dr. Frank's diet did actually work, the dieter would tend to develop fins, gills and other fishy characteristics.

Family Circle promoted the article heavily. And the *New*

York Times accepted a full-page ad for the book, headlined, "Eat and grow younger!"

Much weight was given to the preface of the book, written by one Dr. Hendler, who was identified as a University of California professor. He is quoted by *Family Circle* as saying, ". . . we probably have a greater need for nucleic acid than the cells can make. Dr. Frank is the first to realize this . . ."

But noted nutritionist Dr. Harold Harper, dean of graduate faculties at the University of California in San Francisco, told a reporter from *New York* magazine, "This diet is absolute, sheer quackery . . . It is totally unscientific from A to Z."

The *New York* writer, William Stuckey, began to look for Dr. Hendler, who had prefaced Dr. Frank's book. But no one by that name had ever been a professor in the University of California system. Reporter Stuckey quotes a university official as saying that Hendler had been a part-time tutor. And Stuckey quotes Hendler himself:

" 'Who the hell knows whether Frank's diet is a no-aging diet? I just wanted to help the old guy out . . . and what the hell, he may be right about nucleic acids . . . Sardines? I haven't the slightest idea why he stresses them . . .' "

How did the book get through the editors of Dial Press? Stuckey quotes an editor there as saying she just realized the diet was "slimming, low cholesterol." (It is neither.) "One person in the office tried the sardine and it worked."

Stuckey quotes a *Family Circle* editor as saying, "No checking was done, as we assumed the publisher, Dial, had done that."

In fact, one of the most important points of this story is that— while there are vicious promoters who circulate nutrition untruth out of the coldest profit motives—the greatest impact is probably had by the well meaning. Arthur Hettich, the chief editor of *Family Circle,* like many other editors, honestly believes there is a valid debate going on about many basic facts of nutrition.

In a letter to Dr. Thomas Jukes, who had complained of the magazine's nutrition stories, Hettich writes of an argument "between the scientific establishment and the popular nutritionists." He says he tries to "balance the material from both sides."

This, of course, implies that there is a meaningful struggle between science and some populist philosophers of eating. Hettich says, he is, ". . . aware of 'scientific' viewpoints that have been changed by the mavericks . . . Dr. Pauling and his struggle over vitamin C, the impetus that health food stores have had in bringing more nourishing foods to the supermarket shelves . . ."

There is no doubt that he means what he says.

A final note. It is fashionable among food activists to cite the huge sums spent in advertising by the food industry. These sums, we shall see, are supposed to fill a conspiratorial trough—from which science, government and media feed and are thereby corrupted. Is there really a conspiracy?

The reader might check the pages of magazines which carry stories that attribute much of our disease to the consuming of ordinary, popular foods. You will find millions spent in these pages, by people who sell cornflakes and noodles, white bread and sweet cereal, cokes and candies and all the other items that the miracle diets forbid. These food makers buy the ads, while the editorial matter instructs readers to disdain the products.

It is a puzzling kind of conspiracy. It may not even exist.

21

The Red-Faced
Confession

*And Other Tales of
Food Cures and Law*

The mail-order ad opened with what was called "my red-faced confession." And the confession was blunt. "It all began when my 'holding power' started to grow weak . . . and finally limp . . . In desperation, I confessed my problem to a buddy on our local bowling team . . ."

The buddy said he too, had been, "shamefully LIMP." What had helped him was a mix of, "over 25 ALL-NATURAL AND ORGANIC INGREDIENTS . . . It could work its VIGOR-RESTORATION in a matter of moments . . ." In two days, the buddy was, "like a bridegroom, with the 'POWER OF A STALLION.'"

The red-faced confessor tried the remedy. "By the end of the third week," he reports, "I could hardly wait for my wife to wash the dinner dishes."

The compound offered in the ad was NATURE-VITE, and you could get a whole year's supply for $40. What was in NATURE-VITE that made our correspondent so eager for clean dishes? The ingredients were vague, except for "Famed vitamin E." Others were listed as:

"An unusual substance from raw wheat . . . able to electrify enzyme processes."

". . . Special all natural ingredient .   . to stimulate the nerve senses . . . upon slight contact . . ."

"Concentrated substances that . . . strengthen the inter-cellular cement to provide hard strength."

And so on. On the assumption that this compound was not likely to have the effects claimed, except by psychological suggestion, what might the law have done? (As far as the author knows, it did nothing.)

In terms of Federal regulation, one of three agencies might have acted, the Food and Drug Administration, the Federal Trade Commission or the Post Office. But there are some limitations.

FDA gets involved mainly on one of two general grounds. The first is that the ingredients themselves are dangerous or unapproved. The precedents concerning dangerous ingredients were set long ago. Between January of 1906 and February of 1907, the *Journal of the AMA* reported nine infant deaths due to use of *Kopp's Baby's Friend*, "King of Baby Soothers." It contained morphine sulphate.

· Finally, in 1915, FDA seized a shipment of *Kopp's*. After a court fight, the judge cracked down. He fined the firm $25, plus some $25 more in costs.

The pattern of somewhat slow action and somewhat weak penalty continues to this day. Because the law is simpler and clearer in such matters, action on unapproved substances is prompter. Late in 1975, ads began to appear: "NEW STAR-TLING VITAMIN . . . Vitamin B-15 in its safest most effective form!" Nutritionists were startled especially. For they do not know of a vitamin B-15. In May of 1976, an order to seize 12 cartons of the stuff was issued by FDA.

As is often the case nowadays, no direct claim was made for the "vitamin" in ads or on the package. The claims were all made in magazine reports and the like. The author of an article in *Let's Live*, "Will the Government Suppress Vitamin B-15?" said he could breathe better for taking it. He says the stuff is something called "pangamic acid."

"No doubt," the article continues, "pangamic acid can be used as a treatment for a number of illnesses, just as cabbage can be used as a treatment for ulcers and garlic can be used to lower blood pressure." However, this does not make pangamic acid a drug or additive; it "is a natural food ingredient." Therefore, the conclusion goes, the Government has no right to control it.

The chemical is supposed to increase the oxygen in the blood. *Let's Live* says this helps to explain, "why pangamate helps people with heart disease . . . how it helps aging athletes, overcomes gangrene and maintains cellular health to prevent premature aging . . . Indeed, one Russian scientist has been quoted . . . that he can foresee the day when a bottle of pangamic acid will routinely be found on every dinner table just like a salt shaker."

FDA acted first on technical grounds, saying that when B-15 was labeled for therapeutic use, it was a new and unapproved drug; when it was offered as a food supplement, that food was considered adulterated, since it contained an unapproved food additive.

It has also acted on grounds of "mislabeling." This is a broader term than it may seem. It covers errors in statements about a product's use and effectiveness. And most important, since a 1938 amendment, the "label" need not be on the container itself. As in the case of *Calories Don't Count* and the safflower capsules, a book, leaflet, or oral statement can be considered a label, if statement and product come together at some point in interstate commerce.

Mislabeling is harder to prove when a scientific fact or nonfact is at issue. Defenders of B-15 and the like often howl loudly at FDA's use of such weapons as lack of approval for a new drug or additive. But approval is not a technicality; it means that there is proof of safety and value. The seizure of B-15 was scarcely on a purely technical basis. Witness a complaint filed against three makers of the stuff:

"(a) sodium pangamate is not an identifiable substance and is not a vitamin or pro-vitamin;

"(b) there is no accepted scientific evidence which established any nutritional properties for sodium pangamate;

"(c) there is no accepted scientific evidence which identifies a deficiency of sodium pangamate in man or other animals;

"(d) the safety of sodium pangamate has not been demonstrated . . ."

FDA had a special concern about B-15. It was supposedly discovered in apricot kernels. So was a substance called *Laetrile* (actually a chemical known as *amygdalin*). The line between B-15 and Laetrile is not incidental. (The latter is now being called vitamin B-17 by some, though there is no more evidence that this is a vitamin or has any role in human nutrition than there is about B-15.)*

E.T. Krebs and some others have long asserted that the two chemicals used together are an effective treatment for cancer. Krebs has said that it is "possible to double the number of recoveries of cancer, when Laetrile and chymotrypsin are given with vitamin B-15 . . ."

This treatment has been supported in a highly organized way by the small, but very vocal International Association of Cancer Victims and Friends (I.A.C.V.F.). Members maintain that the cure works and that organized medicine, along with the American Cancer Society, refuse to give it a test, and conspire to suppress it, for selfish reasons.

In truth, in 1953, the Cancer Commission of the California Medical Association reported that in 44 cases treated with Laetrile, no anti-cancer activity could be found. At that time, the stuff could be bought for about 20 cents a gram; some healers were charging $50 to inject this much.

Such medical views—by the National Cancer Institute and the Canadian Medical Association, for example—have never shown value for treating cancer. As early as 1961, E.T. Krebs, Jr. and the John Beard Memorial Foundation pleaded guilty to FDA charges that vitamin B-15 was misbranded. In 1963, Krebs applied for new drug approval for Laetrile. FDA declined, on grounds that the data were "inconclusive and insufficient to demonstrate either

*The American Institute of Nutrition's Committee on Nomenclature "finds no scientific evidence for the existence of a nutrient" called B-17.

efficacy or safety." By this time, a thriving business of diagnosing cancer and selling Laetrile had sprung up in Tijuana, Mexico, just across the California border from San Diego—together with what has been called (by investigative reporter Ralph Lee Smith) "the Cancer Underground Railroad." Laetrile has long been classed as contraband both in Canada and in the U.S. in interstate commerce. Yet its use is still extolled in such books as Glenn Kittler's *Laetrile—Control for Cancer.*

In this light, the reader may wish to appraise the conclusion of the *Let's Live* article on B-15: "All we want is simple fairness and justice. We have *a new product* [emphasis added], pangamate, that can be supplied to us at reasonable prices and that we are eager to use. It is good for us. There is no danger in it for anyone and there is no reason whatsoever why the FDA should choose to deprive us of it."

The Federal Trade Commission's interest in nutrition is mainly in its advertising. Since 1914, when it was created largely to deal with anti-trust violations, FTC has derived from its mission of preventing "unfair competition," a long history of guarding against unfair methods of getting the consumer to buy something. Unfortunately, this has never been anything like FTC's central role. And since, like most of our protective agencies, it is given inadequate staff and funds to carry out all of its assigned activities, it puts its emphasis where White House and Cabinet policies direct.

For real policing, FTC would have to look not only at all the newspapers, magazines and other publications which carry advertising in the U.S., it would have to watch or listen to over 4,000 radio and television stations round the clock. At the White House Conference on Nutrition in 1969, panelists on deception and misinformation questioned FTC about its work with food advertising. A key official said two people spent half time checking advertising. Neither had any background in nutrition. (About this time, FTC did hire one very capable young woman nutritionist. But following her tragic death in an accident, no replacement was sought for several years. At this writing, FTC has only some consulting help, again but one person.) The lack of nutrition expertise was one reason why the Conference proposed that nutrition advertising supervision be transferred, like drug advertising, to FDA.

The deception-panelists were most concerned with the ways in which advertising misinforms Americans about how to choose good nutrition. They were also concerned, though less so, about economic cheats. But in practice, the two often go together.*

For example, consider an ad for Sue Bee Honey. "Ounce for ounce . . ." it says, "our honey has fewer calories than refined sugar." This is substantially true. But what impression is left? Honey has more water, since sugar has virtually none. Thus, if we look at a tablespoon of each, the honey has 64 calories and the sugar only 46.

"As a source of quick energy, our honey is unexcelled. Ask any top athlete or coach." Honey supplies no quicker energy than sugar. Essentially, each is one molecule of glucose and one of fructose. Either has to be broken down to simple sugars—in mouth, stomach and intestine—before it can enter the blood. So either the sugar from a grape, an apple or a piece of Danish pastry would be used as quickly. Sweet drinks, put into an empty stomach, get into the blood fastest. And as for turning to coaches and athletes for nutrition advice, they might well be too busy opening their protein supplements and eating their pre-game steaks in the false hope of building more muscle.

"Natural minerals are important," the ad says. It points to "body builders" such as calcium and iron, "Plus nine others." A tablespoon of honey offers .1 mg. of iron and 1 mg. of calcium. So a typical young woman could get her iron from only 180 tablespoons of honey a day, and her calcium from 1,000 tablespoons. To get her calcium from honey, she would have to eat 64,000 calories a day.

Many nutritionists are much more tolerant of mass-market advertising than they are of ads which run in the smaller publications which cater to foodists. In discussions of some recent FTC proposals for better control of nutrition advertising, many experts tended to discriminate between the ads of "major, responsible

*In general, the author is disposed to say that the vast majority of food advertising which uses nutrition as an inducement, ends by misinforming, either directly or indirectly. Hence, the motivation to buy is false.

corporations" and smaller companies which offer special nutrition products. The author, having studied both, does not always find it easy to tell the difference.

For example, consider two advertising programs. One ad appeared in *Let's Live*. It offers *Theradophilus* for, "intestinal gardening." It says the product contains, "the only true *Lactobacillus acidophilus*—a friendly bacteria that inhibits the growth of putrefying microorganisms which cause digestive disturbances . . . [and] curbs protein stagnation." The ad is reminiscent of John Harvey Kellogg and other long deceased medical friends of the colon.

Less serious in tone, but equally serious in impact is a pamphlet put out by one of the West's biggest dairy producers, to go with a multi-media advertising campaign for a new product. Knudsen ("the dairy best") tells us that the product is, "more than just a funny name that no one (not even us) can pronounce. It's a new kind of milk . . . with something special added. The lactobacillus acidophilus culture. A lot of people think that this new additive for milk is a breakthrough."

In fact, the addition is compared to the adding of vitamins A and D to milk, except that we see a different purpose: it is supposed to put back, "some of the natural digestive aids you may be losing because many of today's foods are over-refined."

We find parallels among some ads that deal with supposed deficiency problems. In a recent *Family Circle*, we find an ad for "the 7 vitamins and 5 minerals our hair desperately needs for health." Or we might look at an ad in *Family Weekly*—a supplement distributed with millions of Sunday newspapers—which offers, "Megavitamin Therapy . . . for your Hair." This ad says that, "Scientists recently discovered that [zinc sulphate] is an absolute essential to hair growth, but . . . sadly lacking in our natural diet."

How different are these ads from one which appeared in *Bestways:* "LOW BACK PAIN! Can be Due to Calcium Deficiency."? Calcium deficiency is an extremely unlikely cause of low back pain among Americans. But additional vitamins and minerals aren't likely to grow or groom Americans' hair, either.

Nutritionists are much more likely to be critical of ads such as the latter, however—possibly because *Bestways* carries more extreme editorial matter. In this issue, for example, one finds, "Magnesium—Cell Regulator and New Hope for Cancer Prevention." But is the editorial matter of big magazines really so different when it comes to nutrition?

Differences are also claimed between big drug companies and small ones. For example, in the same issue of *Bestways* is an ad for "Ultra-Stress, B Complex & Vitamin C," from Essential Organics. The ad says that if you are "under physical or mental stress and want to meet your body's increased needs," you should take a certain compound. Its vitamins come from such things as yeast and rose hips.

Since the total effective vitamin content of a product is shown on the label, whether a vitamin comes from a "high potency" source (such as acerola berries or rose hips) or is made in a factory, the total vitamin activity is just what the label says and no more.

"Natural and synthetic vitamins have the same effect on the body. And while it is possible that some stress and disease states may increase our needs for nutrients, such increase is usually very small. But the "Ultrastress" product contains 300 mg. of vitamin C. For most of us, this is seven days' supply, the vast majority of which will just wash away in the urine.

However, in 1975, Lederle, a major pharmaceutical house, bought a full page in *Time*, headlined, "Stress. Time for a Different brand of vitamin." Saying that, "stress can rob you of vitamins," Lederle offers to replace them. Do they provide a week's vitamin C in a pill? No indeed. They give us 600 mg., *two* weeks' vitamin C. Obviously, in this case, our urine will contain a lot more vitamin C than it would if we bought the product of the small organic firm.

Another major drug house, Squibb, in a *Ladies' Home Journal* ad for *Golden Bounty Vitamins,* makes a big point of reliability. "When you buy vitamins," they say, ". . . you're making an investment in confidence." *Golden Bounty* gives us "natural-source" ingredients, such as "wheat germ oil, rose hips with C, cod liver oil, brewer's yeast, protein tablets . . . and protein powder."

Squibb stresses the value of buying from an old-line firm. The ad points out that Squibb, "has marketed vitamin products since 1875." Although specific products are not identified, this was a major industrial achievement—since Casimir Funk did not announce the discovery of the first vitamin until 1911.

What can FTC do about ads which mislead the public? First, the FTC staffer must amass quite a good deal of scientific documentation and expert opinion. For his is the burden of proof. He next serves a complaint on the advertiser, who gets some time to respond, during which he can keep on advertising and selling his product, with the same promotion.

The advertiser may agree to stop the ads or modify them. Or he may appeal, which is the more usual case. Now FTC must hold a hearing, with expert opinions and scientific and legal briefs prepared. The hearing must wait for an opening on the FTC dockets. Meanwhile the advertising and selling continues.

After the hearing, the Hearing Examiner prepares a decision. If the decision is against the advertiser, he may either quit or appeal to the Commission itself. This means more lawyers, briefs, delays and waiting for a docket opening. Finally, the Commission makes a Finding of Fact. This in effect says what the truth is concerning the subject—perhaps that "Snake Milk" does not do anything for tired blood.

Now the Commission can issue a Final Order, to cease and desist. But if Snake Milk has established a good market, the advertiser may want to appeal to the courts. There is a trial, after more delays for preparation, court date and the like. Then there can be appeals of the court decision. These can, and have, gone all the way to the Supreme Court.

Assume that the court upholds the Final Order. The advertiser still has some alternatives. He can design another ad which may make something like the same claims a little differently. He can, and frequently does, create a new corporation, which carries on much the same old business under a new name. Or he can ignore the order.

In the latter case, he is held to be in violation of the order. After all, the advertiser may have spent a lot building up a brisk trade. Another court action must be brought, often slow to come to trial, be decided and perhaps appealed. This violation could be punished with a fine of up to $5,000, very small just compared to the legal costs, and for a promoter who is really onto a good thing, a relatively small cost of doing business.*

In 1955, FTC Commissioner Sigurd Anderson admitted that it took FTC a median time of over four years and six months to go from investigation to a cease-and-desist order. Then all the rest of the delays could begin. The situation is not much improved today. Clearly, the decision to act on such matters is not lightly taken. It will involve much staff time, taxpayer cost and often ultimate frustration.

Often action is almost pointless. Long ago, the National Better Business Bureau estimated that, "usually a promoter who has a year of freedom to work can easily afford to go out of business with huge profits."

Just to give one specific example, FTC acted on the following ad for *Wonder Bread*:

"During the 'Wonder Years'—one through twelve—your children develop in many ways, actually growing to 90% of their adult height. To help make the most of their 'Wonder Years,' serve them nutritious Wonder Bread. Every slice is carefully enriched for body and mind."

It was alleged and ultimately confirmed that the ad implied Wonder Bread had something that was missing from other breads. But it took the FTC some nine years to make this point stick.

The third major entity in consumer protection is the Post Office. It is empowered to act on fraudulent use of the mails. It can move more rapidly than the other agencies, issuing a fraud order, then seeking to get the advertiser to sign an Affidavit of Discontinuance, in which he agrees either to stop using the offending ads or stop using the mails for disseminating the material. But the Post Office also has a serious legal hurdle. It must prove not only inaccuracy, but also *intent to defraud.*

Later, we can look at some possibilities for improved consumer protection. But for the moment, let us consider some further difficulties. One basic problem is that often the spurious claims for a product are being made by sources other than the manufacturer.

---

*However, at this level, advertisers engage some special risks of contempt of court, which stop most reputable firms.

For example, *Advertising Age* reported not long ago, noting a steady boom in vitamin sales: "Vitamin marketers agree that, with few exceptions, they have been getting a free ride on the current wave of publicity given to vitamins in all media. TV and radio programs, magazine and newspaper articles, books and pamphlets on the subject of vitamins continue to gush forth."

The article explains that only a few drug houses spend much on public promotion, almost $9 million a year for One-A-Day products and over $2 million for Unicap, plus a growing budget for Golden Bounty. "There are two basic reasons behind the relative absence of consumer advertising . . . There are few known, "supportable and legitimate uses of vitamins as approved by the FDA . . . and most . . . drug companies avoid advertising to the consumer for fear of arousing the medical profession's hostility." Squibb, the article comments, runs Golden Bounty ads, "that avoid claims other than product description."

But evidently nothing more is needed. In effect, the promotions are carried out by others. In *Let's Live,* Carlson Wade writes an article, "Mongolism: Hope Through Nutritional Therapy." Remembering that mongolism is a problem of heredity, we are surprised to read that one Henry Turkel, M.D. reports his nutritional treatment of a South Dakota girl. Turkel is quoted, "Her entire body has changed in appearance. The facial expression has especially improved . . . We were told that she was not educable . . . Now, however, she is able to work at third grade level . . . and nearly always makes 100 in spelling."

Explains nutrition writer Wade, "The nine nutritional treatments help alter the inborn structural defects . . ."

Such tales condition the reader to buy supplements. Often the copy is much more specific. *Better Nutrition,* for example, in one typical column which answers readers' questions, responds to such as, "I have tiny broken veins in my legs. Any suggestions?" and "I have non-specific vaginitis. Any suggestions?"

Such conditions are extremely common and are most unlikely to have anything to do with Americans' nutrition. But vitamin C is recommended for the broken veins—as it is elsewhere in the issue for "back trouble." And for the irritated vagina, the reader is advised to take yogurt, Lactobacillus tablets, and/or vitamins A and C. These products are then advertised in the magazine without any claims. But none are necessary.

What can the government do about the elusive partnership between commercial products and separately expressed nutrition ideas? Plainly, nothing. Here we have the clear reason why every health-food store has a book rack, a magazine rack, and leaflets scattered among the shelves.

As for publications, they are protected by the First Amendment. And even if ads for the publications should violate the rules of fair trade, by the time FTC can act, the magazine and the ads have long since disappeared.

So it is that the White House Conference report on deception and misinformation in nutrition drew as its first conclusion: ". . . The American people falsely believe that they are well protected, both by Government and by the ethics of commerce."

And the problem does not end here.

22

Quick, Nurse!
The Bean Sprouts!

One of the most popular letters-to-the-expert columns in the nutrition magazines is written by Dr. Alan H. Nittler, M.D., author of the bestselling *A New Breed of Doctor.* The cover of his book features the pocket of a white coat, from which protrude both a stethoscope and a carrot, a pairing which tells us much.

One lady writes to Nittler complaining of a sore, swollen tongue, which medicine has not been able to cure. She says she is taking acidophilus bacteria for it, as well as daily doses of 12,500 units of vitamin A (2.5 days supply), 1,650 units of D (4 days supply), 200 units of E (13 days supply), large amounts of all the B vitamins (apparently up to 50 days supply), 1,000 mg of C (22 days worth), pantothenic acid, folic acid, minerals, hydrochloric acid to digest protein, and two tablets of "natural digestive enzymes." She asks Dr. Nittler what to do.

Dr. Nittler says she has a vitamin deficiency. He urges her to take more A and D.

Medicine generally says that these vitamins can be toxic when taken for a time in doses as little as five or ten times those recommended. But Nittler says, "Any toxicity found from A and D vitamins has always been caused by synthetic forms. The natural forms are non-toxic, and large doses can be taken with impunity." He tells the lady to take 100,000 units of A (25 times the RDA) for three months.

Treating disease with food is much rarer among physicians than among certain other practitioners. After all, it is nice to be able to give medicine to a patient. And if you happen to be a chiropractor, naturopath or similar healer, your license does not permit you to use drugs. The best you can do is to prescribe diets and supplements—then sell the supplements, sometimes at awesome prices. And since most illnesses cure themselves, most of your patients will swear by your methods—even in court.

Linda Clark, who writes the foreword to Nittler's book, hails it as "a breakthrough of courage, help and encouragement." His publisher, Improvement Books, advertises, "Take FOOD, says this doctor, NOT MEDICINE . . . and see PAIN-CAUSING POISONS LITERALLY POUR OUT OF YOUR BODY!"

Actually Nittler's book offers more than this. For example, it features "A do-it-yourself prostate massage that involves a simple motion *with the legs and soles of your feet* . . ."

Dr. Nittler says that he was once an orthodox physician. Then one day he saw a patient who had experienced a mild coronary. "I had followed the usual medical management in his case . . . Among other things used . . . were vitamin B-12 injections and a high potency synthetic vitamin product from the drugstore." The patient had, however, added "natural and organic vitamins," and seemed to feel good. So Nittler spent $24.96 and bought some of his own.

Having spent the money, Nittler said, he thought he should use the pills, although he "was already taking a 5x potency synthetic vitamin-mineral product." He started singing in the shower, tried some more of the supplement on his wife and dogs and was converted. He began to treat his patients with foods.

About a decade later, in March, 1962, he was expelled from his local medical society, "because of unethical conduct." And his hospital privileges were withdrawn.

More recently, Nittler was brought up before the California Board of Medical Examiners on charges of gross negligence, incompetence and unprofessional conduct. As the *San Francisco Chronicle* reported: "The charges were that Nittler failed to diagnose cancer in two of his longtime patients, who later died, and that in a third patient he diagnosed cancer where there was none." Unfortunately, at this writing, the author does not know the final outcome. But some facts from the hearing are interesting.

One lady, whose husband died of stomach cancer, read a list of pills which Nittler had sold her spouse, from what she called, "a little drugstore" in his office—including "mucozyme," raw heart concentrate, prostate tissue and garlic pills—all described by the prosecuting attorney as nonprescription products found in health-food stores.

A number of loyal patients were present, and *Chronicle* reporter Charles Petit, spoke to a few. One 61-year-old woman said Nittler had saved her life. "I was dying, and no orthodox doctor could find out what was wrong with me. I'd been dying for years. They thought it was in my head . . . I had made my will and funeral arrangements when I finally heard about Dr. Nittler."

He said she had hypoglycemia and insufficient hydrochloric acid. Another woman also said Nittler had saved her daughter from hypoglycemia. In the past months, she said, she had paid $1,500, mainly for food supplements and diet advice, but that, "Oh, it was worth it."

Foodists insist that such treatment from "natural" doctors is harmless. But nutritionists are not so sure.

For example, in 1962, S.J. Haught published the book, *Has Dr. Max Gerson a True CANCER CURE?* Haught reports getting a letter from a woman who had cancer, had seen Dr. Gerson at his Park Avenue office in New York, and for five months had been on his special diet. She describes the diet as:

"Orange juice, green juice, liver juice and carrot juice. I take 12 glasses of juice every day made with a special grinder and press. I receive a B-12 shot with liver extract twice a week, and two coffee enemas a day. My meals consist of fresh fruit, cottage cheese skim milk and yogurt . . ."

The woman's problem was that her diet and supplements were costing her 89 percent of her husband's take-home pay. And neither government nor any voluntary health agency would give her the money to continue the treatment. Dr. Gerson told her she would have to be on this diet for about a year longer. And she had given up conventional therapy.

As early as 1946, the *Journal of the AMA* had reported on the diet, and on Gerson's refusal to "reveal the details of his treatment." In 1958, he had been suspended from membership in his local medical society for two years.

Inquiries concerning Gerson were so numerous that the American Cancer Society prepared a printed statement. It noted that Gerson had used the treatment in Austria, before coming to the U.S. in the early 1940's. From 1946 to 1950, he had used it at Gotham Hospital in New York, until, "his affiliation with that hospital was terminated. At present, he treats patients in his own nursing home outside the city. He also maintains an office at 815 Park Avenue."

The statement says that patients must prepare their food in special glass utensils and use, "juicing machines which are offered to his patients for sale at around $150." They are also taught, "to give their own injections of liver at home."

Gerson got much publicity when John Gunther's son—who, we saw earlier, suffered from a brain tumor—became his patient. The Cancer Society also points to a boy who suffered from bone cancer and was taken to Gerson after amputation, and after a long time, "was returned home in a pitiable state of malnutrition." The Cancer Society said that it could ". . . find no acceptable evidence that the treatment . . . produces any objective benefit . . ."

The Gerson treatment still persists, in the hands of others. The laudatory Haught book went into its 9th printing in 1972, and may have gone further. Supposedly "cured" patients—with unorthodox cancer therapy, it is always well to ask whether the patients really did have cancer in the first place—formed the Foundation for Cancer Treatment. One of them was said by the Foundation to have been Mrs. Albert Schweitzer, and her husband was on the board of directors. His testimonial to Gerson is used on the cover of the book:

"Those he cured will now attest to the truth of his ideas . . . a medical genius who walked among us."

In their book for the American Cancer Society, *Unproven Methods of Cancer Treatment,* Dr. Roald Grant and Irene Bartlett comment on the importance of prominent endorsers of cancer "cures." Why Dr. Schweitzer believed in Gerson is hard to say. But certainly anyone who believed that a loved one was threatened by cancer and saw him or her recover might feel convinced. One can only say that cancer is sometimes not an easy, sure diagnosis, and that there appear to be quite a few cases of spontaneous remission in true cases. One can also observe that Schweitzer had an interest in various diet cures of the old Swiss and German schools.

Among the unproven cancer cures that use nutritional methods are:

• George Zuccala's *Anticancergen Z-50,* some of the rationale of which has to do with food additives.

• *Bamfolin,* from a Japanese bamboo grass, supposedly containing some special sugars and minerals.

• *H.H. Beard methods,* including Laetrile and "vitamin" B-15, which holds that cancer is a "chymotrypsin and nutrition deficiency disease."

• *Cancer Lipid Concentrate,* involving a claim that a certain fatty substance is necessary for cancer cells to grow.

• *Carzodelan,* based on the idea that a certain enzyme can break down cancer cells, and used with the "Freund" diet, founded upon fresh vegetables, fruit and powdered (not fresh) eggs.

• *Fresh Cell (Niehans) Therapy,* widely publicized as having been used for German Chancellor Conrad Adenauer and Pope Pius XII, in Switzerland. A special diet and sun baths are used with it. "Trace element" therapy, supposedly including exotic minerals, is also involved. One labeling is "H3." FDA has seized and destroyed supplies of the materials.

• *The Frost method,* originating in Texas, employing a special vaccine combined with "a complete reorganization of the diet to include only organically grown food." The method employs Koch "antitoxins," Krebiozen, and Mucorhicin, all of which have been the subject of much government protective action.

• *Gibson methods* (out of New York City and Brewster, New York) similar to the above: include vitamins and a simple, natural life with faith in God a requisite for cure.

• *Grape Cures,* following Dr. Kellogg's pattern and involving from two ounces to half a pound of grapes every two hours. Most popularly described by Johanna Brandt in her book, *The Grape Cure,* it depends on the idea that the grape has astonishing properties when eaten alone, but is, "chemically converted into poisons when mixed with other substances . . . in the stomach." (When the grapes become repugnant, one has a natural signal to begin a fast, followed by other curious dietary regimes.) In 1951, Macfadden's Physical Culture Library Service agreed with the Post Office to refrain from selling the books through the mail. The book is, however, still available at health-food stores.

• *Polonine,* which is supposed to attack certain B vitamins. The National Cancer Institute, after tests, said that it could discover "nothing . . . to indicate that it would be of use."

• *Revici Cancer Control* theory, asserting that cancer results from an imbalance between two kinds of fatty substance, acid and alkaline. Scientific review showed no value.

• *Spears Hygiene System,* mainly using chiropractic adjustments, enemas to remove "poisons," and special diets.

One of the key problems in trying to restrict the use of spurious nutrition cures by healers of whatever license is that generally the law sees the licensed therapist as immune, as long as he does not trespass into a regulated domain for which he is not licensed, and is not clearly negligent. However, some states have held that physicians must meet current standards of treatment—somewhat akin to the standards by which malpractice suits are judged.

On the other hand, healers of any stripe may write books and leaflets with impunity. For example, not long ago an engineer in San Diego was charged with manslaughter in the death of his only child, Rhea Diane Sullins, 7. The father, a widower, was past president of a local chapter of the American Natural Hygiene Society, which rejects drugs and turns to "natural" cures of fasting, juices and the like.

When little Rhea became ill, her father put her on a water-only fast for 18 days. Then he put her on a diet of fruit juice for 17 days more. The *Los Angeles Times* report said she died of pneumonia and starvation.

Such tragedies are beyond comment. However, they point up the sad truth that "natural" is not synonymous with "harmless." The danger of misconstruing this relationship is evidenced by a 1974 incident in London. Basil Brown, identified in a *New York Times* report as a "scientist" and "health food enthusiast," became convinced that he needed massive doses of vitamin A. He began to take huge amounts of the pure vitamin. In addition, he stepped up his already large ration of carrot juice.

About four average carrots make an eight-ounce glass of the juice. Believers who buy costly juicers commonly drink two or three glasses a day, often on the basis of curative claims by "demonstrators" who hustle the machines in health-food stores. It is nothing for carrot-juice believers to drink a quart a day.

A single carrot, weighing less than three ounces, yields some 8,000 units of vitamin A. Thus, two modest glasses of carrot juice provide 64,000 units of vitamin A—16 times the RDA, and a potentially toxic level, when continued long enough. Basil Brown drank a gallon a day, in the belief that "natural" vitamin A was harmless. So he got over 500,000 units, or some three and a half years' supply daily—plus his consumption of the vitamin in pure form. After ten days of this, he was bright yellow, and he died, of cirrhosis of the liver (the organ in which excess fat-soluble vitamins are stored).*

Such massive and apparently irrational vitamin doses have lately been dignified with the name "megavitamin therapy." "Megavitamin" therapists usually emphasize use of water-soluble vitamins,** which they erroneously declare to be harmless.

*It is doubtful that death would have resulted from vitamin-A rich foods alone. However, such foods are capable of producing ill effects.

**All vitamins except A, D, E and K, which can be stored in the body.

The essential concept of the megavitamin mongers is that all of nutrition science has misread the needs of the body, and that some individuals need incredible amounts of nutrients to function in a normal way. We saw an example of this in Linus Pauling's claims for the "natural" intake of vitamin C.

Science has no sure, simple answer for mental ills—such as schizophrenia, or even for the pain of depression or hysteria. But these entities tend to be, in their ordinary course, remitting. So remissions may be attributed to *any* therapy.

Characteristic of megavitamin thinking is an article by Norman Cousins, longtime editor of the respected *Saturday Review*. The article is summarized by those distinguished science writers, Ruth Adams and Frank Murray, who gave us *Vitamin C, the Powerhouse Vitamin (conquers more than just colds).* It tells the story of Joan.

Having graduated from a "fashionable college," Joan was diagnosed as schizophrenic and hospitalized. "Finally," write Adams and Murray, "the tortured young woman was taken to a psychiatrist who believes that mental illness is a reflection of the physical condition of the body. He told Joan's family that she was suffering from pellagra."

Pellagra is a malady which results from a serious deficiency of the B vitamin, niacin. Adams and Murray explain that Joan's pellagra was of, "only brain and nerve cells."

But vitamin deficiencies are afflictions of the *whole* body. As one medical manual of nutrition puts it, "pellagra . . . is portrayed by the four D's—dermatitis, diarrhea, dementia and death." First skin lesions appear, from which the disease takes its name. The skin, "becomes dry, scaly and cracked . . . occasionally the skin becomes blistered." There is abdominal pain and diarrhea. The tongue becomes raw and red, sore. The nervous system does not function well. Before death, the patient becomes irritable, loses memory, cannot sleep and suffers great anxiety.

The final stage of pellagra, after months of deficiency, is the dementia that megavitamin believers say is the same as schizophrenia. This means that they would have us believe that the last and most desperate symptom of a deficiency appears with no hint of any earlier signs.

In America, niacin deficiency is precluded first by the typical American diet, which supplies plenty of the vitamin. Second, the body can make its own niacin from one of the most common amino acids found in good protein foods, tryptophan. And the typical American consumes so much tryptophan that he can manufacture all the niacin he needs.

The niacin recommended by all authorities totals some 17 mg. a day. Much less than this will prevent all sign of pellagra. Megavitamin people not only claim that a kind of "hidden pellagra" is the real cause of schizophrenia, but that it takes 4,000 mg. a day to cure it—about an eight months' supply each day, according to the RDA.

The distorted idea began to take hold in about 1954, advanced by the Canadians, Hoffer, Osmond and Smythies. Then, when Pauling advanced his concepts of super-vitamin intakes in 1968, he added the term "orthomolecular medicine," which he defines as "the preservation of good health and the treatment of disease by varying the concentrations in the human body of substances that are normally in the body and are required for health."*

If we read this line carefully, we see that it is really only another way of expressing the old "natural" health idea. It is a way of saying that all the substances needed for cure are to be found in the body or its food. Pauling disdains treatment by "the use of powerful synthetic substances or plant products." Mental illness is no exception.

The therapists who were using wholly unphysiologic amounts of vitamins to treat schizophrenia and other emotional problems loved the idea. Overnight, they became "orthomolecular psychiatrists."

The therapy can be costly (though certainly not because of the dollar worth of the vitamins), and it is today used in small

---

*Actually the term derives from *ortho*, meaning right or straightening (as in orthopedics), and *molecular*, referring to an aim of making sure all the right molecules are in the body. (The author feels that semantically the term fails. He proposes the use of a new term for such work—*orthovernacular therapy*—meaning the rearranging of new words for old ideas in order to create the right financial environment for the therapist.)

hospitals and clinics for all sorts of emotional problems, including alcoholism. Reviewing psychiatrists observe that the therapy does have one value. It helps to remove the stigma of true diagnosis. One is not disturbed; one merely has a problem with one's "chemical balance."

A few years ago, psychiatrists became concerned about the growing belief, carefully encouraged by publicity, that treating "chemical imbalance" with vitamins could cure psychoses. For example, the Retail Clerks Union Local 770 in Los Angeles once had a fine mental health program for its members. It dropped the program for one that centered on nutrient pills and capsules.

The American Psychiatric Association appointed a task force to study the megavitamin claims and treatments. They found a bleak absence of anything like controlled studies. For example, one of the most basic rules of scientific investigation is to bend every effort to get rid of unwanted variables—so that if either good or harm is done, one has a chance of knowing why. But the "orthomolecular" therapists offer hodge-podges of evidence.

The task force found that along with massive doses of niacin, there might be any or all of massive doses of vitamin C, pyridoxine, vitamin E, thyroid, vitamin B-12, "low blood sugar" diets, cereal-free diets, physical exercises, lithium, phenothiazines, "and also the commonly used tranquilizers and antidepressants, . . . Electroconvulsive therapy is still frequently used. Nothing is said . . . as to how the biochemical peculiarities (of individuals) are elucidated, nor corrected . . . There is nothing orthomolecular about the electroconvulsive therapy or the psychotropic drugs . . ."

The task force report goes into great detail. It says that, "serious and major attempts to demonstrate the value of nicotinic acid (a form of niacin) have been . . . uniformly negative." It observes that such tests have shown, "no dramatic individual recoveries"—which might have indicated that a few schizophrenics could be helped in this way.

The report treats, "the nagging question of how many people have been diagnosed as schizophrenic and treated successfully by orthomolecular means when they may not have been schizophrenic at all."

It concludes that the, "credibility of the megavitamin proponents is low . . . further diminished by a consistent refusal over the past decade to perform controlled experiments and to report their results in a scientifically acceptable fashion."

The megavitamin tale has been promoted more and more intensively, through such new organizations as the American Schizophrenia Association, the Huxley Institute for Biosocial Research, the hypoglycemia organizations and the rather new Feingold Association. (The latter derives its name from a California doctor named Ben Feingold, who thinks that food flavors, colors and other additives are the cause of hyperactivity in young children.)*

The literature of the megavitamin proponents is pretty strong. It claims a cure rate of 90 percent among acute schizophrenics (within two years) and of 75 percent among chronic schizophrenics (within five years). These numbers, which supposedly derive from the work of Hoffer and Osmond, are buttressed by such ideas as the contention that schizophrenia is really just a step in evolution. *Bestways* proposes this in a recent article, saying that schizophrenics are "more attractive," that the disease "has been considered the affliction of genius," that patients "rarely have asthma and can walk through fields of pollen without a sniffle," have "more resistance to disease," and "lower sex drives."

The bookshelves and pamphlet racks continue to fill with the megavitamin hard sell. There are such standard references as Adams and Murray's *Body, Mind and the B Vitamins, Hope Giving Stories of Schizophrenic Patients,* Judge Tom Blaine's *Mental Health Through Nutrition,* Cheraskin's *New Hope of Incurable Diseases, The Journal of Orthomolecular Psychiatry* (published by the Schizophrenia Association), Abram Hoffer's *New Hope for Alcoholics and How to Live with Schizophrenia,* Vic Pawlak's *Megavitamin Therapy and the Drug Wipeout Syndrome* and of course, the writings of Dr. David Hawkins, who says he has treated over 2,000 patients in a New York suburb.

Hawkins, in his introduction to the Adams and Murray book on megavitamins (billed as offering "NEW HOPE FOR: AL-

*Feingold's arguments for his case are largely based on anecdotes in his popular book. At this writing, there is no controlled experimental research.

COHOLICS, . . . SCHIZOPHRENICS, HYPERACTIVE CHILDREN"), says that the diet pattern which he calls, "the final All-American-Supermarket-Madison-Avenue-TV-Ad-Teen-Age-Diet," is that of the average American. He says that this, "is the diet which is supported by establishment nutritionists who have the nerve to make public statements that the American Supermarket provides an adequate, nourishing diet." He says also that this is, "the typical diet of most of the patients I have seen with alcoholism, schizophrenia, drug abuse problems, as well as obesity and a variety of other social and medical afflictions."

This sounds pretty startling at first. Then one wonders. Is it really surprising that physical and emotional difficulties which encompass tens of millions of people in America tend to be experienced by people who eat typical American diets? The logic is a little like saying that most of the nation's sick have worn underwear—and blaming underwear for our health problems.

Small wonder that when Dr. Hawkins wrote his book on megavitamins, *Orthomolecular Psychiatry, Treatment of Schizophrenia,* the text which is promoted as *the* serious medical treatise on the subject, he was glad to get a little basic scientific help. So the book has a co-author, Linus Pauling.

The food-and-health folk, long individualists, were banding together.

23

Meanwhile, Back at the Organic Ranch . . .

The family photo is unremarkable—just Mom, Dad and the three kids—but the headline is a bit jarring:

> "Just a typical American mother.
> And her victims."

The ad is for *Prevention*, and it is the kind of message that built this publication. Founded in 1950, by the mid-1960's it had only a few hundred thousand readers. In the last decade its circulation has zoomed toward two *million*.

"Each and every issue brings you . . . *natural* health and living 'secrets,' " says a newer ad. It offers articles on "How you can prevent aging symptoms," "A change in diet can banish crippling arthritis," "What to do to increase sexual vigor," and "Mayonnaise—the amazing beauty aid!"

The magazine is the creature of Jerome I. Rodale, whose eclectic fascination with foodism has dotted these pages. Born in 1899, Rodale started out as an accountant and then made electrical devices. But he loved to write.

By the 1930's, he was mostly writing about crossword puzzles, but he also tried plays and musical comedies. Then, as he is quoted by Herbert Bailey (one of Carlton Fredericks' co-authors), he became worried about his heart "condition," of which he had known "since boyhood." He read the 1940 *Time* article which told about the Shutes and vitamin E, and says, "I bought my first bottle of vitamin E capsules in 1940."

The effect? "I am sure that the Shutes saved my life."

He had been worried about a family history of heart disease. "My father died of it at age 51, my oldest brother at 51, my next oldest at 62, Joe at 56, Tina at 64 and Sally at 60." He is writing this much later, in 1961. He says that he is about to be 63 and, "can walk miles with ease, thanks to my vitamin E, and of course also to my whole Prevention program . . . There is no reason why I can't reach 100 unless I am killed in an accident."

At about the same time that Rodale got interested in vitamins and health, he was developing a business idea. In the late 1930's he read about the work of Sir Albert Howard, then a British agricultural adviser to the Indian state of Indore. Howard had been trying to increase farm yields to feed the Indian hungry. His first effort was to send out for some ordinary fertilizer. But it turned out there was no money for it.

So Howard turned to the old idea of composting, piling up organic (substances derived from life forms) matter, so that it broke down and made a weak fertilizer. Fertility rose in the formerly unfertilized fields. And of course, with more food, local health improved. It was easy for unscientific readers to infer that something in the compost had led to improved health. But the only difference was (and is) that people who have some food to eat are a lot healthier than people who don't.

By 1942, Rodale had turned his Howard-inspired thinking to a magazine, *Organic Gardening and Farming*. The 1930's Dust-bowl had just taught farmers that they could not strip their soils, but should plough back remaining portions of the plants to help keep the soil in place and tillable. The attendant publicity certainly helped the magazine find acceptance.

Gradually, as Rodale's son Robert tells us, his father began to draw connections between farming methods, health and philosophy. "He proclaimed that to be *organic* was to know . . . the lessons of nature in all ways . . . In fact, not caring whether he was called an extremist or crackpot, J. I. Rodale created . . . a *strict* constructionist interpretation of natural life under the banner of organiculture. If it is synthetic, avoid it, he said. If it goes through a factory, examine it with special care."

It is really only the same old theme of "natural" living, with the old promise of extraordinary health. As usual, the person to whom the idea occurs is sure that *he* knows what is natural. So it was with Rodale. In eight years he began to publish *Prevention,* scouring all the nutritional pigeonholes of history for secrets of life and then pouring them out to his believers.

There seems little doubt of Rodale's sincerity. The reader may, for example, remember his interest in walking barefoot in the dew and handling growing plants, to get electricity. He meant it. According to Dr. Edward Rynearson of the Mayo Clinic, "he believed that people do not get enough electricity from the atmosphere, owing to the presence of steel girders and insulation, [so] he would sit . . . under a machine that gave off . . . radio waves, which . . . he believed . . . boosted his body's supply of electricity."

Did Rodale really think that our food was nutritionally insufficient for health? "He used to take," writes Dr. Rynearson, "70 food-supplement tablets a day."

His tracts poured out. He wrote two encyclopedias, *The Health Builder* and *The Encyclopedia for Healthful Living.* His shorter works are typified by *Rodale's System for Mental Power,* ("J. I. Rodale . . . offers startling evidence of why . . . you can grow smarter by eating the smart way.") His style is suggested by some chapter titles from this book: "Vegetarianism's Effect on Sex," "A Case of Low Blood Sugar . . . Adolf Hitler," "Salt and Baldness," "Destruction in the Kitchen," "Destruction in the Factories," "Mental Patients Are Low in Vitamin C," "The Miracle of Vitamin E . . . Helps Reduce Stammering," "Bread

Chemical Gives Fits to Dogs," "How to Keep Your Driving Record Clean . . . Sugary Sweets Not Advisable," "Millions Need Chiropractic," and a good deal more information about why citrus can be eaten, but not drunk, and how dangerous it is to let food make contact with plastic or aluminum.

But aside from the many minor fancies about health and eating, the essence of the Rodale program was that foods grown without the use of commercial fertilizers and sprays had something that ordinary foods lacked—and that this something could prevent much ill health.

Is this idea true? Instead of looking to the usual experts, let us first hear opinions from the Rodale people. It is December 1, 1972, in New York City. A public hearing is being held before New York's attorney general, a hearing about "organic" foods. On the stand is Dr. Mark Schwartz.

SCHWARTZ: . . . I am a director of research for Rodale Press and I have a Doctor's Degree in Food and Nutrition and a Master's and Bachelor's Degree in Agriculture.

MINDELL (Assistant Attorney General): Tell us something about Rodale?

SCHWARTZ: Rodale Press is a publishing company located in Emmaus, Pennsylvania. It is a forum for organic foods, health foods, nutritional foods, writing and publishing articles concerning health foods . . . [He gives the names of publications.]

MINDELL: Does it generally take the position . . . that organic foods are nutritionally superior to ordinary foods?

SCHWARTZ: I think to make that statement certainly upon the basis of what has been said before, I think from an ecological point of view that must be considered. I believe that types of foods we have talked about here, there is a misconception of what Rodale Press particularly has talked about when you talk about organic foods.

MINDELL: Can you define what you mean then?

ATTORNEY GENERAL: Tell us what Rodale Press means.

SCHWARTZ: I don't think organic foods are any different from the foods that we ordinarily eat. The thing we are talking about is the method of producing these foods.

ATTORNEY GENERAL: Growth?

SCHWARTZ: Growing these foods.

ATTORNEY GENERAL: That's what you're talking about?

SCHWARTZ: That is without the use of chemical fertilizers and pesticides.

MINDELL: What are the benefits you see in organic food?

SCHWARTZ: Well, there has certainly been enough in the past year about DDT and PCB and the effect on the environment and the effect on people as well as sodium nitrate and DES in organic foods produced without these chemicals.

ATTORNEY GENERAL: You are going on the assumption, per se, that there are no chemicals in organic foods?

SCHWARTZ: Well, I should say that we have—in order to better define this organically grown that we have put forth, we have a laboratory in California . . . looking at foods from the standpoint of pesticide residue we have come to the conclusion that it is almost impossible to come up with foods that are not, do not, contain pesticides.

* * *

(There is discussion of reasons why pesticide fallout contaminates organic and ordinary farms alike. Very little of the very tiny pesticide residue found in foods is traced to farming practices. Any amount which is found in the constant FDA surveillance of markets around the country is well within the safe limits set by United Nation expert panels. Schwartz talks about a certification program and agrees that the program does not give the consumer much assurance of what he is buying.)

MINDELL: What steps would you think should be taken in order to insure that the public is not being deceived when they go in and buy organic foods, as to representations regarding prevention of diseases and cure of diseases or nutritional superiority . . . ? What would you like to see?

SCHWARTZ: I think there certainly should be some substantiation of these claims. I don't really know in what form that takes.

MINDELL: Would you have objection to labeling requirements that organic foods are not, per se, nutritionally superior?

SCHWARTZ: I certainly don't think it should say that. I don't know whether you can really make that statement . . . That's very difficult to just say that it's conceivable that fresh produce grown locally and locally consumed would be of better nutritional value or high nutritional value than a product coming in from halfway across the country. So that would be very difficult to say . . ."

At the same hearing, Robert Rodale, who had by then succeeded to the command of the Rodale enterprises, also testified.

THE ATTORNEY GENERAL: Are you prepared to say that organic food has a nutritional superiority over ordinary food?

RODALE: Well, there are many factors that influence the nutritional value and many of these factors are part of the organic system . . . The sunlight on an apple affects the spraying of plants in a row, the selection of varieties that are used, the amount of irrigation used, the type of fertilizer, the type of soil.

Now, if a farmer wants to produce food that is nutritionally superior he can use all varieties of methods and do that . . . and it is absolutely incorrect as some people have said here this morning that there is no difference in the nutritional value.

ATTORNEY GENERAL: Do you disagree with these people . . . ? They are doctors. What is your background?

RODALE: I am trained as an English major in journalism. I admit I don't have the background.

In their publications, the Rodales have been much more explicit: "Organically fed animals will provide more minerals to whoever eats the meats that come from them," the editors write. And asking themselves the question that New York officials were asking, they say, "Won't foods grown by ordinary agricultural practices fill the same need as organically grown foods? Unfortunately," they answer in their *Organic Directory*, ". . . most foods raised today are likely to be short in minerals." Vitamin differences are also claimed in various publications.

At the New York organic food hearing, there was overwhelming evidence that this was not so. Consider the statement of Dr. Ruth Leverton, one of the nation's most respected nutrition educators. Speaking for the U.S. Department of Agriculture's Agricultural Research Service, she says:

"There is no proven, substantiated basis for claiming that plants grown with only organic fertilizer have a greater nutrient content . . . The type of fertilizer used . . . is not a determining factor in the nutritive value of the plant.

"The nutrient content of a plant is based on its genetic nature. The genes in a carrot cause it to develop a relatively large amount of Vitamin A-value, just as the genes in an orange are responsible for its high vitamin C . . .

"Nutrient material must be in the *inorganic* form to be

absorbed by the plant . . . Organic fertilizer must be broken down into its inorganic components before the elements are absorbed . . ."

(Organic is used by Dr. Leverton in the scientific sense, referring to substances built upon a chemical skeleton of carbon atoms. When the nutrients come from life forms, such as manure or garbage, they tend to be linked to carbon compounds and have to be broken away before the plant can use them. Bacteria do this.)

"Maintaining 'freshness' is the key to maintaining nutritive value [of fruits and vegetables] . . . But maintaining freshness, including the desirable flavor . . . has nothing to do with the manner in which the vegetables or fruits are fertilized or grown . . ." [Note the reference in Dr. Schwartz's testimony to "fresh produce," when asked about nutritional superiority. His answer said nothing about "organic" farming.]

Commented FDA Commissioner Dr. Charles C. Edwards: ". . . The agency is not aware of any information that food produced in the manner described has any nutritional quality differing from foods produced by usual agricultural practices . . ."

In recent years, science's ability to detect extremely tiny amounts of substances in foods has been sharpened until fractions of one part per *billion* can be identified. So any nutrient peculiar to "organic" food could be found by analysis—if any were there.

In his testimony, FDA's Dr. Edwards explained that the most sophisticated techniques of chemical analysis had not detected any difference between "organic" and ordinary foods. For this reason, he said, "The FDA has not established any definition for 'natural' or 'organic' food and is of the opinion that any attempt to define such products would have limited value."

Nevertheless, the Rodale publications hold out that organic food is better for health. Say the editors: "The ill effects of trace mineral deficiency are so many and varied that *practically any illness that takes you to the doctor might be caused by one."* (Emphasis added.)

Is there any real possibility that—as a host of authors such as Rodale, Carlton Fredericks and Adelle Davis have claimed—the nation's soils are deficient, causing foods grown in those soils to contain less nutritive value? No chance. This is what Dr. Leverton emphasized. Since heredity dictates the food needs of plants, the soil must be able to meet those needs or the plant simply will not grow. So all the fruits and vegetables you see are nutritively complete.

If soils are only *partly* deficient in nutrients which the crop needs, individual plants will be either smaller or fewer. The total crop yield will be poor. So will the farmer. This is why farmers have their soils analyzed and spend small fortunes on fertilizers to keep them up to full production.

Agriculture scientists see the organic theorists as naive in their pleas for a changeover in farming technique. The organic fans like to say that such experts are tools of the makers of fertilizer and sprays. But the facts are plain. Dr. Norman Borlaug (who won the Nobel Prize for his work in improving food production in "the green revolution" and was responsible for developing new strains of wheat that have saved many lives) comments: "If the use of pesticides in the United States were to be completely banned, crop losses would probably soar to 50 percent, and food prices would increase fourfold to fivefold."

The U.S. Department of Agriculture acknowledges that some small farms have been able to "go organic." But its experts observe that this success is heavily dependent on the fact that insects and plant diseases are carefully controlled by the government and by the conventional farmers around them. U.S.D.A. says that one percent of U.S. farms produce some 35 percent of our poultry, 45 percent of our fruits and nuts and some 60 percent of our vegetables. These farms could not function without modern fertilizers and sprays. U.S.D.A. officials have estimated that if the nation turned to organic farming, some 50 million Americans would face starvation—not to mention the cutoff of any U.S. food to the rest of the world.

Some organic enthusiasts point to shortages of trace elements in certain soils, pointing to the incidence of goiter in the iodine-poor soils of certain portions of the country. But logic tells us, and science confirms, that organic farming methods provide no answer. Suppose iodine is low in some of our midwestern soils. Plants which have grown on those soils and manures from animals which have fed on the plants grown in those soils are now used as fertilizer. Where would the needed iodine come from?

Organic farming sets up a tight closed circle. Its methods insure a kind of agricultural isolation, like that of the 19th century.

Indeed, signs of iodine deficiency due to low-iodine soils took a sharp downturn as foods began to be exchanged between various parts of the country. A Michigander living in a low-iodine area today gets his lettuce from California, oranges from Florida, beef from Nebraska, seafood frozen in New England, beans canned in Texas, and so on. While organic fans decry the long-distance shipping of foods and the processing which makes it possible, insisting on local foods instead, modern methods are among our best guarantees of good nutrition.

J.I. Rodale became more and more antagonistic to the food industry as time went on. For one thing, his claims that industry was robbing the food supply of nutritive value made him a lot of friends. After all, if ordinary food had been depleted, wasn't that a good reason for buying the special foods and supplements which were his main sources of advertising revenue?

With all the down-home image cultivated by the enterprises at Emmaus, they were actually big business. Rodale had become a multimillionaire. The more he attacked the food supply, the louder the cash register rang. And attack he did.

In an article called "Our Daily Poison," we get a typical taste of the venom. Once food has been grown, the article tells us, ". . . Food manufacturers must process their food, preserve it for long shelf life, color it an attractive ripe color, sweeten it, emulsify it, cure it, stabilize it, salt it, irradiate it, bleach it, blanch it, polish it, de-germ it, de-bran it, gas it . . . not to mention accumulating sex hormones, antibiotics, tranquillizers, disinfectants, antispoilants, anti-sprouting agents, desiccants, and sex-sterilants."

Some of this is true, and some is absurd. But by 1971, the word "organic" had become synonymous with "healthful." As we have seen, government surveys showed that a majority of Americans bought at least some of Rodale's ideas about the food supply and its effects on health. He was not only at war with industry, but also with such government health programs as fluoridation. He didn't care whether fluoridation would save half the nation's dental cavities; fluoride was a poison, he said, ignoring the fact that some parts of the country have far more fluoride in their water naturally than is added to drinking water.

On a Sunday in June of 1971, he left his 63-acre experimental organic farm and went up to New York to explain organics on the Dick Cavett television show. "I'm going to live to be 100," he said, "unless I'm run over by a sugar-crazed taxi driver."

On Monday night, he began taping the show. As the Associated Press story reports: "Rodale was explaining his secrets when he slumped over, appeared to be snoring and became unconscious . . . The multimillionaire farmer publisher was pronounced dead on arrival at Roosevelt Hospital."

He was 72 years old.

24

Organic Politics
Or
Gloria Swanson
Goes to Washington

In 1951, Bess Truman was hosting the Congressional Wives' Club, and everyone thought it would be nice if Gloria Swanson came to talk to them about food and staying young.

As she told beauty reporter Lydia Lane, she had learned the secrets of eating, back, "in the 20's, when I was ill. I was brought back to health by the wonderful doctor, Henry Bieler, and I have been his disciple ever since."

From this we know that Miss Swanson must surely have had her liver detoxified, watched her sodium and potassium, and swallowed diets of thin soup, zucchini squash and the like. We recall that Bieler didn't believe germs caused disease, but that food did, as in his claims about polio being caused by ice cream. Basically, Gloria ate organic. Lydia Lane tells us that, "Miss Swanson does not abuse her body with foods that are sprayed with insecticides, processed or contain chemicals."

This suggests a very limited diet, since all foods *are* chemical compounds, and life itself is a chemical process. Presumably, Gloria told the Congressional wives how to avoid chemicals. And then she terrified them. She said food additives caused cancer. She said there ought to be a law.

"I'll do anything to stop these bad things from going into food," she says today. "It is criminal! They're like murderers! And I hold the medicals responsible for retardation, epilepsy, dwarfed babies."

Some of the wives set out to get a law, and Gloria tried to keep whatever pressure she could on the situation. Rep. James J. Delaney (Dem., N.Y.) seemed to feel it was simple. All we needed was a law that said that anything that caused cancer couldn't be put in food.

Gradually, other Congressmen, "would buttonhole me in the hall," says Delaney, "and say, 'What's this all about? My wife has been giving me the devil about this bill of yours.'"

In 1958, Congress passed a new Food Additives Amendment, aimed at putting the burden of proving safety upon the manufacturer. For 52 years it had been up to the government to prove danger. Delaney got his clause into it. It read, "No additive shall be deemed to be safe if it is found to induce cancer when ingested by man or animal, or if it is found, after tests which are appropriate for the evaluation of the safety of food additives, to induce cancer in man or animals."

The vast majority of all the fuss about additives since then has centered on extrapolations from these few words. And the result has been much doubt and distortion in public thinking. One false popular impression stands out: while scientists do not want to cause a lot of cancer with food chemicals, they think a little bit is all right.

The problem begins with a misunderstanding much like that about general toxicity—the belief that compounds are either toxic or nontoxic, when in fact toxicity is a matter of amount. So it is with the potential to cause cancer. One can say that smoking causes cancer. But does this mean that one puff on a cigarette will increase your chance of malignancy in the slightest? Emotionally, this is a hard truth to deal with. But to reject the fact is to put ourselves to incredible trouble, expense and sacrifice—all needlessly, as we shall see.

There are enormous numbers of chemicals, some of which occur naturally in foods, which could cause cancer if the exposure to them were great enough and long enough. And yet these chemicals are not only harmless in moderate quantity, they are most useful and sometimes irreplaceable.

Let us look at a couple of examples. Until recently, most of the decaffeinated coffee drunk in America was made with the help of a compound called trichlorethylene (TCE). Only tiny amounts of TCE got into the coffee. But because it is a good solvent for grease, because it is used as cleaning fluid, and because it is a useful anesthetic, TCE was also *breathed* in quantity by a few workers in other industries. Its chemical structure suggested that such quantity intake might predispose to cancer.

The National Cancer Institute (NCI) *gavaged* mice and rats with TCE; that is, huge quantities of TCE were forced into the stomachs of the animals every day for their lifetimes. In the end, a few mice showed liver tumors. After the tests, NCI noticed that TCE was also used to decaffeinate coffee. But a coffee drinker might reach the demonstrated cancer-causing level only if he drank some *50 million cups a day* for many years.

More significantly, other research had shown no harmful effect from TCE ingested in amounts equal to about 100 cups of coffee a day (which the coffee maker deemed a safe upper limit of "reasonable expected use"). But Ralph Nader's Health Research Group petitioned FDA to remove the TCE-containing coffee from the market.

The TCE makers spent millions to change over to another caffeine solvent, the one which all the other coffee makers use. Not for safety. Their research made them confident about the safety. But to deal with possible consumer fear.

Was this a valuable health precaution? At first glance it might seem worthwhile, no matter how unlikely the danger—although there was less TCE in the coffee than in the water of most Eastern cities tested. But the new solvent was chemically close to the old—so much so that it is scheduled for similar testing by the Government. Again, neither compound was to be tested in amounts meaningful to food safety, but rather in quantities related to heavy industrial uses.

Technically, under the Delaney Clause, TCE should have

been banned from food although there was no realistic reason to do so. For while the Clause represents an understandable desire, it makes no scientific sense. Potential carcinogenic agents are all about us in the world—from the earth we stand on to substances in our own saliva. But the crucial question is, at what level, at what intensity do they actually cause harm?

A good example is the sun. Its radiation is a known cancer-causer. Radiation is, under the law, an additive. Therefore, it follows theoretically that all food which has been exposed to sunlight ought to be banned under the Delaney Clause, leaving us with a diet of nothing but foods which have never known the sun, such as mushrooms and bat meat. The example is, of course, as absurd as would be the conclusion that we ought never to step outdoors.

The 1958 Amendment did sensibly except substances which had been used safely in the past, and which were Generally Recognized As Safe (GRAS), from new proofs of safety. About 1,000 substances were on the GRAS list. But any "proof" of cancer "hazard" can reopen the question.

At the White House Conference of 1969, it was recommended that GRAS substances be reviewed, and this is going forward. When the reviewers get to checking out the sun, FDA may hear from activists again.

Actually, most of the news you have heard about "cancer-causing" additives has similarities to the TCE case—the matters of Red Number 2, DES, cyclamates, and the like. And sometimes the needless cost to all of us has been substantial.

Take DES (diethyl stilbesterol). Senator Kennedy introduced some hearings on it by saying the subject, "DES, a known cancer-causing agent, is appearing on thousands of American dinner tables." Naturally, Federal agencies jumped.

So did scientists. For DES had been valuable in the beef cattle industry—by speeding the growth of lean meat. DES is an estrogen compound, estrogen being among the hormones produced by the sex glands of women. Estrogens are important in the reproductive functions of women and seem to have some protective effects against aging and heart disease. Actually, there was precious little DES in the meat by the time it reached the market.

From 1940, it was known that estrogens could predispose to cancer under certain conditions and at certain levels. But no one thought that the levels remaining in meat were unsafe.

However, in 1971, some young women were reported to have developed a form of vaginal cancer; their mothers had been given DES during pregnancy to prevent miscarriages—an average of some 65 mg. a day. But Senators Kennedy, Proxmire, Nelson, and well-meaning others apparently did not look carefully at the science involved. The Senate passed a bill in 1972 to ban DES in beef raising. (Eventually the courts reversed the ban.)

What had been the danger? Virtually all the remaining DES in marketed meat was in the liver. This amounted to about an eighth of a part per billion in liver and about an eightieth of a part per billion in muscle. To get the amount of DES given to the pregnant women in the study, you would have to eat some 10.4 million pounds of boneless beef roast, day after day, for months.

Women's bodies produce much more estrogen than this. Even men's bodies produce far more. Dr. Thomas Jukes estimates that even wheat germ has an estrogenic potency about *2,000 times* the level in beef liver.

In 1973, the *New York Times* printed an editorial which said, "Such sensitivity in measuring infinitesimal quantities is a respectable scientific feat, but how meaningful is it as a guide to the public? Is there a significant—even an appreciable—risk of anyone getting cancer from eating meat containing so tiny a quantity of DES?"

What was the purpose of keeping DES? When the ban was lifted, one agricultural expert, K. Monfort, estimated the savings in feed its use would make. He figured it would be the same as adding between three and five million acres to that year's corn crop.

The fact is that our cancer experts really do not look to our food as either important cause or cure for this terrifying illness. Indeed, scare-talk tends to divert scarce research dollars from more fundamental studies which are our real hope of prevention and cure. As one suggestive note, consider that cancer of the stomach has declined. Now a minor cause of illness and death (after our use of food additives increased), it was once one of our worst cancer killers.

Last year, Congressman Delaney received an award for his Clause. It came from the National Health Federation. Gloria Swanson gave it to him. "Appreciative of her role in winning Congressional support," reports the Federation's *Bulletin*, ". . . he sent Miss Swanson a letter, which she framed. She calls it her 'Oscar—his letter saying I was responsible for passage of the Amendment.' "

Miss Swanson continues on with her career of public service. For a new book by Maurice Messegue (hailed by his publisher as "the world's most famous natural healer") Gloria wrote the ad headline: "We cannot survive unless we go back to natural foods and natural cures . . ."

And she married William Dufty—though in television interviews with the happy couple, she has said that she would not be his bride until he changed his eating habits. He even wrote a book (which is why the two have been seen on television lately). It is called *Sugar Blues*. It reveals the astonishing discovery that refined carbohydrate foods can make us feel depressed.

Congressman Delaney goes on protecting us. In 1975, he rose on the floor of the House and pointed out that he had always fought against fluorides as, "an unnecessary health risk." He mentions in a letter to the *Times* that there was, "nothing holy or infallible in the opinions of . . . public health officials." Then he quoted research of the National Health Federation: ". . . Their study . . . indicates that 25,000 excess cancer deaths occur annually in U.S. cities subjected to imposed water fluoridation . . . I now recommend immediate suspension of all artificial fluoridation pending further investigation."

Fortunately, Delaney did not get his way. But since he, Senator Proxmire of Wisconsin and other officials seem to get a lot of their information from the NHF, it may be worth a look.

Formed in 1955, NHF now styles itself, "America's largest organized, noncommercial health consumer group." It is a focal point for action groups, such as the Federation of Homemakers, which fights to ban DES again. It musters mail support for such measures as Delaney's attempt to ban fluorides and for such bills as Kennedy and Schweiker's S.963 to keep DES out of cattle production. It runs appeals such as, "Dr. Nittler Needs Help—

Letters, Money, Now!" And it is locked in perpetual struggle with the FDA and its policies.

A typical story in its *Bulletin* suggests the character of its interests and beliefs. "FDA Finds Another Villain" tells how surprising it is that FDA would seize shipments of Bio Snacky "seeds and sprouting apparatus." The article says: "To those of us who know and respect the power of new-born cereals and grasses—it seems incredible that an agency of the U.S. government would be involved in such book burning."

What had been FDA's nitpicking charges? That the packages and booklets distributed with them said, ". . . that the articles will grow good health, and supply one with health and wellbeing; that the wheat seed in Bio Snacky kits would provide a significant amount of wheat germ . . . ; that such wheat germ is an essential nutritional supplement containing the anti-sterility and fertility vitamin E, and Vitamin F, of . . . value for a healthy and beautiful skin; that wheat germ is nature's tonic; that a daily intake of freshly-grown wheat germ is essential where there are nutritional deficiencies . . . ; that ingestion of enzymes is necessary for digestion; . . . that soya sprouts in a salad give health; that the Bio Snacky kit would provide all the nutritional substances your family needs. . . ."

The origins of NHF may help to explain its *Bulletin*'s attitude toward Bio Snacky and FDA. About a decade ago, FDA issued a release that began: "The National Health Federation was founded in 1955 by Fred J. Hart, shortly after he consented to a federal court injunction prohibiting . . . shipments of 13 electrical devices which had been widely distributed for the diagnosis and treatment of disease. Hart had for many years been president of the Electronic Medical Foundation . . .*

"He was prosecuted for criminal contempt of the injunction and on July 27, 1962, he was fined . . . at which time the court was informed that the Electronic Medical Foundation had been discontinued . . . leaving Hart free to devote his efforts to NHF.

". . . A number of the leading officers, directors and

---

*This Foundation was the outgrowth of the long-distance diagnosis and cure deceptions of Albert Abrams, from whom Hart took over. (See pp. 106–7.)

members of NHF have been involved in court actions under the Federal Food, Drug and Cosmetic Act."

Listed along with Hart are:

"V. Earl Irons, chairman of the board of governors . . . a food supplement distributor who served a one-year sentence in 1957 for misbranding . . . a vitamin mixture sold by house-to-house agents . . .

"Royal Lee, director . . . and one of the founders . . . is a non-practicing dentist at Milwaukee who has twice been convicted for violating the Federal Food and Drug Law. On April 23, 1962, he was given a one-year suspended prison sentence and put on probation for three years . . . His firm, Vitamin Products Co., was fined $7,000. A court order prohibited it from continuing to ship 115 special dietary products misbranded by false claims for the treatment of more than 500 diseases and conditions.

"Roy F. Paxton, director . . . is the twice convicted promoter of 'millrue,' a worthless cancer remedy . . . He was fined $2,500 and is now serving a three-year prison sentence . . .

"Andrew G. Rosenberger, listed as 'Nutrition Chairman' . . . a food faddist and spieler operating under the name Nature Food Centres at Cambridge, Mass., was recently convicted of misbranding dietary food products . . . Andrew Rosenberger and his brother Henry were each fined $5,000 and the corporation was fined $10,000 . . . Each of the Rosenbergers received a six-month suspended prison sentence and was put on probation for two years . . ."

Lately the cast has changed somewhat, but the sympathies are essentially the same. V. Earl Irons is still vice chairman of the board of governors. But Charles Crecelius is president. Betty Lee Morales—proprietor of Organic-ville—is secretary. Dorothy B. Hart is vice president. Kurt Donsbach is chairman of the board. Clinton R. Miller is vice president of the Washington office.

How NHF becomes a focal point for what we might call dissident nutrition ideas is reflected in its efforts when Senators Proxmire and Schweiker offered S. 548 early in 1975. Its object was to block FDA from regulating as drugs, nutrient supplements which contained more than 150 percent of the RDA.

FDA's point of view was that, if a vitamin is intended as a

food supplement, then it is effective as such when it supplies the requirements for that vitamin; it allowed a 50 percent excess for the many who thought they needed extra. Beyond such levels, FDA and nutrition scientists held, the vitamin or mineral is being used as a drug—there being no rationale for extreme intakes of vitamins.

Apparently thinking that Americans *want* to believe in super-nutrition, more than a third of the Senate joined Proxmire and Schweiker as sponsors of the bill, which Proxmire said was, "to prevent the FDA from regulating safe vitamins as dangerous drugs . . . Vitamins are not drugs. They are foods . . . Under the FDA's proposed regulations, relatively small amounts of very common vitamins would have to be sold either as over the counter . . . or prescription drugs. Vitamin C is a good example of what could happen. The new RDA . . . is 45 milligrams. But vitamin C is routinely sold in 100, 250, or 500 milligram tablets. Since it is nontoxic and harmless (sic) there is no reason why that should not continue."

Cosponsors included: Senators Abourezk, Allen, Chiles, Church, Cranston, Domenici, Eastland, Fannin, Goldwater, Gravel, Hansen, Hartke, Inouye, Johnston, Leahy, Mansfield, McClellan, McClure, McGee, Moss, Nunn, Packwood, Pell, Randolph, Hugh Scott, William Scott, Sparkman, Stafford, Stevenson and Thurmond. It is hard to imagine this group in concert on any proposition other than vitamins, except perhaps the preservation of Mother's Day.

What was really at stake was "megavitamin therapy." And super-nutrition interests closed ranks. How much were they listened to by lawmakers? Congressmen reported that in 1974 they received more mail about vitamins than about Watergate.

In the House, California Congressman Hosmer introduced a bill similar to Proxmire's. 11 other representatives then entered similar bills. In the end, the bill of Randall of Missouri won out.

In the Senate, the Proxmire bill won 81-10. Rep. Paul Rogers, chairman of the House Subcommittee on Health and Environment, began to work on a compromise between Senate and House views of the matter. Previously, Rogers and his committee had thrown out all the House bills in favor of a new

Kyros bill. As NHF's president Crecilius reports, "The NHF expressed its strong opposition to this cleverly-worded piece of legislation conceived by FDA and 'midwifed' by Rogers." He says that NHF was now joined by the Federation of Homemakers and the National Nutritional Foods Association (NNFA) representing the health-food business.

According to the NHF *Bulletin,* "Following a four-hour session between Milton Bass, counsel for NNFA and Congressman Paul Rogers, with telephone communication with Attorney Kirkpatrick Dilling, representing the NHF, Congressman Rogers . . . agreed to include five of six amendments . . . with partial agreement on the last amendment."

When the final legislation passed, NHF's Crecilius said: "We have won the consumer's right to buy high-potency, multivitamin-mineral products . . . We only wish that Fred J. Hart, our founder . . . could have known of this victory before his recent passing. Our deep appreciation to each member of the NHF who helped with the over-one-million communications that reached Congress urging passage."

On April 22, 1976, Gerald Ford signed the bill to restrict FDA's protective limitations on vitamin and mineral sales.

In the meantime, what had become of Maine's Rep. Peter Kyros, who offered a more moderate bill? In December of 1974, Kyros filed formal charges with the House that Republican David Emery had conspired with two "paid lobbyists" (Clinton Miller of NHF and Dr. Carlton Fredericks) to disseminate "false and misleading statements" which had led to Emery's taking Kyros' seat. Kyros provided photostats of press reports, which included a photo of Fredericks holding an "anticonsumer" award for Kyros.

Our representatives in Congress had taken counsel and voted. They had turned a deaf or disbelieving ear to the nation's physicians, to the Consumer's Union, to Nader's minions, to the National Nutrition Consortium (representing the American Institute of Nutrition, the American Society for Clinical Nutrition, the American Dietetic Association, the Institute of Food Technologists, the Society for Nutrition Education and the American Academy of Pediatrics), together with the American Association of Retired Persons, the ethical pharmaceutical industry and the National Academy of Sciences.

To whom had they listened? To the national organization of health-food store owners, to the "nutrition" magazines, and to Fred Hart's National Health Federation.

"Proxmire Liberates Vitamins," was the headline in *Business Week* of March 29, 1976. "The removal of restraints," said the magazine, "will represent a major victory for the industry and for . . . 'vitamin freaks.' It should also lead to the introduction of numerous new health food products and to increased sales of raw vitamins.

"A number of major products . . . will no longer be forced to . . . comply with . . . FDA's version of what is rational." *Business Week* quotes a Geritol executive, Roger Schulz. The magazine also cites Schulz' opinion that, "The removal of FDA control . . . will encourage the introduction of more and higher-potency combination products."

"Under present law," says *Business Week*, "the FDA has the power to seize . . . food supplement products that cannot prove their claims to improve health . . . The new law would put the burden of disproving health claims back on the FDA."

"Somebody," FDA's Commissioner is quoted, "could bottle sawdust and sell it as a food supplement."

As NHF's president Crecilius observed, it really is a shame that Fred Hart, who in 1924 succeeded Albert Abrams in the electronic healing and diagnosis business and 37 years later gave it up to create NHF, didn't know. NHF had beaten all those serious scientists hollow.

Perhaps he did know. And if he did, perhaps suddenly he realized how many kindred spirits there were back in Washington. And then he must have slapped his thighs.

25

How the Poison Gets
into Your Health Food

When Dr. Robert Atkins and his "Diet Revolution" first came to
notoriety, his attention was almost solely on carbohydrates. But
within a couple of years, he was back with a new "Super Diet."
And something had been added.

In the *National Enquirer,* he said that the new diet would
remove weight, "But now you're getting a terrific bonus. This diet
will leave you bursting with energy at the same time . . . You'll
learn to live again . . ."

What was new? "Because many of today's foods are over-
processed and over-refined, they don't have the nutrients necessary to balance metabolism . . ." Atkins had thrown in a formidable batch of vitamins, including some non-nutrients such as
bioflavonoids, cut out some preservatives and recommended that
we buy "chelated" minerals at our health-food stores.

The shift is typical of a pronounced trend in foodism during recent years. It is understandable that people who advance ideas which are sharply criticized by orthodox scientists are likely to turn to sympathizers—to other proponents of unorthodoxy. What happens is a kind of organic log-rolling—"You scratch my vitamin and I'll scratch yours."

The result is that some curious and formidable coalitions have been forming. Some are formalized, as in the new Academy of Orthomolecular Psychiatry, the Academy of Preventive Medicine, the International College of Applied Nutrition, and the Academy of Metabology. Meetings have brought these people together, not only nationally, but internationally, as with the recent International Congress of Sciences for Natural Medicine in France. Among the topics were such as naturopathy, vitamin therapy, auriculotherapy, electromagnetism, chromotherapy (with colored lights), and even "aromatherapy."

We have seen, with the Proxmire-Schweiker bill on vitamins, when a million letters were mustered by the coalition, that there is political clout here. Some legislators, for example, perceive a vote block or a source of campaign money; others see a way to identify with liberal and ecological feelings; and conservative politicians perceive the issue as freedom of choice threatened by government.

In any case, the coalition is effective. When the Canadian Province of Alberta denied government health insurance payments for megavitamin therapy, saying it was ineffective, the Alberta Citizens Supporting Orthomolecular Therapy formed. A hot battle ended in the physicians being over-ridden and the payments made.

Let us look at some examples of the new alignments. We might begin with a scene set for us by *Family Circle*. It is 4:30 A.M. in posh Pacific Palisades, in California. Actor Eddie Albert is in his front yard, which is a small organic farm. He is gathering breakfast. "He digs out a couple of carrots . . . washes them off with a hose and eats them. Then he eats some fresh lettuce and radishes."

Why should Eddie Albert's health practices concern us? Haven't actors always been susceptible to such eccentricities?

The scene changes, and we see Eddie in a Hollywood television studio, doing a show called *Viewpoint on Nutrition.* Seated with him are Carlton Fredericks and Linus Pauling. Eddie talks about his early use of vitamin C, and his hypoglycemic reactions to his snacks of orange juice and honey. Fredericks and Pauling confirm the scientific validity of what he says.

The emcee smiles approvingly. He is Dr. Arnold Pike, D.C. Once he was known, as "the 89-pound weakling . . . at Brooklyn's Boys High." Then his cousin showed him Macfadden's *Physical Culture* magazine and took him to hear Gayelord Hauser. Some years later, he was West Coast editor of *Physical Culture.* He did broadcasts, and in 1970 was asked by the National Nutritional Foods Association to do this syndicated "public affairs" show. His closing credits say the program is done, "in cooperation with the President's Council on Physical Fitness."

Another scene. Eddie again, but now in Rome at the World Food Conference, a genuine world effort to deal with hunger. In the U.S. delegation, appointed by the Governor of Pennsylvania to represent the State (a state which can boast some of the finest nutrition educators in the nation) is Eddie.

Some of the new linkages can be seen on the Pike show. There is always a celebrity. It may be Liberace, describing his supplement as, "the equivalent of eating a steak, liver or six eggs." It may be Chloris Leachman, the actress, telling about her family's "natural" diet. We see Steve Allen and Marty Allen, basketballer Wilt Chamberlain and Olympic gold medalist Micki King, Barbara Feldon and tennis pro Jack Kramer, quarterback Roman Gabriel and Miss America Mary Ann Mobley. And don't forget California Senator Alan Cranston, who staves off colds with vitamin C and was hailed by Robert Rodale for introducing a bill for certifying organic foods, since organic farming is the only "non-polluting" agriculture.

Joining these celebrities, there is always a technical man, such as Pauling, Hauser, Dr. Alan Cott, Dr. Wilfred Shute or various officials of the new "academies" of food medicine.

Elsewhere, another factor is joining in, the consumer movement. For example, the National Health Federation *Bulletin* reprints an article from "A Report to the Consumer." The author is California consumerist Ida Honoroff. She argues for food controls, basing the need on technical data from Cheraskin and Ringsdorf and from England's Dr. John Yudkin, who recommends low-carbohydrate consumption for weight control and the prevention of heart disease.

Much of American consumerism had been suspicious of the food supply since the late 1960's. In 1968, a Ralph Nader Summer Study Group began a project which became a book, *The Chemical Feast*, by James Turner.

In his introduction, Nader talks of fraud and of the degradation of the food supply. He writes: "The failure of . . . regulation to insure safe, pure and nutritious food . . . has been in step with each new ingenious technique for manipulating the content of food products as dictated by corporate greed and irresponsibility."

Such suspicion appeared in the Consumer Reaction Panel reports from the White House Conference in 1969. For example, moved by opinions which originated with Rachel Carson's *Silent Spring* and Daniel Longood's *Poisons in Your Food,* there was a demand for perfect safety in food production.

As Turner expresses the feeling, "The primary purpose of food additives to industry is to increase profits." Additives, he says, "should not be tolerated if there is the slightest indication that a hazard to consumers might exist."

No one argues with this hope. But as we have seen—with Delaney's Clause, with the DES story, and with the fact that toxicity is a potential characteristic of *anything* we eat—safety is only relative, no matter how "natural" our food. One can design an experiment to prove any substance "toxic."

As the National Academy of Science comments, "No method is at hand—and none is in sight—for establishing, with absolute certainty, the safety of a food chemical under all conditions of use."

And remember, all food substances are chemicals.

As FDA puts it, "It is quite human to think of desired safety—in anything—in the realm of 100 percent only. Such 'perfection' is literally impossible."

While the consumerists were often scientifically misinformed, at first many nutritionists welcomed their help toward practical action. Biochemists are poorly equipped for the political arena. And they were delighted to be asked to supply information.

So when the Nader-related Center for Science in the Public Interest, led by Dr. Michael Jacobson, proposed a national Food Day to create nutrition awareness, the prospect was appealing. Scientists lent their names and offered to take the podium.

Then, late in 1974, some of the Food Day literature began to appear. One example that troubled nutritionists was a list of "The Terrible Ten" foods, which were to be attacked.

Sugar, for example, was one. True, sugar probably took too large a part of the daily caloric allowance for some Americans. But it was not a poison. There was no scientific logic by which, as Yudkin had demanded, it ought to be banned. There was no evidence, as some consumerists claimed, that feeding a little sugar to children created a lifelong craving. In fact, it had been shown that the taste for sweetness was present, not only at birth, but even in the womb. And biologically, this made some sense—that there is an innate taste recognition of sources of energy, the body's most basic need.

But CSPI literature held that, "Eating junk baby foods may lead a baby down a lifetime path of junk foods and ill health."

Wonder Bread was on the proscribed list. True, many, including this author, had objected to some advertising of the product. But not because the bread was bad food; rather because it was only ordinary bread and the ads seemed to imply it was more. Moreover, CSPI's reasons focused on the fact that it was "made by Continental Baking, a division of ITT which also owns Sheraton Hotels and makes military supplies." Table grapes were similarly condemned. Why? Because, "The United Farm Workers are conducting a nationwide boycott, because growers refuse to sign UFW contracts."

Gerber Baby Food Desserts were on the list because (said CSPI), "The major ingredient of these baby foods is water, which costs 40 cents per pint."

The major component of fruits and vegetables is water. For example, many baby food desserts are sweetened fruit dishes. Fresh fruit is usually about 90 percent water. Thus, when a fresh peach costs 49 cents a pound, we pay 44 cents a pint for the water in it, which means that the water in a fresh peach costs 10 percent more than that in a peach baby food.

CSPI ignores the fact that baby foods are often needfully fortified. One important such fortification is with vitamin C, which is low in milk (of either human or cow). Another is iron.

Also, some Food Day literature condemned baby foods because they were not high in protein. Yet a baby on a milk-based diet gets all the protein it needs from the milk. The key aim in the feeding of the first solids to infants is to provide missing vitamins and minerals, not protein.

Coca-Cola was also on the Food Day list, though it is nutritionally identical with other sugared soft drinks. And while Coke is not defended by nutritionists as nutritionally valuable, it is not helpful (or accurate) to say that Coke "peddles its wares in under-developed countries, where the beverage is a cause of economic hardship . . ."

Bacon was listed as, "perhaps the most dangerous food in the supermarket. Bacon," continued CSPI, "contains nitrosamines, which the government admits . . . 'have been shown to cause cancer in test animals.' "

Wrong. Bacon does not contain nitrosamines, but nitrites. The latter are used to prevent botulism in virtually all cured and preserved meats. True, nitrites *could* react with certain body chemicals to form nitrosamines. Because of this, FDA has tried to keep nitrites to the lowest practical amounts.

FDA notes that there is a much higher level of nitrites in our own round-the-clock saliva than in the bacon we eat. "By anyone's calculation," say FDA's Commissioner, "whatever risk there might be of nitrosamine forming . . . is far less than the risk of botulism in unpreserved meat."

Again, pure nitrosamines can predispose to cancer in test animals. But only at *high levels*. There is no evidence that bacon is related to cancer in any population of humans.

Gradually, CSPI also began to condemn "chemical" farming methods. Two scientists on the Food Day Advisory Board had made comments on these ideas which typify expert thinking. Said Dr. Michael Latham, "half the population of the world would starve to death if artificial fertilizers were not used." Said Dr.

George Briggs, "Our phenomenal agricultural production would be impossible without pesticides."

Scientists began to withdraw from Food Day. Harvard's noted Dr. Jean Mayer had perhaps been CSPI's most luminous scientific supporter. By January of 1975, he wrote to Jacobson, "I am disturbed about the tone of the statements that come with Food Day announcements . . ."

A few weeks later, he wrote: "You have driven me to the point where I want to dissociate myself completely from any activity you are organizing in relation to Food Day. The inane material you have on agriculture on your Food Day pamphlet is obviously going to make organic nuts very happy, but it has nothing to do with feeding the world and cheaper costs of food. If you don't understand modern agriculture, just stay out of it and don't encourage people to believe that small organic farms are going to give us all the food we need for the world."

In brief, nutritionists who had looked hopefully to a consumer-action boost for nutrition education saw instead another kind of emphasis. They saw a campaign of negativism—a suspicion of the food supply and a back-to-nature naturalism that merely fueled the deceptive fires of the foodists. As Dr. Phillip White summed it up, ". . . The informed consumer can make judgments; the uninformed consumer makes accusations."

How have consumerists dealt with the disappointment of scientific rejection? Many seem to have turned to other bases of support. Especially, they have aligned themselves with a growing trend of the last two decades.

In part that trend is philosophic. At the turn of the century, each technical advance and new product was hailed as evidence of science's promises for a better life. Today that view is commonly reversed, and many see each technological change as another step toward the destructive and dehumanizing. (Some philosophers of science believe that such fears were given great impetus by the atom bomb—although they can be traced back at least to the 1920's, to plays such as *R.U.R.*, in which clever robots took control of the earth, and to novels such as *Brave New World.*)

Whatever the root of this attitude, science has lost much of its beneficent image and for many has become a threat. Technical improvements are commonly seen as signs of an increasingly *ersatz* and depersonalized society, in which resources are squandered and nature defiled, in which personal identity is erased by computer codes, in which Thanksgiving dinner comes from a vial. And along with the threat of an increasingly "plastic" world, goes a sense of hopelessness about stopping the process.

The foodist cult thrives on this fear and negativism. The loss of a milligram of calcium here or a microgram of B-12 there has seemed the realization of vague fears. Words such as "natural" and "organic," though undefined, have acquired great value for many, especially the young. We have come full circle. The 19th century view *(Naturphilosophie)* that Nature is the true scientist, and that philosophy is the true guide to scientific fact, has been restored.

This trend could be perceived some years ago. In 1971, I served as a participant at a meeting on "food faddism and cultism," convened by the Council on Foods and Nutrition. The conference immediately faced the question of who was accepted by the public as authoritative on food and health. What I said then seems equally valid today:

"Originally, the health-food movement discredited industry (starting out with Sylvester Graham, who wanted to put bran back into wheat). Next, the movement discredited government (i.e., the attacks on permissiveness, such as the refinement of sugar and flour) . . . Recently there are attempts to discredit medicine. Also, there is a current trend to discredit the scientist, especially the biochemist, by statements that the biochemical data which comes from the universities with application to food products cannot be trusted. Having discredited the credibility of industry, government, medicine and science, no authority exists for the public which, in a satisfactory way, could combat nutrition nonsense . . ."

The resulting "authority gap" may account for some of the interesting coalitions of effort which appear to be taking shape. Witness the happenings in connection with the Proxmire-Schweiker Bill on FDA's control of vitamin products.

There are also important implications for the consumerist. For by definition of his role, the consumerist is the advocate of the popular interest. How will the consumerist manage his increasingly influential position in nutrition, when scientific research can find no support for many of his concepts? Three recent occurrences give us a basis for speculation.

On the masthead of a recent issue of a publication called *Caveat Emptor*, we find three editors and a short list of official "contributors." The magazine is published by The Consumer Education Research Group, which in press releases describes itself as "Nader-related." Among the regular contributors are Ralph Nader, Michael Jacobson and Robert Choate. (Choate is an engineer who in 1970 made an analysis of breakfast cereals, comparing their nutritive value by adding their content of nine nutrients into one total. It caused a flurry in the press, until scientists explained that such a totaling had little meaning.)*

Associate editor and nutrition authority for *Caveat Emptor* is Gary Null, billed as Executive Director of the Nutrition Institute of America. In a mid-1976 issue, he has a report on meat. ". . . The meat industry," he says, "is constantly looking for ways to shirk its responsibility to the public," and must be forced to, ". . . provide us with healthy foods, instead of empty, even poisonous products."

Scientifically, he notes that his Institute has found that hot dogs contain, "an astounding 60 percent moisture . . ." Alas, as any food-composition table will tell us, so do beef steaks and roasts fresh from the butcher.

Null is identified by his book publisher, Dell, as "gaining ever greater renown as one of the leading nutritional authorities and spokesmen for organic living . . . In addition, Gary Null is proprietor of one of the country's most successful health food stores."

From one of his books, we might take some typical answers to nutrition questions:

"Hearing problems? Don't forget the importance of vitamin A."

---

*Scientifically, there were other flaws. Two of the nutrients used were calcium and vitamin D. Grains are very poor sources of these; for example it would take over 300 slices of whole wheat bread to provide a day's calcium. Moreover, we eat cereal with milk, which is a very fine source of calcium and vitamin D.

"Colds are shortened . . . if you take natural vitamin C."

"Why not give a natural remedy like garlic a chance . . ."

"Max Gerson . . . brought with him another dietary 'cure'—this time for cancer . . . The ghost of Dr. Gerson hangs over the entire question of cancer research today . . ."

". . . Many patients . . . should be given a diet to overcome low blood sugar conditions."

"We do not know what causes muscular dystrophy, but all research has pointed to the fact that it is nutritional . . . Make sure that it is certified raw milk that the patient is being administered . . . Plenty of vitamin E as well as desiccated liver . . ."

A second item: In 1975, an "official food day handbook" appeared, under the title, *Food for People, Not for Profit.* It was edited by Catherine Lerza, former editor of *Environmental Action,* and Michael Jacobson of CSPI.

The book covers diverse areas. Its acknowledgments begin with thanks to people at Rodale Press. It recommends only six periodicals on food issues, two of which come from Rodale. When it offers recipes from food activists, it also chooses only six, one of which is *Robert Rodale's Corn Pone.*

A third item: In 1976, the *Washington Star* reported: "Food scientists are accused of becoming advocates for industry practices or deliberately keeping mum on controversial issues . . ."

The story concerned a report issued jointly by Rep. Ben Rosenthal (Dem., N.Y.) and the Center for Science in the Public Interest. The tone of the report was bitter. Consider the title, *Feeding at the Company Trough,* and such conclusions as, ". . . Many professors are, quite frankly, on the take . . ."

The report centered on the truths that the food industry gives some money to universities for research, and that some companies ask nutritionists for advice and pay them for their time. None of this was very revealing.

Virtually every nutrition department in the world has some industry grant support. The report chose 17 professorial examples. And they have some common characteristics. They either (1) declined to give their names and support to Food Day and other CSPI activities, (2) withdrew their names and support or (3) challenged one or more principles of consumerist attacks, such as the amount of water in baby food or the need for organic farming.

Dr. Jean Mayer, for example, is listed because of an association with Monsanto, "which manufactures food flavorings, preservatives . . . pesticides, fertilizer and other food industry chemicals." Yet in 1972, Dr. Mayer wrote the introduction to Jacobson's own book on food additives. In this, Mayer renewed the call for a review of the GRAS (Generally Recognized as Safe) list of additives.*

Dr. Frederick Stare of Harvard was cited for statements that sugar is not dangerous and that food chemicals are not immediate sources of peril. He also "has refused to disclose to the authors of this report the companies which currently employ him."

Actually, Dr. Stare does not accept fees from industry. Even royalties for his books and columns are all signed over to Harvard.

Dr. E. M. Foster of the U. of Wisconsin's Food Research Institute is singled out. Why? ". . . He believes that consumer advocates 'hold the uncompromising view that industry and the regulatory agencies are in league to rip off the consumer . . . The chief tools of these self-styled consumer advocates . . . are exaggeration and facts taken out of context . . . ' "

Professor Paul Kifer of Oregon State is also chosen. Why? Because he has said that, "There has never been a single proven case of humans being hurt from eating normal quantities of food containing additives." The authors of the report refute this. They even cite a case. "One young boy who was sensitive to peanuts died a few years ago after eating ice cream that contained a little peanut butter."

Dr. Fergus Clydesdale of the U. of Massachusetts is accused of "moonlighting." The report says that his prejudice is revealed in his statement, "In order to supply wholesome, high-quality food in today's over-populated, urbanized world, nearly all foods must be processed and preserved."

Dr. Theodore Labuza of the U. of Minnesota is indicted for his statement: "Let's face it, the food industry has to make a profit, otherwise it will not be able to keep providing us with food."

*(Incidentally, the White House Conference on Nutrition, which Dr. Mayer chaired, strongly urged this review. And to clarify his own position, the author wrote one of those demands for GRAS review into the report.)

And the report concludes: "In sharp contrast to the pervasive and multifarious links between professors and industry, professional associations with consumer groups are rare . . . Professors should examine current practices with a critical eye, cooperating with citizens' groups."

The author refrains from conclusions.

So, curiously, do the lines continue to be drawn.

But such lines are not always apparent. And both the public and its officials tend to regard consumer organizations as sources of truth without prejudice. In 1976, the Nader-sponsored Public Citizen Forum invited presidential candidates to speak. One of them who did had earlier said, "I would like to be known as the foremost protector of consumers." He reaffirmed this statement and laid out some specifics for reaching the goal, among them the needed strengthening of regulatory agencies, to which, he said, "I will appoint consumer or citizen advocates . . . One of the goals that I have for my own appointees is that they would be acceptable to Ralph Nader."

The candidate's name was Jimmy Carter.

Through such avenues and through such people of good intention have some of the oldest errors about food and health acquired astonishing force in our own time. Thus has the need to clarify truth and fiction in nutrition acquired new urgency.

* * *

As we have noted, some years ago, *Poisons in Your Food* was one of the first books to play upon food fears with the threat that the nation's nutriment was a veritable cup of hemlock. Organic farming and "natural" foods were the answers.

(In 1971, Signet Books issued *Beware of the Food You Eat,* "the revised, updated edition of *Poisons in Your Food.*" The new edition was graced by an introduction from then Senator Walter F. Mondale.)

But there are poisons far more deadly than those envisioned by these authors and their friends. These are the poisons of greed and ambition and unreasoning fear. They are the poisons of false hope and impossible promise that now powerfully misdirect not only tens of millions of individuals but also the efforts of the state to deal with the critical problems of health and hunger.

A liberal dose comes free with every strange scheme of eating, with every package of health-food you buy.

*   *   *

"The use of the word 'health' in connection with foods constitutes a misbranding under the Food and Drug Act. The use of this word implies that these products have health-giving or curative properties, when in general, they merely possess some of the nutritive qualities to be expected in any wholesome food product."

—U.S. Food and Drug Administration.

Bibliography

Some Controversial Books in Nutrition

Abehsera, Michel, *Zen Macrobiotic Cooking*, University Books, New Hyde Park, New York, 1968 (also Avon Books, 1970).

Abrahamson, E.M. and Pezet, A.W., *Body, Mind, and Sugar*, Holt, New York, 1951 (also Pyramid Books, 1971).

Adams, Ruth, *The Complete Home Guide to All the Vitamins*, Larchmont Books, New York.

Adams, Ruth and Murray, Frank, *Megavitamin Therapy*, Larchmont Books, New York, 1973.

——, *The Good Seeds, The Rich Grains, The Hardy Nuts for a Happier, Healthier Life*, Larchmont Books.

——, *Vitamin E, Wonder Worker of the 70's?*, Larchmont Books.

——, *The High Risks of a Low Calcium Diet*, Larchmont Books.

——, *Body, Mind and the B Vitamins*, Larchmont Books.

——, *Vitamin C, the Powerhouse Vitamin, Conquers More than Just Colds*, Larchmont Books.

——, *Is Low Blood Sugar Making You a Nutritional Cripple?* Larchmont Books.

——, *A New Look at Vitamin A*, Larchmont Books.

Ahlson, Charles B., *Health from Sea and Soil*, Exposition-Banner, New York, 1962.

Airola, Paavo O., *Sex and Nutrition*, Award Books, New York, 1970.

——, *Health Secrets from Europe*, Arco, New York, 1971.

Alexander, Dan Dale, *Arthritis and Common Sense*, Witkower, Hartford, 1956.

——, *The Common Cold and Common Sense*, Nash, Los Angeles.

Allen and Lust, *Royal Jelly Miracle*, Lust's Publications, Health Book Service, Beaumont, Cal.

Amend, Eleanor, *Health Can Be Yours Naturally*, Greenwith, New York, 1958.

Amon-Wilkins, J., *About Cocoanuts and Constipation*, Lust's Publications, Health Book Service, Beaumont, Cal.

Atkins, Robert C., *Dr. Atkins' Diet Revolution* (with Ruth West Herwood), David McKay, New York, 1972 (also Bantam, New York).

Bailey, Herbert, *Vitamin E, Your Key to a Healthy Heart*, Arc, New York, 1964. (See also, Fredericks, Carlton).

Barker, J. Ellis, *Miracles of Healing* (Homeopathy), Maxwell Love, London.

Bates, W.H., *Better Eyesight without Glasses*, Pyramid, New York.

Bauer, W.W., *Eat What You Want*, Greenberg Press.

Bernard, R.W., *Secret of Rejuvenation*, Health Research, Mokelumne Hill, Cal.

Bicknell, Franklin, *Chemicals in Your Food and in Farm Products, Their Harmful Effects*, Emerson Books, New York, 1961.

Bieler, Henry G., *Food Is Your Best Medicine,* Random House, New York, 1966 (also Vintage Books).

Bircher-Benner, M. *The Prevention of Incurable Disease,* James Clarke and Co., England.

Blaine, Judge Tom R., *Goodbye Allergies,* The Citadel Press, New York, 1965.

——, *Mental Hygiene Through Nutrition,* The Citadel Press, New York, 1969.

Bragg, Paul, *Toxicless Diet Body Purification and Healing System,* Health Service, Inc.

——, *Building Powerful Nerve Force,* Health Service, Inc.

Brandner, Gary P., *Vitamin E: Key to Sexual Satisfaction,* Nash, Los Angeles.

Brandt, Johanna, *The Grape Cure,* Beneficial Books, Beaumont, Cal.

Burtis, C. Edward, *The Fountain of Youth,* Arco, New York, 1972.

——, *The Real American Tragedy,* Lee Foundation for Nutritional Research, Milwaukee.

Cantor, Alfred J., *Dr. Cantor's Longevity Diet,* Award, New York.

Cayce, Edgar, *Secrets of Beauty Through Health* (ed. by L.M. Steinhart), Berkley, New York, 1975.

Chapman, Esther, *How to Use the 12 Tissue Salts,* Pyramid, New York.

Cheraskin, E. and Ringsdorf, W.M., *Psychodietetics,* Bantam, New York, 1974 (also Stein and Day, New York).

——, *New Hope for Incurable Diseases,* Arco, New York, 1971.

——, *Preventive Medicine; a Study in Strategy,* Pacific Press, Mountain View, Cal., 1973.

Clark, Linda, *Get Well Naturally,* Devin-Adair, New York (also Arc Books, New York).

——, *Stay Young Longer,* Devin-Adair, New York, 1961 (also Pyramid, New York, 1968).

——, ed., *Light on Your Health Problems,* Pivot/Let's Live (Keats Publishing), New Canaan, Conn., 1972.

Clymer, R. Swinburne, *The Medicines of Nature—The Thomsonian System,* The Humanitarian Society, Quakertown, Pa., 1960.

——, *Nature's Healing Agents,* Dorrance and Co., Philadelphia, 1963.

Cocannover, Joseph, *Organic Gardening and Farming,* Arco, New York.

Cosmopolitan (See Seligson, Marcia).

Cott, Alan, *Orthomolecular Treatment: A Biochemical Approach to Treatment of Schizophrenia,* American Schizophrenia Assn., New York.

Crile, George Jr., *Cancer and Common Sense,* Viking, New York, 1955.

Davis, Adelle, *Let's Get Well,* Harcourt Brace Jovanovich, New York (also Signet Books, New York).

——, *Let's Have Healthy Children,* Harcourt, Brace, New York (also Signet Books, New York).

——, *Let's Cook it Right,* Harcourt Brace Jovanovich, New York (also Signet Books, New York).

——, *Vitality Through Planned Nutrition,* Harcourt, Brace, New York.

——, *You Can Stay Well,* Harcourt, Brace, New York.

Davis, Francyne, *The Low Blood Sugar Cookbook,* Grosset and Dunlap, New York.

Davis, Helen A., *The No Willpower Diet,* David McKay, New York, 1969.

DeGroot, R., *How I Reduced with the New Rockefeller Diet,* Horizon, New York, 1956.

Donaldson, B.F., *Strong Medicine,* Doubleday, New York, 1962.

Dufty, William, *Sugar Blues,* Warner, New York, 1976.

——, and Ohsawa, George, *You Are All Sanpaku,* Award Books, New York.

Dunn, Joan, *The Career Girl's Diet and Beauty Book,* Award Books, New York.

Ehret, Arnold, *Rational Fasting,* Beneficial Books, Beaumont, Cal.

——, *Mucusless Diet Healing System,* Beneficial Books, Beaumont, Cal.

——, *Instructions for Fasting and Dieting,* Beneficial Books, Beaumont, Cal.

——, *The Internal Uncleanliness of Man,* Lust's Publications, Beaumont, Cal.

Eichenlaub, John, *A Minnesota Doctor's Home Remedies for Common and Uncommon Ailments,* Prentice-Hall, Jersey City, 1960.

Eiteljorg, S., *The Sweet Way to Diet,* Doubleday, Garden City, New York, 1968.

Elwood, Catharyn, *Feel Like a Million!,* Devin-Adair, New York (also Pocketbooks, New York).

Evans, Isabelle W., *Sugar, Sex and Sanity,* Carlton Press.

Feingold, Ben F., *Why Your Child Is Hyperactive,* Random House, New York, 1974.

Fiore, E.L., ed., *The Low Carbohydrate Diet,* Ridge Press, New York.

Fitzgerald, W. and Bowers, E., *Zone Therapy or Relieving Pain at Home and Zone Therapy,* Health Research, Mokelumne, Cal., 1952.

Fletcher, Horace, *Fletcherism, What Is It?* Ewart, Seymour, London (also reprint by Lee Foundation, Milwaukee).

Fredericks, Carlton, *Dr. Carlton Fredericks' Low-Carbohydrate Diet,* Award Books, New York, 1965.

——, *The Carlton Fredericks Cookbook for Good Nutrition,* Lippincott, Phila., 1960.

——, *Nutrition, Your Key to Good Health,* London Press, N. Hollywood, Cal. (a revised version of *Eat, Live and Be Merry,* 1964).

——, *The Eat-More-to-Lose-More Diet Book,* Award Books, New York.

——, *Eating Right for You,* Grosset and Dunlap, New York, 1972.

——, and Bailey, H., *Food Facts and Fallacies,* The Julian Press, New York, 1965 (also Arc Books).

Galton, Lawrence, "Why Young Adults Crack Up," reprint from 1967 *Family Circle,* dist. by American Schizophrenia Assn., New York.

Gerardi, Victor, *Sexual Power* (Nutritional Approach), Nash, Los Angeles.

Gerson, Max, *A Cancer Therapy, Results of Fifty Cases,* Dura Books, New York, 1963.

Gjerde, Mary, *Organic Make-Up,* Nash, Los Angeles.

Goodman, Herman, *Your Hair: Its Health, Beauty and Growth,* Emerson Books, New York.

Grant, Doris, *Your Bread and Your Life,* Faber and Faber, London.

Haught, S.J., *Has Dr. Max Gerson a True Cancer Cure?*, London Press, N. Hollywood, Cal., 1962.

Hauser, Gayelord, *Gayelord Hauser's Treasury of Secrets*, Farrar, Straus and Giroux, New York (also Fawcett, Greenwich, Conn.).

——, *Look Younger, Live Longer*, Fawcett Crest, Greenwich.

——, *Be Happier, Be Healthier*, Fawcett Crest, Greenwich.

——, *Mirror, Mirror on the Wall*, Fawcett Crest, Greenwich.

——, *New Guide to Intelligent Reducing*, Fawcett Crest, Greenwich.

——, *Keener Vision without Glasses*, Beneficial Books, Beaumont, Cal.

——, *The New Diet Does It*, G.P. Putnam's Sons, New York.

——, *New Guide to Intelligent Reducing*, Farrar, Straus, New York.

——, and Ragnar Berg, *Dictionary of Foods*, Beneficial Books, Beaumont, Cal.

Hawkins, D. and Pauling, L., *Orthomolecular Psychiatry, Treatment of Schizophrenia*, W.H. Freeman, San Francisco, 1973.

Hay, William Howard, *How to Always Be Well*, Groton, Island Park, New York.

Hazzard, L., *About Scientific Fasting*, Lust's Publications, Beaumont, Cal.

Hewitt, Jean, *The New York Times Natural Foods Cookbook*, New York.

Hoffer, Abram, *New Hope for Alcoholics*, University Books, New Hyde Park, New York, 1968.

——, and Osmond, Humphrey, *How to Live with Schizophrenia*, University Books, New Hyde Park, New York, 1966.

Howard, Sir Albert, *An Agricultural Testament*, Oxford University Press, New York.

Hunter, Beatrice Trum, *Consumer Beware! Your Food and What's Been Done to It*, Simon and Schuster, New York, 1971.

——, *The Natural Foods Cookbook*, Simon and Schuster, New York, 1961.

——, *The Natural Foods Primer*, Simon and Schuster, New York, 1972.

Hunter, Kathleen, *Health Foods and Herbs*, Arc, New York.

Jacobson, Michael and Lerza, Catherine, *Food for People, Not for Profit*, Ballantine, New York, 1975.

James, Claude, *Herbs and the Fountain of Youth*, Amrita Books, Alberta, Canada.

Jameson, Gardner and Williams, Elliott, *The Drinking Man's Diet*, Cameron, San Francisco.

Jarvis, D.C., *Folk Medicine*, Holt, New York, 1958.

——, *Arthritis and Folk Medicine*, Holt, New York, 1960 (also Fawcett, New York).

Keller, Jeanne, *Healing with Water*, Award Books, New York.

Kirschner, H.E., *Live Fruit Juices*, Kirschner, Monrovia, Cal.

——, *Nature's Healing Grasses*, H.C. White, Yucaipa, Cal.

Kittler, Glenn, *Laetrile, Control for Cancer*, Paperback Library, New York, 1963.

Kloss, Jethro, *Back to Eden*, Beneficial Books, Beaumont, Cal.

Kordel, Lelord, *Health the Easy Way*, Award Books, New York.

——, *Eat Your Troubles Away*, World, Cleveland (also Belmont Books, New York).

———, *Eat Right and Live Longer,* Health Today.

———, *Health Through Nutrition,* Macfadden-Bartell, New York, 1971.

Korth, Leslie O., *Some Unusual Healing Methods,* Health Science Press, Surrey, England, 1960.

Kraus, Barbara, *Calories and Carbohydrates,* Grosset and Dunlap, New York.

LaLanne, Jack, *The Jack LaLanne Way to Vibrant Good Health,* Arc, New York, 1970.

La Leche League, *The Womanly Art of Breastfeeding,* La Leche League International, Franklin Park, Ill.

Lappé, Frances Moore, *Diet for a Small Planet,* Ballantine, New York, 1975.

Larson, Gena, *Better Food for Better Babies,* Pivot/Let's Live, Keats, New Canaan, Conn.

Lee, Royal, *How and Why Synthetic Poisons Are Being Sold As Imitations of Natural Foods and Drugs,* Lee Foundation, Milwaukee.

Levitt, E. *The Wonderful World of Natural-Food Cookery,* Hearthside Press, Great Neck, New York, 1971.

Lindlahr, Victor, *The Natural Way to Health,* Newcastle, Hollywood, California.

———, *You Are What You Eat,* Newcastle, Hollywood, Cal.

———, *Vitamin Cookbook,* Newcastle, Hollywood, Cal.

———, *Eat and Reduce,* Newcastle, Hollywood, Cal.

———, *Calorie Countdown,* Prentice-Hall, Englewood Cliffs, N.J.

Little, B., *Recipes for Allergics,* Vantage, New York, 1968.

Longgood, William, *The Poisons in Your Food,* Simon and Schuster, New York (also Pyramid Books, New York).

Lopez, L., *Hope for the Arthritic,* Lust's Publications, Beaumont, Cal.

Lucas, Richard, *Common and Uncommon Uses of Herbs for Healthful Living,* Arco, New York.

Lust, Benedict, *Your Memory,* Lust's Publications, Beaumont, Cal.

———, *The Blood Washing Method,* Lust's Publications, Beaumont, Cal.

Lust, John, *Drink Your Troubles Away,* Beneficial, Beaumont, Cal.

———, *Fifteen Years Younger in 4 Weeks,* Beneficial, Beaumont, Cal.

———, *The New Raw Juice Therapy,* Lust's Publications, Beaumont, Cal.

Lust, V., *Grandma's Kitchen Was Her Drugstore,* Lust's Publications, Beaumont, Cal.

Marcus, Rory, *The Organic Health Food Cookbook,* Award Books, New York.

Marsh, A., *How to Be Healthy with Natural Foods,* Arc, New York.

Martin, Clement G., *Low Blood Sugar and Your Health,* Arco, New York.

Martin, W. Coda, *A Matter of Life,* Devin-Adair, New York, 1964.

McKie, Mildred, *Natural Aids for Common Ills,* Northboro, Iowa.

Miller, Marjorie, *Introduction to Health Foods,* Nash, Los Angeles.

Newman, L., *Make Your Juicer Your Drug Store,* Beneficial, Beaumont, Cal.

Nichols, J.D., *Please, Doctor, Do Something,* Natural Food Associates, Atlanta, Texas, 1972.

Nittler, Alan H., *A New Breed of Doctor,* Pyramid, New York, 1974.

Nolfi, Kirstine, *The Raw Food Treatment of Cancer and Other Disorders,* The Vegetarian Society, London.

Norris, P.E., *Everything You Want to Know about Wheat Germ*, Pyramid, New York, 1972.

——, *About Nuts and Dried Fruit*, Thorsons Publishers, London.

Null, Gary, *The Complete Question and Answer Book of Natural Therapy*, Dell, New York.

——, *The Complete Handbook of Nutrition*, Dell, New York.

——, *Grow Your Own Food Organically*, Dell, New York.

Nyoiti, Sakurazawa (George Ohsawa) and Dufty, William, *You Are All Sanpaku*, Award Books, New York, 1965.

Ohsawa, George, *Zen Macrobiotics, The Art of Longevity and Rejuvenation*, Ignoramus Press, Los Angeles.

——, *The Philosophy of Oriental Medicine*, Ignoramus Press, Los Angeles.

——, *The Book of Judgment*, Ignoramus Press, Los Angeles.

Page, Melvin and Abrams, H.L. Jr., *Your Body Is Your Best Doctor*, Keats, New Canaan, Conn.

Pauling, Linus, *Vitamin C and the Common Cold*, W.H. Freeman, San Francisco (also Bantam Books, New York).

Pendergast, Chuck, *Introduction to Organic Gardening*, Nash, Los Angeles.

Perlman, Dorothy, *The Magic of Honey*, Nash, Los Angeles.

Petrie, Sidney and Stone, Robert, *Martinis and Whipped Cream*, Parker, West Nyack, New York (also Warner, New York).

Pike, Arnold, *Viewpoint on Nutrition*, Newcastle, Hollywood, Cal., 1973.

Price, Weston A., *Nutrition and Physical Degeneration*, Price-Pottinger Foundation, Santa Monica, Cal.

Pyramid Healthful Living Series includes volumes on Honey, Yogurt, Soya Beans, Garlic, Fasting, Vitamins, Molasses, Yeast, Sea Foods, Slimming, etc., Pyramid Books, New York.

Quigley, D.T., *The National Malnutrition*, Lee Foundation for Nutritional Research, Milwaukee.

Reuben, David, *The Save Your Life Diet*, Random House, New York, 1975.

Rienzo, G.R., *Slim Down*, Vantage Press, New York, 1964.

Righter, Carrol, *Your Astrological Guide to Health and Diet*, G.P. Putnam's Sons, New York, 1967.

Ringsdorf, W.M. Jr. (see Cheraskin, E.).

Rodale, J.I., *Rodale's System for Mental Power and Natural Health*, Rodale Press, Emmaus, Pa. (also Pyramid Books, New York).

——, *Natural Health, Sugar and the Criminal Mind*, Pyramid Books, New York.

——, and Ruth Adams and Charles Gerras, *The Health Builder* (Vol. II of *The Health Finder*), Rodale, Emmaus, Pa.

——, and Harald J. Taub, *Magnesium, the Nutrient That Could Change Your Life*, Pyramid Books, New York.

——, and Staff, *Encyclopedia for Healthful Living*, (Ruth Adams, ed.), Rodale Press, Emmaus, Pa.

——, and Staff, *Our Poisoned Earth and Sky*, Rodale Books, Emmaus, Pa.

Rodale, Robert et al., *The Organic Directory*, Rodale, Emmaus, Pa.

Rose, I.F., *Faith, Love and Seaweed,* Prentice-Hall, Englewood Cliffs, N.J.

Scott, Cyril, *Crude Black Molasses,* Benedict Lust Publications, New York.

———, *Victory over Cancer,* Health Science Press, New York.

Seligson, Marcia and Cosmopolitan, *Cosmopolitan's Super Diets and Exercise Guide,* Avon, New York, 1973.

Shelton, Herbert M., *Health for the Millions,* Natural Hygiene Press, Chicago.

———, *Fasting for Health and Long Life,* Natural Hygiene Press, Chicago.

———, *Hygienic Care of Children,* Natural Hygiene Press, Chicago.

———, *Superior Nutrition,* Natural Hygiene Press, Chicago.

———, *Hygienic System* (Three Volumes), Natural Hygiene Press, Chicago.

———, *Human Beauty; Its Culture and Hygiene,* Natural Hygiene Press, Chicago.

Shute, E.V. and W.F., *Your Heart and Vitamin E,* Devin-Adair, New York.

Shute, Wilfred E. and Harald Taub, *Vitamin E for Ailing and Healthy Hearts,* Pyramid Books, New York.

Smith, Lendon, *Improving Your Child's Behavior Chemistry,* Prentice-Hall, Englewood Cliffs, N.J.

Steincrohn, Peter, *Your Life to Enjoy,* Prentice-Hall, N.J., 1963.

Stillman, Irwin Maxwell and Baker, S.S., *The Doctor's Quick Teenage Diet,* David McKay, New York, 1971.

———, *The Doctor's Quick Weight Loss Diet,* Prentice-Hall, N.J. (also Dell, New York).

Taller, H., *Calories Don't Count,* Simon and Schuster, New York, 1961.

Taylor, Eric, *Fitness After Forty,* Arc, New York, 1966.

Taylor, Renee, *The Hunza-Yoga Way to Health and Longer Life,* Lancer Books, New York, 1969.

Thompson and Thompson, *Healthy Hair,* Arc Books, New York.

Toms, Agnes, *Eat, Drink and Be Healthy—The Joy of Eating Natural Foods,* Devin-Adair, New York, 1963.

Trimmer, Eric, *Rejuvenation,* Award Books, New York.

Trop, J.D., *You Don't Have to Be Sick,* Julian Press, New York, 1961.

Turner, James S., *The Chemical Feast,* Grossman, New York, 1970.

Verrett, Jacqueline and Carper, Jean, *Eating May Be Hazardous to Your Health,* Simon and Schuster, New York, 1974.

Wade, Carlson, *Instant Health the Nature Way,* Award Books, New York, 1968.

———, *The Rejuvenation Vitamin,* Award Books, New York.

———, *Vitamins and Other Food Supplements,* Pivot, New Canaan, Conn., 1972.

Walker, N.W., *Raw Vegetable Juices,* Norwalk Press, Phoenix, Arizona.

Warmbrand, Max, *Encyclopedia of Natural Health,* Groton, New York.

Watson, George, *Nutrition and Your Mind,* Harper & Row, New York, 1972.

Webster, James, *Vitamin C—The Protective Vitamin,* Award Books, New York.

Weller, C. and Boylan, B., *How to Live with Hypoglycemia,* Award Books, N.Y.

West, Ruth, *Stop Dieting, Start Losing,* E.P. Dutton, New York, 1956.

Whitehouse, G.T., *Stop Poisoning Yourself!* Award Books, New York.

Williams, Roger J., *Nutrition Against Disease,* Pitman, New York (also Bantam Books, New York).

Wilson, M., *Double Your Energy and Live Without Fatigue,* Prentice-Hall, N.J., 1961.
Winter, Ruth, *Beware of the Food You Eat,* Signet, New York, 1971. (Originally published as *Poisons in Your Food.*)
Wood, H. Curtis, *Overfed But Undernourished,* Exposition, New York, 1962.

The Factual Resources for This Book

Adams, C. *Nutritive Value of American Foods: in Common Units,* Agriculture Handbook No. 456, USDA, Washington, 1975.
Alfin-Slater, A. and Aftergood, L. *Nutrition for Today,* William C. Brown, Dubuque, Iowa, 1973.
Beeson, P. and McDermott, W. *Cecil-Loeb Textbook of Medicine,* esp. section, "Diseases of Nutrition," pp. 1187–1229, Saunders, Philadelphia, 1963.
Bogert, L., Briggs, G. and Calloway, D. *Nutrition and Physical Fitness,* Saunders, Philadelphia, 1973.
Calhoun, A. *A Social History of the American Family,* Vol. I, 1607–1776, Vol. II, 1776–1865, Vol. III, 1865–1919, University, New York, 1960.
Deutsch, R. *Family Guide to Better Food and Better Health,* Meredith, Des Moines, 1971.
——. *The Realities of Nutrition,* Bull, Palo Alto, California, 1976.
Economic Research Service, USDA, *The World Food Situation and Prospects to 1985,* Foreign Agricultural Economic Report No. 98, USDA, Washington, 1974.
Fomon, S. et al. *Infant Nutrition,* Saunders, Philadelphia, 1974.
Food and Nutrition Board, *Recommended Dietary Allowances,* National Academy of Sciences, Washington, 1974.
Food for Us All, 1969 Yearbook of Agriculture, USDA, Washington, 1969.
Frazier, W. *Food Microbiology,* McGraw-Hill, New York, 1967.
Furia, T. *Handbook of Food Additives,* Chem. Rubber Pub. Co., Cleveland, 1968.
Galdston, I., *Human Nutrition: Historic and Scientific,* New York Academy of Medicine Monograph III, International Universities Press, New York, 1960.
Goldblith, S. and Joslyn, M. *An Anthology of Food Science,* Avi, Westport, 1964.
Goodhart, R. and Shils, M. (eds.) *Modern Nutrition in Health and Disease,* Lea & Febiger, Philadelphia, 1973.
Guthrie, H. *Introductory Nutrition,* Mosby, St. Louis, 1971.
Labuza, T. *Food for Thought,* Avi, Westport, Connecticut, 1974.
Latham, M. et al. *Scope Manual on Nutrition,* Upjohn, Kalamazoo, 1970.
Leverton, R. *Food Becomes You,* Iowa State U., 1965.
Lovelock, Yann, *The Vegetable Book,* St. Martin's, New York, 1973.
Lowenberg, M. et al. *Food and Man,* Wiley, New York, 1974.
McCollum, E. *A History of Nutrition,* Houghton-Mifflin, Boston, 1957.
McWilliams, M. *Nutrition for the Growing Years,* Wiley, New York, 1971.

Mitchell, H. et al. *Cooper's Nutrition in Health and Disease*, Lippincott, Philadelphia, 1968.

Montagne, P. *Larousse Gastronomique, The Encyclopedia of Food, Wine and Cookery*, Crown, New York, 1961.

National Nutrition Consortium and Deutsch, R. *Nutrition Labeling*, Bethesda, Maryland, 1975.

Pyke, R. and Brown, M. *Nutrition: An Integrated Approach*, Wiley, New York, 1967.

Report of the White House Conference on Food, Nutrition and Health, 1969, USGPO, Washington, 1970.

Robinson, C. *Fundamentals of Normal Nutrition*, Macmillan, New York, 1973.

Stare, F. and McWilliams, M. *Living Nutrition*, Wiley, New York, 1973.

Stewart, G. and Amerine, M. *Introduction to Food Science and Technology*, Academic, New York, 1973.

Tannahill, R. *Food in History*, Stein and Day, New York, 1973.

U.S. Senate, *National Nutrition Policy Study*, Vols. I–VII, Washington, 1974.

Watts, B. and Merrill, A. *Composition of Foods*, USDA Agriculture Handbook No. 8, USDA, Washington, 1963.

White, P. ed. *Let's Talk About Food: Answers to Your Questions about Foods and Nutrition*, AMA, Chicago, 1970.

Williams, S. *Nutrition and Diet Therapy*, Mosby, 1973.

Index